# Emotion Regulation and Well-Being

Ivan Nyklíček · Ad Vingerhoets
Marcel Zeelenberg
Editors

# Emotion Regulation and Well-Being

Springer

*Editors*
Ivan Nyklíček
Center of Research on Psychology in
Somatic Diseases (CoRPS)
Tilburg University
P.O. Box 90153, 5000 LE Tilburg
The Netherlands
I.Nyklicek@uvt.nl

Ad Vingerhoets
Department of Clinical Psychology
Tilburg University
P.O. Box 90153, 5000 LE Tilburg
The Netherlands
vingerhoets@uvt.nl

Marcel Zeelenberg
Department of Social Psychology and
Tilburg Institute for Behavioral
Economics Research
Tilburg University
P.O. Box 90153, 5000 LE Tilburg
The Netherlands
M.Zeelenberg@uvt.nl

ISBN 978-1-4419-6952-1 e-ISBN 978-1-4419-6953-8
DOI 10.1007/978-1-4419-6953-8
Springer New York Dordrecht Heidelberg London

Library of Congress Control Number: 2010938910



Printed on acid-free paper

Springer is part of Springer Science+Business Media (www.springer.com)

*This book is dedicated to our children:*
*Milan, Jonas, and Cato Nyklíček*
*Rens, Bregje, and Meike Vingerhoets*
*Jimmie and Storm Zeelenberg*

# Contents

## Part II Social Perspective



## Part III Clinical Perspective

# Contributors

**Henk Aarts, PhD**
Utrecht University, Psychology Department, P.O. Box 80140,
3508 TC Utrecht, Netherlands
h.aarts@uu.nl

**Pär Bjälkebring, PhD**
Department of Psychology, Göteborg University, P.O. Box 500,
40530 Gothenburg, Sweden
par.bjalkebring@psy.gu.se

**Seger M. Breugelmans, PhD**
Department of Social Psychology, Tilburg University, P.O. Box 90153,
5000 LE Tilburg, Netherlands
s.m.breugelmans@uvt.nl

**Jos F. Brosschot, PhD**
Leiden University, Institute of Psychology, Clinical, Health and Neuropsychology
Unit, P.O. Box 9555, 2300 RB Leiden, Netherlands
brosschot@fsw.leidenuniv.nl

**Lauren M. Bylsma, PhD**
Mood and Emotion Laboratory, University of South Florida,
4202 E. Fowler Avenue, PCD4118G, Tampa, FL 33620, USA
lmbylsma@gmail.com

**Nathan S. Consedine**
Department of Psychological Medicine,
The University of Auckland, Auckland, New Zealand
n.consedine@auckland.ac.nz

**Filippo Cordaro, PhD**
School of Psychology, University of Southampton, Southampton,
SO17 1BJ, England, UK
fc8@soton.ac.uk

**Arden Corter, PhD**
Department of Psychological Medicine, Faculty of Medical and Health Sciences, University of Auckland, Private Bag 92019, New Zealand
ac_leigh@hotmail.com

**Beatrice de Gelder, PhD**
Department of Medical Psychology and Cognitive Neuroscience, Tilburg University, and Harvard Medical School, P.O. Box 90153, 5000 LE Tilburg. Netherlands
b.degelder@uvt.nl

**Ilona E. de Hooge, PhD**
Rotterdam School of Management, Erasmus University, Burgemeester Oudlaan 50, 3062 PA Rotterdam, Netherlands
IHooge@rsm.nl

**Catharine Evers, PhD**
Department of Clinical and Health Psychology, Utrecht University, P.O. Box 80140, 3508 TC Utrecht, Netherlands
c.evers@uu.nl

**Agneta H. Fischer, PhD**
Department of Psychology, University of Amsterdam, Roetersstraat 15, 1018 WB Amsterdam, Netherlands.
A.H.Fischer@uva.nl

**Winifred A. Gebhardt, PhD**
Leiden University, Institute of Psychology, Clinical, Health and Neuropsychology Unit, P.O. Box 9555, 2300 RB Leiden, Netherlands
gebhardt@fsw.leidenuniv.nl

**Alexa Ispas, PhD**
School of Philosophy Psychology and Language Sciences, The University of Edinburgh, 7 George Square, Edinburgh EH8 9JZ, UK
Alexa.Ispas@ed.ac.uk

**Patrick Kanyangara, PhD**
National University of Rwanda, Rwanda, and University of Louvain, Place Cardinal Mercier 10, B 1348 Louvain-la-Neuve, Belgium
patrick_kan2000@hotmail.com

**Mariska E. Kret, MSc**
Department of Medical Psychology and Cognitive Neuroscience, Tilburg University, P.O. Box 90153, 5000 LE Tilburg, Netherlands
m.e.kret@uvt.nl

**Anja Laan, MSc**
Reinier van Arkel Groep, P.O. Box 70058, 5201 DZ s-Hertogenbosch, Netherlands
a.laan@rvagroep.nl

**Colin W. Leach, PhD**
Department of Psychology, University of Connecticut, Bousfield Psychology Building 172, 406 Babbidge Road, U-1020, Storrs, CT 06269-1020, USA
colin.leach@uconn.edu

**Joyce Maas, MSc**
Radboud University Nijmegen, Nijmegen, Netherlands
j.maas@psych.ru.nl

**Michael Macht, PhD**
Institute of Psychotherapy and Medical Psychology, University of Würzburg, Klinikstr. 3, 97070, Würzburg, Germany
macht@psychologie.uni-wuerzburg.de

**Manstead, A.S.R.**
Cardiff University, School of Psychology, Tower Building, Park Place, Cardiff CF10 3AT, UK
MansteadA@Cardiff.ac.uk

**Iris Mauss, PhD**
Department of Psychology, University of Denver, 2155 South Race Street, Denver, CO 80208, USA
imauss@psy.du.edu

**Ivan Nyklíček**
Center of Research on Psychology in Somatic disease (CoRPS), Tilburg University, P.O. Box 90153, 5000 LE Tilburg, Netherlands
i.nyklicek@uvt.nl

**Dario Paez, PhD**
Grupo de Investigacion in Psicologia Social, Universitad del Pais Vasco, Paseo de la Universidad 7, E 01006 Vitoria, Spain
Dario.paez@ehu.es

**Ellen Peters, PhD**
Decision Research, 1201 Oak St, Suite 200, 97401 Eugene, Oregon, USA
empeters@decisionresearch.org

**Keith J. Petrie, PhD**
Department of Psychological Medicine, University of Auckland, Private Bag 92019, New Zealand
kj.petrie@auckland.ac.nz

**Bernard Rimé, PhD**
Department of Psychology, University of Louvain, 10, Place Cardinal Mercier, B 1348 Louvain-la-Neuve, Belgium
Bernard.Rime@uclouvain.be

**Jonathan Rottenberg, PhD**
Mood and Emotion Laboratory, University of South Florida, 4202 E. Fowler Ave, PCD4118G, Tampa, FL P.O. Box 33620, USA
jrottenb@cas.usf.edu

**Kirsten I. Ruys, PhD**
Utrecht University, Psychology Department, P.O. Box 80140, 3508 TC Utrecht, Netherlands
k.i.ruys@uu.nl

**Constantine Sedikides, PhD**
School of Psychology, University of Southampton, Southampton, SO17 1BJ, England, UK
cs2@soton.ac.uk

**Gwenda Simons, PhD**
Department of Experimental Psychology, University of Oxford, South Parks Road, Oxford OX1 3UD, UK
gwenda.simons@psy.ox.ac.uk

**Charlotte B.A. Sinke, MSc**
Department of Medical Psychology and Cognitive Neuroscience, Tilburg University, and Maastricht University. P.O. Box 90153, 5000 LE Tilburg, Netherlands
c.b.a.sinke@uvt.nl

**Russell Spears, PhD**
School of Psychology, Cardiff University, Tower Building, 70 Park Place, Cardiff, CF10 3AT, UK
SpearsR@Cardiff.ac.uk

**Diederik A. Stapel, PhD**
Tilburg University, Tilburg Institute for Behavioral Economics Research (TIBER), P.O. Box 90153, 5000 LE Tilburg, Netherlands
d.a.stapel@uvt.nl

**Claudia Subic-Wrana, PhD**
Clinic for Psychosomatic Medicine and Psychotherapy, University of Mainz, Untere Zahlbacher Str.8, 55131 Mainz, Germany
subic-wrana@psychosomtik.klinik.uni-mainz.de

**Joseph Sweetman, PhD**
School of Psychology, Cardiff University, Tower Building, 70 Park Place Cardiff, CF10 3AT, UK
sweetmanjp@Cardiff.ac.uk

**Maya Tamir, PhD**
Department of Psychology, Boston College, 140 Commonwealth Ave., Chestnut Hill, MA 02467, USA
tamirm@bc.edu

**Nicole Tausch**
School of Psychology, Cardiff University, Tower Building, 70 Park Place, Cardiff, CF10 3AT, UK
tauschn@Cardiff.ac.uk

**Julian F. Thayer, PhD**
The Ohio State University, Department of Psychology, 133 Psychology Building, 1835 Neil Avenue, Columbus, OH 43210, USA
thayer.39@osu.edu

**Martijn van Zomeren, PhD**
Department of Social and Organizational Psychology, University of Groningen, Grote Kruisstraat 2/1, 9712 TS Groningen, Netherlands
m.van.zomeren@rug.nl

**Daniel Västfjäll, PhD**
Decision Research, 1201 Oak St, Suite 200, 97401 Eugene, Oregon, USA
daniel.vastfjall@psy.gu.se

**Bart Verkuil, PhD**
Leiden University, Institute of Psychology, Clinical, Health and Neuropsychology Unit, P.O. Box 9555, 2300 RB Leiden, Netherlands
bverkuil@fsw.leidenuniv.nl

**Ad J.J.M. Vingerhoets**
Department of Developmental, Clinical, and Cross-Cultural Psychology, Tilburg University, P.O. Box 90153, 5000 LE Tilburg, Netherlands
vingerhoets@uvt.nl

**Tim Wildschut, PhD**
School of Psychology, University of Southampton, Southampton, SO17 1BJ, England, UK
timw@soton.ac.uk

**Andreas Wismeijer, PhD**
Department of Developmental, Clinical, and Cross-Cultural Psychology, Tilburg University, P.O. Box 90153, 5000 LE Tilburg, Netherlands
a.a.j.wismeijer@uvt.nl

**Vincent Yzerbyt, PhD**
Departement of Psychology, University of Louvain, Place Cardinal Mercier 10, B 1348 Louvain-la-Neuve, Belgium
Vincent.yzerbyt@uclouvain.be

**Marcel Zeelenberg**
Deaprtment of Social Psychology, Tilburg University, P.O. Box 90153, 5000 LE Tilburg, Netherlands
m.zeelenberg@uvt.nl

# Abbreviations

| | |
|---|---|
| AAI | Adult Attachment Interview |
| AAP | Adult Attachment Prototypes |
| ACT | Acceptance and Commitment Therapy |
| ANS | Autonomic Nervous System |
| BAS | Behavioral Activation System |
| BIS | Behavioral Inhibition System |
| (C)CBT | (Computer-assisted) Cognitive Behavioral Therapy |
| DBT | Dialectical Behavioral Therapy |
| DSM-IV | Diagnostic and Statistical Manual of Mental Disorders, 4th Edition |
| ECG | Electrocardiogram |
| EEG | Electroencephalograph(ic) |
| EER | Emotion and Emotion Regulation |
| EMA | Ecological Momentary Assessment |
| EMG | Electromyograph(ic) |
| ER | Emotion Regulation |
| ESM | Experience Sampling Method |
| EW | Expressive Writing |
| FTP | Future Time Perspective |
| GAD | Generalized Anxiety Disorder |
| HIV+ | Human Immunodeficiency Virus seropositive |
| KMS | Keeping a Major Secret |
| LEAS | Levels of Emotional Awareness Scale |
| MBSR | Mindfulness Based Stress Reduction |
| MDD | Major Depressive Disorder |
| PC | Perseverative Cognition |
| RCT | Randomized Controlled Trial |
| RQ | Relationship Questionnaire |
| SC | Self-Concealment |
| SIT | Social Identity Theory |
| STS | Superior Temporal Sulcus |
| SWB | Subjective Well-Being |
| TAS | Toronto Alexithymia Scale |
| ToM | Theory of Mind |

# Chapter 1
# Emotion Regulation and Well-Being: A View from Different Angles

**Ivan Nyklíček, Ad Vingerhoets, and Marcel Zeelenberg**

## 1.1 Emotion

Emotion is a basic phenomenon of human functioning, normally having an adaptive value enhancing our effectiveness in pursuing our goals in the broadest sense. On the inter-individual level, emotions help inform others about one's internal states and behavioral intentions (Frijda, 1986). Interchange of such information between people is essential for human relationships, a crucial determinant of social and psychological well-being. In addition, important intra-individual functions of emotions have been hypothesized and demonstrated. One example of an important function is gaining insight into one's personal values, which is a crucial motivational factor in adequate decision making (Bechara, Damasio, & Damasio, 2000).

Emotions are generally the result of the appraisal of events. Dependent on the outcome of appraisal, a coordinated set of responses involving behavioral and physiological systems is triggered (John & Gross, 2004; Scherer, Schorr, & Johnstone, 2001). Thus, emotions trigger specific action tendencies and the necessary physiological support, facilitating overt action. A well-known example of this process is the fight-flight reaction involving increased heart rate and blood pressure, dilation of the bronchi and increased blood flow to the muscles, preparing the body for action. Conversely, depressed affect and grief are characterized by a quite different physiological reaction pattern, aimed at the conservation of energy. This is expressed in a passive reaction, often accompanied with a reduced muscle tone with the head directed downward (Henry & Stephens, 1977). This passive condition may be adaptive, because it saves energy and it may act as a signal to indicate that the person is in need of emotional or instrumental support from others (Nesse, 2000). In addition, it may reduce aggression in possible assaulters.

There is little doubt that emotions have played an essential role in survival and adaptation of the human species (Ketelaar, 2004; Nesse & Ellsworth, 2009).

I. Nyklíček (✉)
Center of Research on Psychology in Somatic disease (CoRPS), Tilburg University,
P.O. Box 90153, 5000 LE Tilburg, Netherlands
e-mail: i.nyklicek@uvt.nl

I. Nyklíček et al. (eds.), *Emotion Regulation and Well-Being*,
DOI 10.1007/978-1-4419-6953-8_1, © Springer Science+Business Media, LLC 2011

However, for an adequate understanding, one has to be aware of the distinction between the short-term and long-term effects of emotions and of the major changes in living conditions of our ancestors and modern man.

## 1.2 Emotion Regulation and Well-Being

Emotion regulation (ER) is regarded as a crucial factor in well-being, in the popular literature, clinical psychological practice, and scientific research alike. Regulation of emotions is essential for adaptive functioning, and suboptimal or dysfunctional ER is perceived as counterproductive and resulting in adverse consequences including a poor well-being (Gross & Muñoz, 1995), and sometimes even somatic disease (for recent reviews, see Denollet, Nyklíček, & Vingerhoets, 2008; Gross & John, 2003).

ER and well-being are both broad concepts that can be viewed from different angles and at different levels of analysis: from a microlevel of firing neurons in certain brain areas to a macrolevel involving overt behavior of people in social interaction with others (e.g. sharing emotional experience and expression, being active in a satisfactory way in the contexts of one's social networks and society at large). In addition, they range between different points on the continuum from optimal functioning to dysfunction such as seen in psychopathology (psychological level), social isolation (social level) and somatic disease (physical level).

ER is defined here as regulation of affective states, in its broadest sense, covering all points on dimensions such as: overt (perceivable by others) to covert (internal regulation not perceivable by others), explicit (conscious) to implicit (unconscious), and voluntary to automatic (Gross, 1998).

### *1.2.1 Two Examples*

As stated above, cognitive appraisal is an important factor influencing the quality and intensity of the resulting emotion. Changing the way we appraise a potentially emotion-eliciting event, is one important example of *antecedent-focused* ER aimed at modifying the emotional impact of a situation (Gross, 1998). If one expects that another person plans to do harm, this may induce anxiety or anger; if an unpleasant situation is considered as being caused by one's own behavior, this will probably result in remorse, shame or guilt. If a situation is appraised as involving danger, fear is a likely emotional outcome, whereas loss experiences generally evoke sadness. Cognitive reappraisal may be applied to decrease negative feelings and increase positive feelings and adaptive behavior, which is manifested by increased interpersonal functioning and positive mood (Gross & John, 2003).

ER not only depends on our appraisal of the emotion-eliciting event. *Response-focused* ER involves behavior that manifests itself once the emotion process is already underway and response tendencies have already been generated (Gross, 1998). A common and widely studied form of this category of ER is emotion suppression, which refers to consciously inhibiting ongoing expression of emotion-related behavior. Emotion suppression may negatively influence one's self-image: it may make individuals feel inauthentic about themselves, facilitating negative emotions and depressive symptoms. In addition, while suppression decreases the behavioral expression of negative emotions, it does not affect subjective experiences (Gross & John, 2003). Importantly, there is increasing evidence that ER styles aimed at not expressing emotion, either consciously or unconsciously – in the latter case often called repression – may have adverse effects on not only subjective well-being, but also physical health (John & Gross, 2004; Jorgensen, 1996; Nyklíček, Vingerhoets, & Denollet, 2002).

### *1.2.2 Conceptual and Methodological Issues*

The effects of emotions and ER on well-being is depending on various factors, such as consequences of emotion experience and emotion expression for one's self-image, physiological consequences of the expression of emotions, the nature of the relationship with the person one expresses to, and his or her overt or expected reaction. For example, crying has been shown to elicit emotional support. It may be this social support or the fact that an opponent becomes less aggressive that makes one feel better rather than the shedding of tears per se (Hendriks, Nelson, Cornelius, & Vingerhoets, 2008).

When studying the relationship between ER and well-being, several methodological issues must be considered, before being able to draw valid conclusions regarding the specific nature of the association (Nyklíček et al., 2002). The first issue is a conceptual one. What is the conceptual model one is investigating? If the hypothesis is that ER influences well-being, what are the underlying mechanisms? Is the expected association a direct psychophysiological one (i.e. direct internal psychoneuroendocrine effects) or an indirect one? In the latter case, which factors mediate this association? These may involve intermediate effects such as changes in interpersonal relationships or changes in one's living environment (e.g. working environment), which subsequently influence one's psychological well-being. However, one should also take into consideration the possibility of a reverse causal path; more precisely, psychological well-being influencing the way one regulates emotions. One can imagine that when being in a positive mood, other ER strategies may be applied than when in a state of anger, sadness, or anxiety. Finally, the "third variable" option should also not be overlooked. For example, personality (e.g. neuroticism, extraversion) may influence both the preferred ER tactics as well as psychological well-being, potentially resulting in a spurious association between ER and well-being. This complexity emphasizes the need for the inclusion of basic psychological factors, such as personality characteristics, when investigating the association between factors that are at least partially dependent on them, such as ER and well-being.

Further, ER and well-being are dependent on the situational context, which possibly may also influence the association between ER and well-being (Kennedy-Moore & Watson, 1999). Another potential context ER and its relation with well-being is influenced by is phase of life. ER strategies may not be equally effective in enhancing well-being across all life phases (Consedine, see Chap. 2). All such interactions imply statistical moderation effects that should be taken into account. ER itself may act as a moderator in a relationship between environmental challenge and psychological well-being. An example of this would be the case that only in certain stressful situations ER strategies are associated with well-being, not in situations without any challenge (Nyklíček et al., 2002). One step further, certain behavioral strategies that are generally associated with negative well-being, may simultaneously have positive psychological consequences (e.g. sense of personal growth) in certain challenging situations.

Needless to say that the study design is crucial concerning the issue to what degree causal inferences can be made. While only experimental designs allow conclusions concerning causality, prospective cohort studies with follow-up periods that are long enough and with adequate control for possible confounding variables are the second best, leaving correlational studies at the other extreme of complete inadequacy regarding attempts for answering the question of causality, no matter how advanced the statistical analysis one employs may be.

## 1.3 Contents of this Volume

This volume brings together various approaches to ER and it makes clear how they may relate to well-being. This allows the readers to view and examine this association and its fundaments from different perspectives, complementing each other and thus making the resulting picture more detailed and complete. Well-being in this volume refers mainly to psychological well-being, but some chapters also discuss the relation between ER and well-being in the social context. For example, the chapter by De Hooge et al. (Chap. 12) reviews work on interpersonal behaviors that follow experiences of guilt and shame, whereas Rimé et al. (Chap. 9) discuss the effects of sharing one's emotions with others. In other chapters, the focus is more on physical well-being (physiological functioning or physical disease; Chaps. 1 and 6).

The volume is organized along three major perspectives: (1) basic psychological processes involved in the link between ER and health, (2) the social, lifespan, and gender contexts in which the associations between ER and well-being take place and which influence the nature of the associations, and (3) views and applications in the clinical context.

### *1.3.1 Basic Psychological Processes*

In the first part, psychological processes are discussed that may be fundamental for the phenomenon of ER, especially in its relation to well-being, ranging from unconscious processes to conscious tactics and even a certain deliberate lack of volitional regulation as seen in mindfulness.

In the first chapter, Consedine considers ER from a broader perspective of the functional context the different stages of life provide. The often heard claim that ER may improve with age is challenged by Consedine who argues that (1) not much evidence exists in favor of this view and (2) the reality is far more complex. It is argued that ER capacities and its relation to well-being depend on three main categories of factors, namely psychophysiological capacity, targets of ER, and tactics used to attain them, which all change during life.

ER from a social cognitive perspective is discussed by Tamir and Mauss in the second chapter. They argue that two important factors determining ER, namely one's beliefs about controllability and self-efficacy, and values and goals of ER, have not received adequate attention from theorists and researchers to date. They provide a theoretical framework emphasizing the relevance of these factors, in addition to strategies and competencies. They also review the empirical literature on these factors with their relation to well-being.

Ruys et al. address whether people need not be consciously aware of the eliciting events for emotions to unfold. They propose a global-to-specific unfolding view on emotional responding, analogous to the contention that perception typically unfolds from global to specific. They also demonstrate that both global moods and specific emotional reactions can be triggered unconsciously and contrast this view with appraisal theories of emotion.

Wildschut et al. address the possible role of positive emotions, in particular nostalgia, for one's well-being. Recent evidence is presented suggesting that nostalgia may occur in particular when one feels lonely, which makes sense, because nostalgia appears to have the capacity to increase perceived social connectedness. The authors further discuss how this effect may be moderated by personality characteristics, in particular resilience and attachment style.

The potentially central role of perseverative cognition in dysregulation of both mental and physiological processes is the focus of the chapter by Verkuil et al. Perseverative cognition, such as worry and rumination, substantially extends the period of experienced distress with its concomitant load on both the nervous system and the other systems of the body (e.g. endocrine, immune, cardiovascular). Evidence is reviewed for this hypothesis as well as for the role of excessive goal commitment in trait perseverative thinkers in the relation with well-being and health.

Mindfulness and its relation to ER and well-being is discussed by Nyklíček in the last chapter of this section. Mindfulness is a state of open and nonjudgmental attention to phenomena occurring in the present moment. Although its positive association with well-being is well established, the role of ER in this association is still unclear. It is claimed that mindfulness enhances adaptive ER, but that the effect is indirect, via effects such as decreased experiential avoidance and decreased perseverative cognition. A new theoretical model and preliminary evidence is presented.

### *1.3.2 ER and Well-Being in the Social Context*

In the second part of this volume, the social, lifespan, and gender contexts of emotional regulation and more general emotional processing is discussed. Traditional emotion research has focused primarily on intra-individual processes, while many emotions are elicited and experienced in social contexts. Moreover, many emotions and emotional phenomena are highly social in nature. This is apparent in all chapters in this section, but is central in the chapter by Spears et al. They review research on intergroup emotions and group-based emotions. Spears et al. argue that taking into account ER processes when studying intergroup behavior extends our understanding of intergroup relations but also feeds back into emotion theory. They build on the concept of social appraisal, the idea that emotional reactions of others inform people about their own emotional experience (Manstead & Fischer, 2001).

One intriguing aspect of emotional behavior is the human need to engage in the social sharing of emotion. Rimé et al. argue that social sharing of emotion and collective rituals are markedly similar. Both lack the capacity to bring emotional recovery, and are more likely to induce the reactivation of the emotional episode. However, both also elicit empathic processes and bring those interacting closer together and may hence buffer the potentially destabilizing effects that emotional events may have.

Västfjäll et al. focus on the regulation of a specific emotional experience, namely regret (cf., Zeelenberg & Pieters, 2007). Regret negatively impacts psychological and physical health and understanding how and why we experience regret and how regret influences choices and behaviors is important. Västfjäll et al. start from the premise that little is known about how and if the experience and anticipation of regret changes over the adult life-span. Hence they review the available research and merge existing findings to develop a set of novel hypotheses of how aging and emotional experience and regulation may interact in everyday life.

The relationship between attachment and ER, with a specific focus on adult crying, is explored by Maas et al. They make clear how attachment styles may exert a life-time influence on ER. They further emphasize that crying may be considered an attachment behavior, which implies that not only the exposure to an emotional event is important for crying, but also the availability (and presence) of an attachment figure. They further summarize recent findings consistently demonstrating that an avoidant attachment style is associated with the inhibition of tears and negative emotions.

De Hooge et al. review research on the self-conscious emotions and how they may facilitate or inhibit prosocial behaviors. The gist of their argument is that these emotions, as any other emotion, are best understood if one adopts a pragmatic perspective. That is, predictions about emotional behavior are best made on the basis of the experiential content of the emotions. Such an approach explains why sometimes moral emotions are regulated by means of amoral behaviors.

Evers et al. adopt a social appraisal perspective to understand gender effects in ER. They debunk the general stereotypes about how males and females cope with emotion, more specifically anger. The authors review research showing that gender affects the regulation of anger expressions but only in interaction with the social context. Males and females do behave differently in response to anger. But, this difference can easily be understood in terms of expectations about how others respond to their anger expressions.

Together these chapters are testimony to the importance of interpersonal and more general social aspects of emotion elicitation and regulation. They reveal that emotions and the way in which people cope with them play an important role in how people interact. The chapters also show that these interpersonal processes are crucial for a full understanding of ER.

### 1.3.3 Clinical Perspective

The third part of this volume is devoted to several views and applications in the clinical context. This section starts with a chapter by Bylsma and Rottenberg who aptly review the Experience Sampling Method, a useful approach for the study of emotion and ER in daily life of patients and healthy individuals. The additional value of this method also relates to the fact that it offers the possibility to focus on the dynamics of experiences and behaviors as they develop over time. The authors, who have a wealth of experience with the study of mood and anxiety disorders, put forth suggestions how the method can be used for improving diagnosis and treatment of emotional disorders.

Somatoform disorders and the role of alexithymia and mentalization, also termed psychological mindedness, are discussed by Subic-Wrana. This author argues that deficits in awareness and differentiation of one's own emotional states (alexithymia) and those of others (lack of mentalization) may be etiologically involved in the development of somatization and somatoform disorders. First evidence for a link between these factors and somatoform disorders is presented and discussed.

Kret et al. focus on emotion perception processes in faces as well as whole bodies and their relation to various neuropsychological disorders, such as autism, schizophrenia, and neurodegenerative disorders. The relevance of these processes for psychiatric conditions, including anxiety and depression, and for personality factors that are associated with health risks, is also reviewed. Behavioral, electrophysiological, and neurofunctional data on these associations and their implications are discussed.

Corter and Petrie devote their chapter to the latest findings regarding the evaluation of Pennebaker's expressive writing cure among cancer patients and whether this approach is an accepted and feasible intervention for this group. It is concluded that prostate and breast cancer patients report many positive effects on symptoms and medical care use, which is consistent with results obtained in other cancer patient groups. In contrast, there is no evidence that writing may prolong survival and it neither seems to have a positive effect on emotional distress.

Current theorizing about emotional eating is discussed by Macht and Simon. In particular, they address individual differences in emotional eating behavior and the underlying mechanisms. They emphasize the role of psychological (hedonic) and physiological (more precisely neurochemical) factors, the impact of which depends on the degree of emotional eating. Whereas they consider the hedonic responses as essential in most instances of emotional eating, in some cases positive neurochemical effects may also play a role.

In the final chapter, Wismeijer discusses the intra-individual and inter-individual consequences of secrecy, especially for one's psychological well-being. It is argued that secrecy is a multifaceted phenomenon, consisting of several independent factors that may have different consequences. A theoretical model is presented and the particular example of the sometimes opposite effects of being a secretive person as a trait, usually having a negative impact on well-being, and keeping a specific secret as a state, sometimes having positive consequences, is highlighted.

## 1.4 Conclusion

As can be seen from this overview, the topic of ER in its relation to well-being is discussed from different and often multidisciplinary views, providing both a broad and an in-depth discussion of the topic. The theories, reviews of the evidence, and critical reflections are relevant for both researchers from various disciplines and clinicians working with clients with emotional problems.

## References

Bechara A., Damasio, H., & Damasio, A. R. (2000) Emotion, decision making and the orbitofrontal cortex. *Cerebral Cortex*, *10*, 295–307.

Denollet, J., Nyklíček, I., & Vingerhoets, A. (2008) Introduction: Emotions, emotion regulation, and health. In A. Vingerhoets, I. Nyklíček, & J. Denollet (Eds.), *Emotion regulation: Conceptual and clinical issues* (pp. 3–11). New York: Springer.

Frijda, N. H. (1986) *The emotions*. New York: Cambridge University Press.

Gross, J. J. (1998) Antecedent- and response-focused emotion regulation: divergent consequences for experience, expression, and physiology. *Journal of Personality and Social Psychology*, *74*, 224–237.

Gross, J. J., & John, O. P. (2003) Individual differences in two emotion regulation processes: implications for affect, relationships, and well-being. *Journal of Personality and Social Psychology*, *85*, 348–362.

Gross, J. J., & Muñoz, R. F. (1995) Emotion regulation and mental health. *Clinical Psychology: Science and Practice*, *2*, 151–164.

Hendriks, M. C. P., Nelson, J. K., Cornelius, R. R., & Vingerhoets, A. J. J. M. (2008) Why crying improves our well-being: An attachment theory perspective on the functions of adult crying. In A. Vingerhoets, I. Nyklíček, & J. Denollet (Eds.), *Emotion regulation: Conceptual and clinical issues* (pp. 87–96). New York: Springer.

Henry, J. P., & Stephens, P. M. (1977) *Stress, health and the social environment: A sociobiological approach to medicine*. Berlin: Springer.

John, O. P., & Gross, J. J. (2004) Healthy and unhealthy emotion regulation: personality processes, individual differences, and life span development. *Journal of Personality*, *72*, 1301–1333.

Jorgensen, R. S. (1996) Elevated blood pressure and personality: A meta-analytic review. *Psychological Bulletin*, *120*, 293–320.

Kennedy-Moore, E., & Watson, J. C. (1999) *Expressing emotion: Myths, realities, and therapeutic strategies.*. New York: Guilford.

Ketelaar, T. (2004) Ancestral emotions, current decisions: Using evolutionary game theory to explore the role of emotions in decision making. In C. Crawford & C. Salmon (Eds.), *Evolutionary psychology, public policy and personal decisions* (pp. 145–168). Mahwah, NJ: Lawrence Erlbaum.

Manstead, A. S. R., & Fischer, A. H. (2001) Social appraisal: The social world as object of and influence on appraisal processes. In K. R. Scherer & A. Schorr (Eds.), *Appraisal processes in emotion: Theory, methods, research* (pp. 221–232). London: Oxford University Press.

Nesse, R. M. (2000) Is depression an adaptation? *Archives of General Psychiatry*, *57*, 14–20.

Nesse, R. M., & Ellsworth, P. C. (2009) Evolution, emotions, and emotional disorders. *American Psychologist*, *64*, 129–139.

Nyklíček, I., Vingerhoets, A. J., & Denollet, J. (2002) Emotional (non-)expression and health: Data, questions, and challenges. *Psychology and Health*, *17*, 517–528.

Scherer, K. R., Schorr, A., & Johnstone, T. (2001) (Eds.), *Appraisal processes in emotion: Theory, methods, research*. London: London University Press.

Zeelenberg, M., & Pieters, R. (2007) A theory of regret regulation 1.0. *Journal of Consumer Psychology*, *17*, 3–18.

# Part I
# Basic Psychological Processes

# Chapter 2
# Capacities, Targets, and Tactics: Lifespan Emotion Regulation from the Perspective of Developmental Functionalism

**Nathan S. Consedine**

## 2.1 Current Data and Interpretations Regarding Age Differences in Emotion and Emotion Regulation

Broadly speaking, there are three classes of data that address lifespan emotion regulation. First are self-report data circumscribing a less negative/more positive "affective balance" among older adults (Carstensen, Mayr, Pasupathi, & Nesselroade, 2000; Charles, Reynolds, & Gatz, 2001; Mroczek & Kolarz, 1998) and/or reporting greater emotional control (Gross et al., 1997). In many cases, such data are the basis upon which inferences about differences and/or changes in emotion regulation are made. Second, other self-report studies have assessed emotion regulatory tendencies somewhat more directly, with data showing either greater control in older groups (Labouvie-Vief, Hakin-Larson, DeVoe, & Schoeberlein, 1989; McConatha & Huba, 1999), a preference for conflict avoidance, delayed expression, de-escalation, and/or a wider range of coping/defense strategies in later life (Birditt & Fingerman, 2005; Levenson, Carstensen, & Gottman, 1994).

Finally, there are studies that have *experimentally* manipulated and measured the ability to regulate the visible (facial) expression of emotion in developmentally diverse groups – ironically, no study provides unequivocal support for the notion that there are age related improvements in emotion regulation. One study (Kunzmann, Kupperbusch, & Levenson, 2005) assigned younger and older participants to a control condition or to suppress and amplify emotional expressions during film presentation. No age differences in the effects of the regulatory instruction, or the impact of regulation on experience or physiology were found. Other experimental studies suggest that younger and older adults are equally able to inhibit expression (Magai, Consedine, Krivoshekova, McPherson, & Kudadjie-Gyamfi, 2006; Phillips, Henry, Hosie, & Milne, 2008), and that older adults are more effective in reducing the early experience of negative emotion (Phillips et al., 2008).

N.S. Consedine (✉)
Department of Psychological Medicine, Level 12, Support Building,
Room 12.003, Faculty of Medical and Health Sciences, The University of Auckland,
Private Bag 92019, Auckland, New Zealand
e-mail: n.consedine@auckland.ac.nz

I. Nyklíček et al. (eds.), *Emotion Regulation and Well-Being*,
DOI 10.1007/978-1-4419-6953-8_2, © Springer Science+Business Media, LLC 2011

Taken together, the available work has generally been interpreted as indicating lifespan improvements in emotion and emotion regulation (EER):

> "a growing body of empirical research… points instead to developmental gains in later life" (Carstensen, Fung, & Charles, 2003. p. 103)

> "old age is marked by … improved regulation of emotions" (Carstensen & Charles, 1998. p. 144)

Unfortunately, writers *infer* superior regulation based on greater positive affect and accept self-reported regulatory tendencies as evidence of improved *skill*. The notion of improvement with age is central to leading theories of emotion and aging and forms the entry point into most contemporary empirical work. This interpretation has become so popular that, in the near-absence of experimental and/or longitudinal proof, the notion that emotional functioning improves with age has attained the status of a contemporary dogma. As when a supposedly prestigious wine is purchased on the recommendation of a less than reputable merchant, we are repeatedly told that EER "improve with age." Worse yet, we strive to believe this assertion despite the evidence from our palate and knowing full well that even the best of vintages are subject to the vagaries and vicissitudes of time. Less dramatically, in accepting the consequente (greater positive emotion) as proof of the process (better emotion regulation), the field commits a major logical fallacy. The normative construal regarding lifespan differences in emotion regulation *vastly* exceeds the extant empirical base.

## 2.2 Developmental Functionalism: A Brief Overview

Any theory of emotion regulation must be based in a clear conceptualization of emotions. Developmental functionalism (Consedine, 2008; Consedine & Magai, 2003, 2006; Consedine, Magai, & Bonanno, 2002; Consedine, Magai, & King, 2004; Consedine & Moscowitz, 2007) is a discrete emotions approach to emotions and their links to outcome that pays explicit attention to age related issues. Each emotion represents an adaptation that evolved to facilitate adaptive responding with respect to reliably occurring selective pressures in past environments (Nesse, 1990) – specific classes of adaptive challenge or opportunity (Consedine & Moscowitz, 2007). Emotions are "particular" mechanisms, shaped by natural selection to adjust aspects of the organism's responses in ways that have, on average, given an advantage with respect to particular *types* of situation (Tooby & Cosmides, 2008).

While immediate or future behavioral change is necessary for selection to operate (Consedine, Strongman, & Magai, 2003), emotions accomplish multiple functional ends via multiple componential changes. The components of an emotional response include cognitive changes (Keltner, Ellsworth, & Edwards, 1993), physiology (Levenson, 1994), signals (Brown & Consedine, 2004), experience (Izard, 1991), and behavior (Consedine et al., 2003). Importantly, while the components of an emotion tend to be similar notwithstanding variation in the elicitor and tend to co-occur (particularly in early life), this does not mean that each component is accomplishing the same functional end (Consedine & Moscowitz, 2007). While components share functions with respect to situational classes, each component may have a unique role in facilitating adaptation. This view of emotion implies that the motivations, capacity requirements, and consequences of *regulating* diverse components will vary (Consedine, Magai, & Bonanno, 2002). In particular, because their functions may be quite distinct, we should expect distinct consequences to follow the regulation of *emotion signals* (expressions) versus the regulation of experience.

While emotions are adaptive in general, developmental functionalism suggests that emotions entail both fitness costs and benefits (Consedine & Moscowitz, 2007). Emotions are "many splendored things" (c.f. Averill, 1994), that have multiple effects on bodily and social systems. Adaptations, like the emotions, involve selective trade-offs (Kaplan, Hill, Lancaster, & Hurtado, 2000) and opportunity costs (Bjorklund & Bering, 2002) in terms of investment in other adaptations that might be more adaptive in a different developmental environment. Emotions are almost certainly designed with an eye towards early life (Consedine, Magai, & Bonanno, 2002) for the simple reason that later life suitability is moot if the organism does not survive to reproduce. Thus, the manner in which emotions are capable of functioning in later life is *constrained* by their structure *as they were selected for regarding developmentally earlier challenges*. Although selective pressures on post-reproductive years exist (Carstensen & Löckenhoff, 2003), optimal early life designs will likely be suboptimal in later life, and the earlier design will be favored. Adults of different ages may "inherit" a constellation of emotional systems selected because they facilitated adaptation to early life tasks (Consedine & Moscowitz, 2007).

Perhaps most importantly, developmental functionalism suggests that because individuals from different stages of life are confronted with different challenges and tasks (Consedine & Magai, 2006), and have different capacities and resources, the functions of emotions and their manifestations in organismic systems vary. Changes in EER are powerfully influenced by the interrelated characteristics of the eliciting situation, developmental changes in the primary challenges or tasks facing the organism, as well as by their changing physiological, cognitive, social, and behavioral capabilities.

## 2.3 Organismic Tasks Change with Age

Developmental functionalism asserts that understanding of lifespan changes in emotion regulation is predicated on understanding the adaptive tasks that have normatively confronted organisms at different stages of development. If emotions were selected because of their utility in meeting particular adaptive challenges (Tooby & Cosmides, 2008), then their functions and the manner in which they operate must be found with respect to them. The challenges we have faced as a social species are numerous, immensely complex, and both long- and short-term. A brief list would include: ensuring maternal attention (Bowlby, 1969), internalizing real world physical rules, face recognition, foraging, mate choice and retention, heart rate regulation, sleep management, predator vigilance, alliance and cheater detection (Tooby & Cosmides, 2008), knowledge transmission and conflict resolution (Carstensen & Löckenhoff, 2003), and accommodating reductions in systemic resources (Baltes, 1997).

However, most importantly with respect to the current discussion, *the primary tasks confronting organisms vary developmentally* (Consedine & Magai, 2006). At birth, the human newborn is unformed and helpless (Eibl-Eibesfeldt, 1989), and takes a long time to mature (Bjorklund, 1997). Although there are advantages to this design (Bjorklund, 1997; Kaplan et al., 2000), one consequence is that the most pressing adaptive challenges are (a) to communicate and bond with an caregiver such that the they will provide them with the protection, care, and sustenance they need (Bowlby, 1969), and (b) to develop in such a way as to reduce the fitness costs of events upon repetition – they must be able to learn.

In contrast, young adults are confronted with the challenges involved in selecting, attracting, and securing a mate, in reproduction itself, and in successfully raising offspring. These tasks are, in turn, less relevant to older adults, who have typically raised children and acquired the bulk of the information they require, at least as indexed by the self-reported importance of information seeking goals (Carstensen, 1995). Older individuals must adapt to declining social and cognitive resources (Baltes, 1997), declining physical, motor, or somatic capabilities (Panksepp & Miller, 1995), increases in dependency (Baltes, 1996), and with new roles in the intergenerational transmission of knowledge and resources (Carstensen & Löckenhoff, 2003), conflict resolution, and second generation kin-care.

In short, adaptive challenges and opportunities and the accompanying selective pressures vary developmentally, and the functions of emotions are consequently likely to vary in tandem. There are few data circumscribing lifespan changes in normative life tasks or elicitors of emotion. Nonetheless, it seems likely that emotions assist organisms with respect to different adaptive challenges, in different ways, at different stages of the life cycle (Consedine & Magai, 2006). In developmental functionalism, maintaining an appreciation for an organism's primary tasks is critical to the study of EER because this understanding provides guidance when seeking to determine (a) the situations the organisms will likely find themselves in, (b) the likely targets and purpose of emotion regulatory processes, and (c) the consequences of more and less effective regulatory strategies.

## 2.4 Organismic Capacities Change with Age

The developmental functionalist view suggests that lifespan changes in EER cannot be understood in isolation from changes in the physiological, social, cognitive, and behavioral capabilities of the organism. It seems evident that emotion and emotion regulatory systems require numerous developmentally varying capacities. Importantly, while we can characterize the functions of an emotion like sadness in the broad terms of an "adaptation to irrevocable loss" (Averill, 1968), the *manner* in which an emotion facilitates the accomplishment of functional ends varies depending on capacities (Consedine & Magai, 2006). In developmental functionalism, emotions' functions are differentially manifest in infants, adolescents, younger, and older adults *because* humans have different physical, cognitive, experiential, behavioral, and social resources at different stages.

Among infants, for example, developmental constraints mean the functions of emotions are primarily manifest in signaling channels. With poorly developed cognitive and behavioral capacities, the changes that characterize sadness may facilitate energy conservation (Brehm, Brummett, & Harvey, 1999) and help elicit assistance from the social surround via facial and vocal signaling (Averill, 1968; Izard, 1991) for both infants and older organisms. However, other functions of sadness, including altering of goal relationships (Johnson-Laird & Oatley, 1992), and constructing plans for dealing with losses (Stein & Levine, 1990) suggest certain levels of cognitive-representational development and are unlikely to form part of the functions of sadness in infancy. Thus, in developmental functionalism, as behavioral, cognitive, experiential, physical, signaling, and social systems develop and decline with age, the initial signaling functions of the emotions are progressively supplemented with additional cognitive, experiential/motivational, and social functions.

A similar argument applies in the case of emotion physiology. Changes in physiology are critical to emotion's functions insofar as they create a physiological milieu that supports adaptive action (Levenson, 1994). In developmental functionalism, because physiological resources (Labouvie-Vief, Lumley, Jain, & Heinze, 2003; Levenson, Carstensen, Friesen, & Ekman, 1991; Levenson et al., 1994; Tsai, Carstensen, & Levenson, 2000) and the system's ability to tolerate deviations from baseline (Davidson, 1993; Panksepp & Miller, 1995) decline developmentally, emotions' physiological functions and manifestations are likely to shift to accommodate changes in resource availability. In older adults, reductions in physiological capabilities parallel a reduced capacity for certain types of adaptive action and may index a developmentally graded shift in function *away from behavioral activation*. Consistent with this view, older adults show a lower level of somatic activity in fear (Levenson et al., 1991). Lower somatic activity when afraid may reflect a transition in the primary behavioral manifestations of fear, with "flight" being primary in youth and "freezing" becoming more prominent in older subjects.

At root, the developmental functionalist view suggests that understanding the functions and operations of EER systems is necessarily informed by an understanding of the relevant organismic capacities. Coupled with an understanding of organismic tasks, changes in capacities have profound implications for the individual's *ability* to regulate different aspects of emotions at different points in the emotion process. Lifespan changes in physiological, cognitive, experiential, behavioral, and social capacities are likely to influence (a) situational exposure and selection processes, (b) the targets and purpose of emotion regulation, and (c) the consequences of more and less effective strategies.

## 2.5 Implications for the Study of Lifespan Changes in Emotion Regulation

Following from these assertions are several subsidiary claims, many of which lead to testable predictions about the processes of EER across the lifespan. Below, four areas of theoretical and empirical development are described with the focus resting on how the view of emotion regulation implied within developmental functionalism may provide insights into emotion regulation and its links to outcomes.

### *2.5.1 The Targets of Emotion Regulation May Change with Age*

Task and capacity are critical concepts because they provide a global backdrop to the assessment of lifespan changes and differences in the *targets* of emotion regulation, a content issue that researchers know little about; there are no studies that systematically assess the targets of regulation in developmentally diverse samples. Rather than measure regulatory targets, we equate greater positivity with superior regulation, *assuming* that the primary target of regulation is to maximize felt positive emotion (Charles, Mather, & Carstensen, 2003). Such an undifferentiated, *hedonic* approach that concentrates on experiential and, to a lesser extent, expressive regulation, is inconsistent with models of emotion regulation (Bonanno, 2001; Bonanno, Papa, Lalande, Westphal, & Coifman, 2004; Gross, 2001), with functionalist approaches to emotions (Consedine & Magai, 2006; Tooby & Cosmides, 1990, 2000), and with data showing that both hedonic and instrumental motivations influence emotion regulatory processes (Tamir, Mitchell, & Gross, 2008).

First, any model of regulation is predicated on the notion that the system is seeking a "set point" or "emotional goal state" (Lucas, Clarke, Georgellis, & Diener, 2004) – an emotional target. However, rather than *measure* targets, writers assume that the target of experiential regulation is "greater positive affect/lower negative affect" despite the fact that the human emotional repertoire exists *precisely because* the full range of discrete emotions has generally proven adaptive. Cross-cultural work suggests that the motivation to experience happiness is lower among non-Americans (Izard, 1971) and/or Westerners (Eid & Diener, 2001), and that "ideal" or goal affect varies cross-culturally (Tsai, Knutson, & Fung, 2006). Whether experiential or expressive goals vary developmentally/across cohorts remain open questions, although attachment research – generally showing greater dismissiveness with age – suggests older cohorts have more restrictive expressive and experiential goals (Consedine & Magai, 2003). Theory regarding the signal value of distinct emotional expressions (Brown & Consedine, 2004) implies variation at the level of discrete emotions and the possibility that the consequences of "successful" regulation are influenced by the extent to which processes ensure target states rather than positive affect is worth investigating.

Second, it is noteworthy that data addressing the question of which *particular* emotional expressions and experiences are subject to which forms of regulation by persons from across the lifespan is missing. Developmental functionalism is capable of providing guidance regarding which components of which emotions are likely to be regulated. In the context of expressive regulation, for example, it would seem likely that the preference of older adults for conflict avoidance should lead to a premium on the downregulation of signals that have negative interpersonal consequences. Both benefits and costs accompany disclosures, expressions, and inhibition (Consedine, Magai, & Bonanno, 2002) and while inhibition may have negative effects on health, expressed negativity may produce negative social consequences. Angry expressions, in particular, can be unpleasant and frightening (Kennedy-Moore & Watson, 1999) and may threaten interpersonal relationships (Keltner et al., 1993). Similarly, while sadness expressions have evolved specifically in order to evoke sympathy and helping responses in others (Averill, 1968; Izard, 1971), excessive sadness may lead to rejection from others (Bonanno, Keltner, Holen, & Horowitz, 1995).

Finally, theory of lifespan emotion regulation pays only passing attention to the distinction between regulating experiences versus regulating expressions. Hypothetically, a shift in motivational priorities emphasizing affective over informational goals provides the backdrop for the age related prioritization of positive experience. The view of developmental functionalism is distinct from this hedonic characterization insofar as it suggests that considering the normative *targets* of emotion regulatory processes in conjunction with *organismic capacity* is a necessary precursor to understanding the techniques and tactics used by individuals to attain their regulatory goals as well as the consequences.

### 2.5.2 Diverse Emotion Regulatory Capacities Vary with Age

Emotion regulation has been characterized as a set of *skills or abilities* that are acquired across the lifespan (Gross et al., 1997; Labouvie-Vief et al., 2003). Emotion regulation is a complex, highly nuanced constellation of abilities that requires the capacity to flexibly and strategically adjust aspects of emotions in accordance with goals and situational demands (Bonanno et al., 2004), in both real-time as well as in anticipation (Gross, 2001; Magai et al., 2006) or retrospectively. The capacity requirements for emotion regulation are extensive. Even a simple form of regulation such as expressive suppression during a social exchange requires that the individual represent and assess their current state and its visible signals, the emotional state and signals of one or more others, and evaluate the potential impact and efficacy of a large number of possible alterations in signaling on a moment-by-moment basis.

The fact that emotion regulatory abilities emerge relatively late in child development likewise implies that the capacities needed to enact regulation are not simple (Eisenberg, 2000). Indeed, regulatory abilities in the early years are so primitive that a large proportion of infant and young children's emotion regulation occurs through others. A short list of the "requirements" for emotion regulation would include self-awareness and cultural referencing ability (Saarni, 1989), attentional resources/control (Ochsner & Gross, 2005), linguistic capacities (Eisenberg, Sadovsky, & Spinrad, 2005), and understanding regarding the connection between emotions and internal processes (Thompson & Meyer, 2007).

Making matters more complex is the fact that, by definition, regulation requires effort and depletes a *finite* pool of regulatory resource (Baumeister, Bratslavsky, Muraven, & Tice, 1998). Evidence suggests that the deployment of self-regulatory capacities in one context depletes the amount available for subsequent tasks (Baumeister et al., 1998). It remains unclear how this "pool" should be characterized and/or measured in developmental emotion regulation research although dividing tasks up by their regulatory requirements would seem an obvious starting point. It may be, for example, that the raw "amount" of online regulatory resource declines in later life, but that reductions are offset by an increasing ability to effectively *deploy* the resources that are available (Baltes, 1997) – changes in regulatory tactics.

In the developmental functionalist view, the capacities needed for regulation have complex trajectories of improvement and decline across the lifespan. Several lines of research suggest that older adults are more reflective and conscious of emotions and themselves and have greater knowledge regarding emotions, the links between situational exposures and emotions, and the effects of emotion on others (Labouvie-Vief, Chiodo, Goguen, Diehl, & Orwoll, 1995; Labouvie-Vief et al., 1989; Schieman, 1999). Thus, there is evidence that knowledge based and self-reflective capacities germane to emotion regulation may increase with age, although it is worth noting that emotion recognition ability appears to decline (MacPherson, Phillips, & Della Sala, 2006).

Recent studies examining age differences in aspects of cognitive processing, attention, and memory provide a demonstration of how complex the capacity issue is (for a review, see Mather & Carstensen, 2005). Older adults appear to preferentially recall positive material (Mather & Carstensen, 2005), differentially de-attend to negative stimuli (Mather & Carstensen, 2003), and show greater amygdala activation in response to positive versus negative pictures (Mather et al., 2004). Such data have been interpreted as consistent with improvements in regulation, with the general conclusion being that both cognitive abilities and motivation contribute (Mather & Carstensen, 2005). However, other data show that the attentional avoidance of negative stimuli that characterizes older adults is reversed (with greater attention to negative stimuli) when cognitive load increases (as when they are distracted) (Knight et al., 2007).

More generally, capacities necessary for other forms of emotion regulation appear to decline; older adults have generally fewer adaptive resources. Somatic resource and energy levels decline (Panksepp & Miller, 1995), and there are widespread declines in executive functioning as well as in tasks involving planning, inhibition, abstraction (Gilhooly, Phillips, Wynn, Logie, & Della Sala, 1999), task switching (Kray & Lindenberger, 2000), and selective attention (Maylor & Lavie, 1998). If we accept that resources of this class are sometimes necessary for the "real time" deployment of regulatory resource, it seems likely that such regulation may become more (rather than less difficult) in later life.

There are a number of ways in which the capacities required for various emotion regulatory strategies could be grouped – by regulation's purpose, by the component of emotion that is targeted, or by the temporal stage at which regulation occurs. Although some regulatory techniques target multiple components (such as when we anticipatorily avoid a situation likely to provoke anger because we do not wish to *appear* angry), the approach advocated here suggests a clear demarcation between two interrelated classes of capacity – those necessary for real time regulation of experience, signals, behavior, and physiology and those needed for regulatory techniques that occur prior to an emotion's activation such as avoidance or situational selection.

To return to the question of developmental differences in emotion regulatory capacities, the evidence suggests that resources needed for regulation where an emotional response is already active (e.g., signal regulation), decline with age whereas those germane to anticipatory and retrospective techniques may improve. Developmental functionalism suggests that although online regulatory tasks may become somewhat automatized and thus less resource demanding (see Mauss, Evers, Wilhelm, & Gross, 2006) with repeated use or be expedited through use of developmentally acquired knowledge, *the capability to voluntarily deploy emotion regulatory resources in real time nonetheless relies on cognitive and physiological resources* that decline with age. Examining age differences in the balance of automatic versus voluntary emotion regulatory strategies is a key area for future study.

### 2.5.3 *The Tactics Used to Attain Regulatory Goals Vary with Age*

Closely linked to issues of capacity are questions of technique, strategy, and tactics. Changes in capacity may make certain targets and tactics more and less viable and/or effective for individuals of different ages. Consistent with Baltes' (1997) model of selection, optimization, and compensation, developmental functionalism suggests that changes in regulatory capacities promote changes in both the targets of regulation as well as the strategies used to attain them.

Lifespan research has concentrated on the downregulation of negative emotion and anticipatory techniques such as conflict avoidance and situational selection, an apparent age difference in regulatory targets. Older adults use several tactics to achieve this end; they are less reactive to interpersonal stressors (Birditt, Fingerman, & Almeida, 2005), more flexible in problem solving than younger adults (Blanchard-Fields, Chen, & Norris, 1997), and when stressors revolve around emotionally charged interpersonal issues, deploy emotion-focused strategies (Blanchard-Fields, Camp, & Jahnke, 1995). Older adults use greater distancing and positive reappraisal (Folkman, Lazarus, Pimley, & Novacek, 1987), and report more goals aimed at avoiding losses and fewer at maximizing gains than younger groups, together with greater goal flexibility (Heckhausen, 1997). To this extent, developmentally acquired emotional understanding and knowledge may enable older adults to more effectively seek and manage the environments that further their emotional goals either because they are better capacitated for this form of regulation (in terms of knowledge), or because forms of regulation in response to situations where emotions are already active are too resource demanding in systems with fewer online resources.

More broadly, although it may be tempting on this basis to suggest that older adults are better regulators, the components of emotions can be regulated in an astonishing variety of ways (Bonanno, 2001). Current data circumscribe a restricted range of strategies and targets that have been assessed with retrospective, self-report techniques; the full range of regulatory tactics has yet to be examined. Experiences and expressions can be both up- and down-regulated (experience or expression heightened versus being suppressed), and indeed faked (Consedine, Magai, & Bonanno, 2002). Experiences can be avoided, anticipated, adjusted, and foreclosed. Developmental functionalism emphasizes a distinction between skill based regulation under conditions of authentic emotional arousal and regulatory techniques centered in representational knowledge that impact emotional experience pre-emptively or in anticipation.

Empirically, these distinctions are readily tested. Individuals from different age groups should participate in both up and down regulatory expressive tasks under controlled conditions that systematically vary parameters such as the nature of the elicitor, the presence of social others, the component to be regulated (e.g., experience vs. expression), as well as the degree of task demand. In this way, the "success" of regulation can be objectively determined and skill can be measured separately from differences in emotion understanding or knowledge.

## *2.5.4 The Effects of Regulatory Strategies on Physical and Psychological Outcomes Will Vary Developmentally*

Finally, while regulatory strategies have short and long-term effects on bodily systems as well associations with longer-term psychological and physical health, self-regulatory capacities are a cornerstone for adaptive success (Mauss, Cook, Cheng, & Gross, 2007) and among the most impressive functions of adulthood (Muraven, Tice, & Baumeister, 1998). Although there are few data examining possible age moderation of regulatory techniques on outcomes, developmental functionalism suggests that because of developmental variation in regulatory targets and resources, utilization of regulatory tactics may have different short and long term consequences across age groups (Magai et al., 2006).

### 2.5.4.1 Short Term Effects of Emotion Regulation

Emotion regulation, particularly expressive suppression and reappraisal, has been shown to have acute effects on aspects of physiology, cognition, and experience, as well as having distinct social consequences; deliberate acts of regulation are often costly (Mauss et al., 2006). Expressive suppression predicted greater physiological activation, but did not alter experience, while reappraisal decreased both experience and expression without impacting physiology in younger groups (Gross, 1998). Interestingly, both emotion suppression and enhancement instructions (Bonanno et al., 2004) impair memory. Such data are consistent with suggesting that regulating an emotion that has been "activated" is resource demanding.

Of the few experimental studies examining the effects of expressive regulation across age groups, one did not find differences in the consequences of inhibition (Kunzmann et al., 2005) while the other found that inhibiting reduced both subjective experience and narrative content in the *older* group (Magai et al., 2006). These writers suggest that greater knowledge about emotions and their own capacities together with declining resources among older adults prompted them begin regulating emotion earlier in the process, proactively controlling either their emotional language or the feelings themselves *in order to minimize the resource demand of anticipated signal regulation*. This interpretation is consistent with recent data showing that older adults were more effective than a younger group in using positive refocusing to reduce negative affect (Phillips et al., 2008).

#### 2.5.4.2 Long Term Effects of Emotion Regulation

Consistent with the short-term "costs" of regulation, characteristically or chronically regulating emotions in certain ways has been associated with negative physical and mental health outcomes. Most extensively studied are "restrictive" styles of regulation such as those involving the inhibition of emotion signals and the defensive or repressive regulation of negative emotional experiences. The literature linking emotion inhibition to physical health is quite small, with much work examining the *benefits* of expression rather than the costs of inhibition (see e.g., Nyklíček, Vingerhoets, & Denollet, 2002). Inhibition has been linked to greater health symptomatology (Consedine, Magai, Cohen, & Gillespie, 2002), and as part of the Type D construct, to cancer incidence (Denollet, 1998) and an array of poorer cardiovascular outcomes (Denollet, 2000).

However, in other contexts, work has begun to question the notion that inhibition is detrimental and expression beneficial. In one study, expressions of negative emotion (particularly anger) during a narrative interview predicted increased grief at 14 months and poorer health at 25 months (Bonanno & Keltner, 1997). Other work suggests that the *ability* to flexibly suppress and enhance emotion signals predicts longitudinal reductions in distress (Bonanno et al., 2004) and that inappropriate positive expression predicts poorer adjustment (Bonanno et al., 2007); only genuine expressions of positive emotion predicted better long-term adjustment, while non-Duchenne smiles (which presumably reflect expressive regulation) did not (Papa & Bonanno, 2008).

Data linking repression to health outcomes are equally complex. Repression has been linked with greater cancer incidence in AIDS patients (Cole, Kemeny, Taylor, & Visscher, 1996) and disease progression in HIV (Cole, Kemeny, Taylor, Visscher, & Fahey, 1996), as well as reduced immunocompetence (Jamner & Leigh, 1999). Conversely, repression also predicts better self-reported health (Brosschot & Janssen, 1998), and greater positive emotion and/or life satisfaction (Furnham, Petrides, & Spencer-Bowdage, 2002). Although there are no data that examine whether the relation between dispositional regulatory characteristics and health outcomes varies developmentally, it is worth noting that older samples provide a unique opportunity to examine the "accumulation" thesis in the context of personality-health relations. If regulatory tendencies are relatively stable, it should follow that the damage to physical systems will become progressively more evident over time – age should moderate the effect.

## 2.6 Developmental Functionalism: The Short and Long of It

Patterns of emotion regulation predict outcomes in both experimental studies as well as when assessed as dispositional characteristics. However, changes in resources make it likely that the cognitive, experiential, and physiological effects associated with emotions and their regulation will vary developmentally; somatic resource concerns represent one reason why patterns of emotion regulation vary across age groups (Consedine & Magai, 2006). Theoretically, there may be a greater need to keep systems nearer to baseline (by regulating, by not regulating, or by regulating at different stages) because arousal is "toxic" to older systems or because the effort required to correct deviations is proportionally greater. However, whether developmental differences in systemic resource translate into differences in short-term effects with implications for health and well-being is currently unclear.

It has been suggested that the combination of peripheral or central responding associated with inhibition and its effects on the immune system damage health *over time* (Consedine, Magai, & Bonanno, 2002). However, data directly supportive of this accumulation model are scanty. Developmental functionalism suggests that the relation between inhibition/expression and long-term outcomes varies as a function of variation in regulatory capacities and targets. The effects of dispositional regulatory strategies on health may depend on the form and reasons for regulation, on ethnic "fit," on situational context or the characteristics of the emotion that is being inhibited or signaled.

## 2.7 Concluding Remarks

Although studies examining lifespan differences in emotion regulation and their implications for health and well-being have increased in recent years, the field is still young and considerable work is needed. The current chapter has presented a novel perspective on lifespan differences in emotion regulation – developmental functionalism. At the core of this view are the assertions that because individuals from different stages of life are confronted with different challenges and tasks and have different capacities and resources, the operations of emotions vary. In extending this framework to emotion regulation, four propositions regarding lifespan differences in emotion regulation and their implications for health and well-being have been described. First, the experiential and signal *targets* of emotion regulation vary across age groups. Second, emotion regulatory capacities are both finite and likely to vary developmentally, particularly insofar as the distinction between online and anticipated regulatory tasks is concerned. Third, and perhaps as a part consequence of changes in capacity, the tactics used to attain regulatory goals are also likely to vary developmentally. Finally, it has been suggested that because of variation in capacities, targets, and tactics, the relations between emotion regulation and patterns of short- and long-term effect can be expected to vary across age groups.

## References

Averill, J. R. (1968) Grief: Its nature and significance. *Psychological Bulletin, 70*, 721–748.
Averill, J. R. (1994) Emotions are many splendored things. In P. Ekman & R. J. Davidson (Eds.), *The nature of emotions: Fundamental questions* (pp. 99–102). New York: Oxford University Press.
Baltes, M. M. (1996) *The many faces of dependency in old age*. New York: Cambridge University Press.
Baltes, P. B. (1997) On the incomplete architecture of human ontogeny: Selection, optimization and compensation as foundation of developmental theory. In U. M. Staudinger & U. Lindenberger (Eds.), *Understanding human development: Dialogues with lifespan psychology* (pp. 17–43). Dordrecht, The Netherlands: Kluwer.
Baumeister, R. F., Bratslavsky, E., Muraven, M., & Tice, D. M. (1998) Ego depletion: Is the active self a limited resource? *Journal of Personality & Social Psychology, 74*, 1252–1265.
Birditt, K., & Fingerman, K. L. (2005) Do we get better at picking our battles? Age group differences in descriptions of behavioral reactions to interpersonal tensions. *Journals of Gerontology: Series B: Psychological Sciences and Social Sciences, 60B*, 121–128.
Birditt, K., Fingerman, K. L., & Almeida, D. M. (2005) Age differences in exposure and reactions to interpersonal tensions: A daily diary study. *Psychology & Aging, 20*, 330–340.
Bjorklund, D. F. (1997) The role of immaturity in human development. *Psychological Bulletin, 122*, 153–169.
Bjorklund, D. F., & Bering, J. M. (2002) The evolved child: Applying evolutionary developmental psychology to modern schooling. *Learning & Individual Differences, 12*, 347–373.
Blanchard-Fields, F., Camp, C., & Jahnke, H. C. (1995) Age differences in problem-solving style: The role of emotional salience. *Psychology & Aging, 10*, 173–180.
Blanchard-Fields, F., Chen, Y., & Norris, L. (1997) Everyday problem solving across the adult life span: Influence of domain specificity and cognitive appraisal. *Psychology and Aging, 12*, 684–693.
Bonanno, G. A. (2001) Emotion self-regulation. In T. J. Mayne & G. A. Bonanno (Eds.), *Emotion: Current issues and future directions* (pp. 251–285). New York: Guilford.
Bonanno, G. A., Colak, D. M., Kelner, D., Shiota, M. N., Papa, A., Noll, J. G., et al. (2007) Context matters: The benefits and costs of expressing positive emotion among survivors of childhood sexual abuse. *Emotion, 7*, 824–837.
Bonanno, G. A., & Keltner, D. (1997) Facial expressions of emotion and the course of conjugal bereavement. *Journal of Abnormal Psychology, 106*, 126–137.
Bonanno, G. A., Keltner, D., Holen, A., & Horowitz, M. J. (1995) When avoiding unpleasant emotions might not be such a bad thing: Verbal-autonomic response dissociation and midlife conjugal bereavement. *Journal of Personality & Social Psychology, 69*, 975–989.
Bonanno, G. A., Papa, A., Lalande, K., Westphal, M., & Coifman, K. (2004) The importance of being flexible: The ability to both enhance and suppress emotional expression predicts long term adjustment. *Psychological Science, 15*, 482–487.
Bowlby, J. (1969) *Attachment and loss: Vol. I. Attachment*. New York: Basic.
Brehm, J. W., Brummett, B. H., & Harvey, L. (1999) Paradoxical sadness. *Motivation & Emotion, 23*, 31–44.
Brosschot, J. F., & Janssen, E. (1998) Continuous monitoring of affective-autonomic response dissociation in repressors during negative emotional stimulation. *Personality & Individual Differences, 25*, 69–84.

Brown, W. M., & Consedine, N. S. (2004) Just how happy is the happy puppet? An emotion signaling and kinship theory perspective on the behavioral phenotype of Angelman Syndrome Children. *Medical Hypotheses*, *63*, 377–385.
Carstensen, L. L. (1995) Evidence for a life-span theory of socioemotional selectivity. *Current Directions in Psychological Science*, *4*, 151–156.
Carstensen, L. L., & Charles, S. T. (1998) Emotion in the second half of life. *Current Directions in Psychological Science*, *7*, 144–149.
Carstensen, L. L., Fung, H. H., & Charles, S. T. (2003) Socioemotional selectivity theory and the regulation of emotion in the second half of life. *Motivation and Emotion*, *27*, 103–123.
Carstensen, L. L., & Löckenhoff, C. E. (2003) Aging, emotion, and evolution: The bigger picture. *Proceedings of the National Academy of Sciences*, *1000*, 152–179.
Carstensen, L. L., Mayr, U., Pasupathi, M., & Nesselroade, J. R. (2000) Emotional experience in everyday life across the adult life span. *Journal of Personality & Social Psychology*, *79*, 644–655.
Charles, S. T., Mather, M., & Carstensen, L. L. (2003) Aging and emotional memory: The forgettable nature of negative images for older adults. *Journal of Experimental Psychology: General*, *132*, 310–324.
Charles, S. T., Reynolds, C. A., & Gatz, M. (2001) Age related differences and change in positive and negative affect over 23 years. *Journal of Personality & Social Psychology*, *80*, 136–151.
Cole, S. W., Kemeny, M. E., Taylor, S. E., & Visscher, B. R. (1996) Elevated physical health risk among gay men who conceal their homosexual identity. *Health Psychology*, *15*, 243–251.
Cole, S. W., Kemeny, M. E., Taylor, S. E., Visscher, B. R., & Fahey, J. L. (1996) Accelerated course of human immunodeficiency virus infection in gay men who conceal their homosexual identity. *Psychosomatic Medicine*, *58*, 219–231.
Consedine, N. S. (2008) The health-promoting and health-damaging effects of emotions: the view from developmental functionalism. In M. Lewis, J. Haviland-Jones, & L. F. Barrett (Eds.), *Handbook of emotions* (3rd ed.). New York: Guilford.
Consedine, N. S., & Magai, C. (2003) Attachment and emotion experience in later life: The view from emotions theory. *Attachment & Human Development*, *5*, 165–187.
Consedine, N. S., & Magai, C. (2006) Emotion development in adulthood: A developmental functionalist review and critique. In C. Hoare (Ed.), *The Oxford handbook of adult development and learning* (pp. 209–244). New York: Oxford University Press.
Consedine, N. S., Magai, C., & Bonanno, G. A. (2002) Moderators of the emotion inhibition-health relationship: A review and research agenda. *Review of General Psychology*, *6*, 204–228.
Consedine, N. S., Magai, C., Cohen, C. I., & Gillespie, M. (2002) Ethnic variation in the impact of negative affect and emotion inhibition on the health of older adults. *Journal of Gerontology: Series B: Psychological Sciences*, *57B*, 396–408.
Consedine, N. S., Magai, C., & King, A. R. (2004) Deconstructing positive affect in later life: A differential functionalist analysis of joy and interest. *International Journal of Aging & Human Development*, *58*, 49–68.
Consedine, N. S., & Moscowitz, J. T. (2007) The role of discrete emotions in health outcomes: a critical review. *Journal of Applied and Preventive Psychology*, *12*, 59–75.
Consedine, N. S., Strongman, K. T., & Magai, C. (2003) Emotions and behavior: Data from a cross-cultural recognition study. *Cognition and Emotion*, *17*, 881–902.
Davidson, R. J. (1993). The neuropsychology of emotion and affective style. In M. Lewis & J. M. Haviland (Eds.), *The handbook of emotions* (1st ed., pp. 143–154). New York: Guilford.
Denollet, J. (1998). Personality and risk of cancer in men with coronary heart disease. *Psychological Medicine*, *28*, 991–995.
Denollet, J. (2000). Type D personality – A potential risk factor refined. *Journal of Psychosomatic Research*, *49*, 255–266.
Eibl-Eibesfeldt, I. (1989). *Human ethology*. Hawthorne, NY: Aldine de Gruyter.
Eid, M., & Diener, E. (2001) Norms for experiencing emotions in different cultures: Inter-and intra-national differences. *Journal of Personality and Social Psychology*, *81*, 869–885.

Eisenberg, N. (2000) Emotion, regulation, and moral development. *Annual Review of Psychology, 51*, 665–697.

Eisenberg, N., Sadovsky, A., & Spinrad, T. L. (2005) Associations of emotion-related regulation with language skills, emotion knowledge and academic outcomes. *New Directions in Child and Adolescent Development, 109*, 109–118.

Folkman, S., Lazarus, R. S., Pimley, S., & Novacek, J. (1987) Age differences in stress and coping processes. *Psychology & Aging, 2*, 171–184.

Furnham, A., Petrides, K. V., & Spencer-Bowdage, S. (2002) The effects of different types of social desirability on the identification of repressors. *Personality and Individual Differences, 33*, 119–130.

Gilhooly, K. J., Phillips, L. H., Wynn, V., Logie, R. H., & Della Sala, S. (1999) Planning processes and age in the five-disc Tower of London task. *Thinking & Reasoning, 5*, 339–361.

Gross, J. J. (1998) Antecedent- and response-focused emotion regulation: Divergent consequences for experience, expression, and physiology. *Journal of Personality & Social Psychology, 74*, 224–237.

Gross, J. J. (2001) Emotion regulation in adulthood: Timing is everything. *Current Directions in Psychological Science, 10*, 214–219.

Gross, J. J., Carstensen, L. L., Pasupathi, M., Tsai, J., Goetestam-Skorpen, C. G., & Hsu, A. Y. C. (1997) Emotion and aging: Experience, expression, and control. *Psychology & Aging, 12*, 590–599.

Heckhausen, J. (1997) Development regulation across adulthood: primary and secondary control of age related challenges. *Developmental Psychology, 33*, 176–187.

Izard, C. E. (1971) *The face of emotion*. New York: Appleton-Century Crofts.

Izard, C. E. (1991) *The psychology of emotions*. New York: Plenum.

Jamner, L. D., & Leigh, H. (1999) Repressive/defensive coping, endogenous opioids and health: How a life so perfect can make you sick. *Psychiatry Research, 85*, 17–31.

Johnson-Laird, P. N., & Oatley, K. (1992) Basic emotions, rationality, and folk theory. *Cognition & Emotion, 6*, 201–223.

Kaplan, H. S., Hill, K., Lancaster, J., & Hurtado, M. (2000) A theory of human life history evolution: Diet, intelligence, and longevity. *Evolutionary Anthropology, 9*, 156–185.

Keltner, D., Ellsworth, P. C. E., & Edwards, K. (1993) Beyond simple pessimism: Effects of sadness and anger on social perception. *Journal of Personality & Social Psychology, 64*, 740–752.

Kennedy-Moore, E., & Watson, J. C. (1999) *Expressing emotion: Myths, realities and therapeutic strategies*. New York: Guilford.

Knight, M., Seymour, T. L., Gaunt, J. T., Baker, C., Nesmith, K., & Mather, M. (2007) Aging and goal-directed emotional attention: distraction reverses emotional biases. *Emotion, 7*, 705–714.

Kray, J., & Lindenberger, U. (2000) Adult age differences in task switching. *Psychology & Aging, 15*, 126–147.

Kunzmann, U., Kupperbusch, C., & Levenson, R. W. (2005) Behavioral inhibition and amplification during emotional arousal: A comparison of two age groups. *Psychology & Aging, 20*, 144–158.

Labouvie-Vief, G., Chiodo, L. M., Goguen, L. A., Diehl, M., & Orwoll, L. (1995) Representations of self across the life span. *Psychology and Aging, 10*, 404–415.

Labouvie-Vief, G., Hakin-Larson, J., DeVoe, M., & Schoeberlein, S. (1989) Emotions and self-regulation: A lifespan view. *Human Development, 32*, 279–299.

Labouvie-Vief, G., Lumley, M. A., Jain, E., & Heinze, H. (2003) Age and gender differences in cardiac reactivity and subjective emotion responses to emotional autobiographical memories. *Emotion, 3*, 115–126.

Levenson, R. W. (1994) Human emotion: A functional view. In P. Ekman & R. J. Davidson (Eds.), *The nature of emotion: Fundamental questions* (pp. 123–126). New York: Oxford University Press.

Levenson, R. W., Carstensen, L. L., Friesen, W. V., & Ekman, P. (1991) Emotion, physiology, and expression in old age. *Psychology & Aging*, *6*, 28–35.

Levenson, R. W., Carstensen, L. L., & Gottman, J. M. (1994) The influence of age and gender on affect, physiology, and their interrelations: A study of long-term marriages. *Journal of Personality & Social Psychology*, *67*, 56–68.

Lucas, R. E., Clarke, A. E., Georgellis, Y., & Diener, E. (2004) Unemployment alters the set point for life satisfaction. *Psychological Science*, *15*, 8–13.

MacPherson, S. E., Phillips, L. H., & Della Sala, S. (2006) Age related differences in the ability to perceive sad facial expressions. *Aging Clinical and Experimental Research*, *18*, 418–424.

Magai, C., Consedine, N. S., Krivoshekova, Y. S., McPherson, R., & Kudadjie-Gyamfi, E. (2006) Emotion experience and expression across the adult lifespan: Insights from a multi-modal assessment study. *Psychology & Aging*, *21*: 303–317.

Mather, M., Canli, T., English, T., Whitfield, S., Wais, P., Ochsner, K., et al. (2004) Amygdala responses to emotionally valenced stimuli in older and younger adults. *Psychological Science*, *15*, 259–263.

Mather, M., & Carstensen, L. L. (2003) Aging and attentional biases for emotional faces. *Psychological Science*, *14*, 409–415.

Mather, M., & Carstensen, L. L. (2005) Aging and motivated cognition: The positivity effect in attention and memory. *Trends in Cognitive Sciences*, *9*, 496–502.

Mauss, I. B., Cook, C. L., Cheng, J. Y. J., & Gross, J. J. (2007) Individual differences in cognitive reappraisal: Experiential and physiological responses to an anger provocation. *International Journal of Psychophysiology*, *66*, 116–124.

Mauss, I. B., Evers, C., Wilhelm, F. H., & Gross, J. J. (2006) How to bite your tongue without blowing your top: Implicit evaluation of emotion regulation predicts affective responding to anger provocation *Personality and Social Psychology Bulletin*, *32*, 589–602.

Maylor, E. A., & Lavie, N. (1998) The influence of perceptual load on age differences in selective attention. *Psychology & Aging*, *13*, 563–573.

McConatha, J. T., & Huba, H. M. (1999) Primary, secondary, and emotional control across adulthood. *Current Psychology: Developmental, Learning, Personality, Social*, *18*, 164–170.

Mroczek, D. K., & Kolarz, C. M. (1998) The effect of age on positive and negative affect: A developmental perspective on happiness. *Journal of Personality & Social Psychology*, *75*, 1333–1349.

Muraven, M., Tice, D. M., & Baumeister, R. F. (1998) Self-control as limited resource: Regulatory depletion patterns. *Journal of Personality and Social Psychology*, *74*, 774–789.

Nesse, R. M. (1990) Evolutionary explanations of emotions. *Human Nature*, *1*, 261–289.

Nyklíček, I., Vingerhoets, A., & Denollet, J. (2002) Emotional (non-)expression and health: Data, questions, and challenges. *Psychology and Health*, *17*, 517–528.

Ochsner, K. N., & Gross, J. J. (2005) The cognitive control of emotion. *Trends in Cognitive Sciences*, *9*, 242–249.

Panksepp, J., & Miller, A. M. (1995) Emotions and the aging brain: Regrets and remedies. In C. Magai & S. H. McFadden (Eds.), *Handbook of emotion, adult development and aging*. San Diego, CA: Academic.

Papa, A., & Bonanno, G. A. (2008) Smiling in the face of adversity: The interpersonal and intrapersonal functions of smiling. *Emotion*, *8*, 1–12.

Phillips, L. H., Henry, J. D., Hosie, J. A., & Milne, A. B. (2008) Effective regulation of the experience and expression of negative affect in old age. *Journals of Gerontology: Series B: Psychological and Social Sciences*, *63B*, 138–145.

Saarni, C. (1989) Children's understanding of strategic control of emotional expression in social transaction. In C. Saarni & P. Harris (Eds.), *Children's understanding of emotion* (pp. 181–208). New York: Cambridge University Press.

Schieman, S. (1999) Age and anger. *Journal of Health & Social Behavior*, *40*, 273–289.

Stein, N. L., & Levine, L. J. (1990) Making sense out of emotion: The representation and use of goal-structured knowledge. I. In N. L. Stein, B. Leventhal & T. Trabasso (Eds.), *Psychological and biological approaches to emotion* (pp. 45–73). Hillsdale, NJ: Lawrence Erlbaum.

Tamir, M., Mitchell, C., & Gross, J. J. (2008) Hedonic and instrumental motives in anger regulation. *Psychological Science*, *19*, 324–328.
Thompson, R. A., & Meyer, S. (2007) Socialization of emotion regulation in the family. In J. J. Gross (Ed.), *Handbook of emotion regulation* (pp. 249–268). New York: Guilford.
Tooby, J., & Cosmides, L. (1990) The past explains the present: Emotional adaptations and the structure of ancestral environments. *Ethology & Sociobiology*, *11*, 375–424.
Tooby, J., & Cosmides, L. (2000) Evolutionary psychology and the emotions. In M. Lewis & J. M. Haviland-Jones (Eds.), *Handbook of the emotions* (2 ed.). New York: Guilford.
Tooby, J., & Cosmides, L. (2008) The evolutionary psychology of the emotions and their relationship to internal regulatory variables. In M. Lewis, J. Haviland-Jones & L. F. Barrett (Eds.), *Handbook of emotions* (3rd ed., pp. 114–137). New York: Guilford.
Tsai, J. L., Carstensen, L. L., & Levenson, R. W. (2000) Automatic, subjective, and expressive responses to emotional films in older and younger Chinese Americans and European Americans. *Psychology and Aging*, *15*, 684–693.
Tsai, J. L., Knutson, B., & Fung, H. H. (2006) Cultural variation in affect valuation. *Journal of Personality and Social Psychology*, *90*, 288–307.

# Chapter 3
# Social Cognitive Factors in Emotion Regulation: Implications for Well-Being

**Maya Tamir and Iris B. Mauss**

## 3.1 Introduction

Emotion regulation (i.e., the attempts people make to modify their emotional responses; Gross, 1998) is critical for well-being. As highlighted in this volume, healthy emotion regulation is a cornerstone of mental health and adjustment, whereas unhealthy emotion regulation lies at the core of many mental disorders (for recent reviews, see Gross, 2007; Kokkonen & Kinnunen, 2006; Vingerhoets, Nyklíček, & Denollet, 2008). To understand the implications of emotion regulation for well-being, researchers have examined features that distinguish different types of emotion regulation and factors that influence how people regulate their emotions. Building on social cognitive theories of self regulation (e.g., Mischel, Cantor, & Feldman, 1996), we propose that people's emotion-regulatory attempts are influenced by three key factors: Strategies and competencies, beliefs about controllability, and values and goals. Whereas strategies and competencies have received considerable attention in the emotion regulation literature, this has not been the case with respect to the other two factors. Importantly, these factors appear to determine whether and how people will regulate their emotions. In this chapter, therefore, we examine how beliefs about controllability and how values and goals may contribute to emotion regulation and determine its implications for well-being.

We begin by identifying the role of beliefs about controllability and the role of values and goals in research on self regulation, broadly defined. We then apply this analysis to emotion regulation. With respect to each social cognitive category, we highlight several theoretical predictions, review related empirical research, and discuss implications for well-being. We conclude by pointing to several future directions.

Our discussion of well-being encompasses hedonic and eudaimonic approaches. Hedonic well-being involves experiencing greater pleasant than unpleasant emotions and satisfaction with life (Diener, 1984). Eudaimonic well-being involves a

M. Tamir (✉)
Department of Psychology, Boston College, 140 Commonwealth Ave,
Chestnut Hill, MA 02467, USA
e-mail: tamirm@huji.ac.il

I. Nyklíček et al. (eds.), *Emotion Regulation and Well-Being*,
DOI 10.1007/978-1-4419-6953-8_3, © Springer Science+Business Media, LLC 2011

sense of fulfillment and meaning in life (Ryan & Deci, 2000; Ryff, 1989). We also view mental health as associated, albeit not synonymous, with well-being.

### 3.1.1 Social Cognitive Factors in Self Regulation

Social cognitive theories of self regulation have highlighted several critical factors that can be roughly grouped into three categories: Beliefs about control, values and goals, and strategies and competencies (Mischel et al., 1996; Mischel & Shoda, 1995).[1] Table 3.1 lists these three main categories and the aspects of self regulation they are most likely to impact.

These three social cognitive factors in self regulation operate sequentially. People's beliefs about their ability to control the environment affect whether they initiate self-regulatory efforts and how long they maintain such efforts (Aspinwall & Taylor, 1992; Kuhl, 1984). This category includes beliefs about how amenable versus impervious to control features of the world are as well as beliefs about one's personal capability to exert control (i.e., self-efficacy; Bandura, 1977). Once initiated, personal values shape the goals people pursue and how they assess their progress toward such goals. The goals people pursue, in turn, define the target of self regulation.

The goals people pursue as they self-regulate helps define the relevant set of regulation strategies. The strategies people use and their competencies contribute to the final outcome of self regulation. Clearly, some strategies are more effective than others (e.g., Gollwitzer, Fujita, & Oettingen, 2004) and some individuals are more competent than others (e.g., Baumeister, Braslavsky, Muraven, & Tice, 1998).

**Table 3.1** Social-cognitive factors in self regulation

| Social-cognitive factor | Aspect of self regulation directly impacted | Example from the emotion domain |
|---|---|---|
| *Beliefs about control*: Beliefs about the controllability of attributes and self-efficacy | Initiation | "Can emotions be controlled?" "Can I control my emotions?" |
| *Values and goals*: Desirable outcomes in the self regulation process | Content | "Which emotions do I value?" "How do I want to feel?" |
| *Strategies and competencies*: Potential behaviors, plans, and strategies used for organizing action and for obtaining desirable outcomes, as well as personal abilities and skills | Process | "How do I change my emotions?" |

[1]The original formulation of Mischel and Shoda (1995) involved two additional categories: Encoding and affect. Encoding is greatly influenced by values and goals (see Mischel et al., 1996). For instance, whether a situation is encoded as satisfactory or not depends on the individuals' desired end state (i.e., goal). In this chapter, therefore, we highlighted values and goals as overlapping, albeit not synonymous with, encoding. Another category that was included in the original formulation involves affect. Because this chapter focuses on affect as a target rather than a predictor of self regulation, we chose to omit this category from our analysis for simplicity sake.

In summary, self regulation is shaped by three main categories of social cognition. As summarized in Table 3.1, the beliefs people have about controllability determine whether they initiate self regulation, their values and goals determine the content (i.e., the target) of self regulation, and the ways in which they pursue such goals determine the process (i.e., what people do to attain the desired target) of self regulation.

### 3.1.2 *Social Cognitive Factors in Emotion Regulation*

Although emotion regulation is a subset of self regulation, historically, the two fields have developed somewhat independently. In the broad realm of self regulation, researchers have traditionally focused on the content of self regulation, turning only recently to focus on the process of self regulation (Gollwitzer & Moskowitz, 1996). In contrast, in the realm of emotion regulation, researchers have been primarily focused on the process of emotion regulation, leaving questions of content and initiation relatively unexplored.

Our approach is grounded in the idea that emotion regulation is a subset of self regulation. The present analysis, therefore, is heavily informed by research and theories of self regulation. We believe that the same factors that impact self regulation may impact emotion regulation. As shown in the last column of Table 3.1, beliefs about the controllability of emotion may determine the initiation of emotion regulation; emotional values and emotion regulatory goals may determine the content of emotion regulation; and emotion regulation strategies and competencies may determine the process of emotion regulation.

Emotion regulation strategies and competencies have been the focus of much research. However, the other two categories (i.e., beliefs about controllability, values and goals) have been relatively neglected to date. We believe the time has come to examine these two categories more closely with reference to emotion regulation, beginning with beliefs about controllability.

## 3.2 Can Emotions Be Controlled and Can I Control My Emotions? Beliefs About the Controllability of Emotion

Beliefs about controllability are an important prerequisite for the process of self regulation (Bandura, 1977; Seligman, 1975). In order for people to initiate self-regulatory attempts, they must first believe that the target experience or behavior is controllable (Kuhl, 1984; Mischel et al., 1996). Such beliefs can concern attributes (i.e., is an attribute amenable to control?) as well as one's personal ability to control the attribute (i.e., can I control the attribute?). Beliefs about the controllability of attributes have been referred to as "implicit theories" (e.g., Dweck, 1999). Beliefs about one's personal ability to control an attribute have been referred to as "self-efficacy" (e.g., Bandura, 1977).

People who have a sense of self-efficacy in a particular domain necessarily believe that the domain is controllable, whereas people who have a low sense of self-efficacy may or may not believe that the domain is controllable. Therefore, people who believe an attribute is impervious to control should have lower self-efficacy in that domain, compared to those who believe the attribute is controllable. People who believe they can control an attribute are more likely to try to control it, and therefore, over time, learn to use more adaptive regulation strategies. This, in turn, should ultimately result in more successful self regulation.

The belief that a domain is in principle controllable is a prerequisite for a sense of self-efficacy in a particular domain. However, people can believe that a particular domain is controllable but still have a low sense of personal self-efficacy. Consider height and body weight as an example. People rarely try to modify their height, for instance, because they typically assume that it cannot be controlled. In contrast, people's beliefs about weight differ. If people believe that weight is impervious to control, they are generally unlikely to try to modify their weight. If, however, people believe that weight can be controlled in principle, it doesn't necessary follow that they believe that they personally have the ability to control their own weight. Only if they believe they can control their own weight, would they be likely to take self-regulatory actions to do so. Indeed, many people believe that body weight can be controlled, in principle, yet refrain from doing so because they believe they are personally doomed for failure (e.g., Rimal, 2000; Povey, Conner, Sparks, James, & Sheperd, 2000). Beliefs about the controllability of weight, therefore, whether they apply to the attribute or to the self, carry important implications for weight regulation.

Beliefs about the controllability of personal attributes have been shown to be domain-specific. Carol Dweck and her colleagues (for reviews, see Dweck, 1999; Dweck, Chiu, & Hong, 1995) have studied such beliefs, focusing on the intelligence domain. This research has shown that beliefs about the controllability of intelligence predict important aspects of self regulation. First, they impact self-efficacy. When faced with setbacks, people who believe intelligence is fixed tend to show signs of resignation, whereas those who believe intelligence is controllable engage in greater effort to resolve the problem. Second, beliefs about the controllability of intelligence impact the use of learning strategies. Whereas those who believe intelligence is fixed focus on performance to validate their intelligence, those who believe it is controllable focus on learning to cultivate their intelligence. Third, beliefs about the controllability of intelligence are associated with academic performance, such that those who believe intelligence is fixed tend to show decrements in performance over time, whereas those who believe intelligence is controllable tend to improve in performance over time (Dweck, 1999).

We argue that these principles can also be applied to the regulation of emotion. In order for people to initiate attempts to regulate their emotions, they must first believe that emotions can, in principle, be controlled. Furthermore, they must also believe that they personally can control their emotions. Just as beliefs about the controllability of intelligence impact the regulation of intelligence-related processes, beliefs about the controllability of emotion might impact the regulation of emotion-related processes. People who believe emotion is controllable may have higher self-efficacy in emotion regulation, use more adaptive emotion regulation strategies, and ultimately have more favorable emotional experiences.

In a recent longitudinal study, we provided direct support for the importance of beliefs about the controllability of emotion as well as self-efficacy in emotion regulation (Tamir, John, Srivastava, & Gross, 2007). We found substantial variability in the extent to which individuals believe that emotions can be controlled. Such individual differences, in turn, were associated with important aspects of emotion regulation. First, people who believed emotions are controllable reported higher self-efficacy in emotion regulation, compared to those who believed emotions cannot be controlled.

Second, beliefs about the controllability of emotions were associated with the use of particular emotion regulation strategies. People who believed emotions are controllable tended to use cognitive reappraisal, an adaptive emotion regulation strategy, more frequently than those who believed emotions cannot be controlled. Third, beliefs about the controllability of emotions were associated with more favorable emotional experiences – namely, more positive emotions and less negative emotions over time. Consistent with social cognitive models of self regulation, the associations between beliefs about the controllability of emotion and emotional outcomes were mediated by self-efficacy in emotion regulation.

These findings demonstrate that, as in other domains of self regulation, beliefs about the controllability of emotion may play an important role in the regulation of emotion. Beliefs about the controllability of emotion enable people to develop a sense of self-efficacy in emotion regulation, promoting active attempts at emotion regulation. Through trial and error, people may learn to use more effective emotion regulation strategies and, as a result, be more successful at emotion regulation. Given their potential impact on emotion regulation, beliefs about the controllability of emotion are likely to have important implications for well-being, as reviewed in the next section.

### *3.2.1 Beliefs About the Controllability of Emotions: Implications for Well-Being*

Failure to regulate emotions is involved in emotional disorders (Gross & Muñoz, 1995; Rottenberg & Gross, 2007; Teasdale, 1988). Therefore, to the extent that beliefs about the controllability of emotions contribute to successful emotion regulation, they may also promote mental health. Beliefs about controllability should also promote hedonic as well as eudaimonic well-being. From a hedonic perspective, compared to people who do not try to regulate their emotions, people who try to regulate their emotions are more likely to change unsatisfactory emotional experiences, resulting in greater hedonic well-being. From a eudaimonic perspective, compared to people who believe they cannot change their emotions, those who believe they can do so experience a greater sense of environmental mastery, which is a core aspect of eudaimonia (Ryff, 1989). Therefore, we expect beliefs about the controllability of emotion to impact both hedonic and eudaimonic well-being.

These predictions are consistent with existing evidence. We have shown that the belief that emotion can be controlled is associated with less depression (Tamir et al., 2007). Similarly, self-efficacy in emotion regulation has been associated with lower depressive symptoms, less emotional distress and more efficient coping with life stressors (for a review, see Catanzaro & Mearns, 1990). With respect to hedonic well-being, we found that people who believe that emotion can be controlled and people who have a higher sense of self-efficacy in emotion regulation experience more positive and less negative emotions and report greater satisfaction with life (Tamir et al., 2007). Finally, the belief that emotion can be controlled and higher self-efficacy in emotion regulation were associated with greater psychological (i.e., eudaimonic) well-being (Tamir et al., 2007). Thus, as expected, people who believe emotion can be controlled and that they have the ability to control their emotions tend to experience better mental health and higher levels of well-being

Beliefs about the controllability of emotions precede the initiation of emotion regulation. Once it is initiated, however, emotion regulation might target either the decrease or increase of either pleasant or unpleasant emotions (Gross, 1998). A critical determinant of the content (i.e., the target) of emotion regulation involves the values people hold, which in turn, determine the goals they pursue as they engage in emotion regulation. We turn to these constructs in the next section.

## 3.3 Which Emotions Do I Value and What Do I Want To Feel? Values and Goals in Emotion Regulation

People engage in self-regulation to obtain outcomes that they value, where value refers to the abstract subjective worth or importance (Higgins, 2006). For instance, people may value pleasure, social conformity, or health. Values, in turn, often give rise to the goals people pursue as they self-regulate, where goals refer to the desired outcome of self regulation that direct specific actions (e.g., lose weight; become a vegetarian; lower blood pressure). The specific goals people pursue define the set of relevant regulation strategies (e.g., exercise to lose weight, change one's diet to become a vegetarian; take medication to lower blood pressure).

What determines whether an outcome is viewed as valuable or not? There are different sources that contribute to value (for an in depth analysis, see Higgins, 2006, 2007). One prominent source of value involves pleasure (e.g., "losing weight could increase value by making me feel better"). However, pleasure is not the only source of value. For instance, value can be derived from adhering to cultural norms (e.g., "becoming a vegetarian could increase value by helping me conform to my culture's norms") and from satisfying personal needs (e.g., "lowering my blood pressure could increase value by increasing my chances of survival"). Regardless of whether it is derived from hedonic sources (i.e., pleasure and pain) or nonhedonic sources (i.e., sources that are not primarily concerned with pleasure or pain), the value of outcomes shapes the goals people pursue and defines the direction of self regulation.

In stark contrast to research in self regulation, where values and goals have been of primary interest, these social cognitive constructs have received relatively little attention in the context of emotion regulation. This may be due to the unique nature of emotions as states of pleasure and pain. Given that immediate pleasure is a prominent source of value, it might seem obvious that pleasant emotions are typically viewed as valuable, whereas the opposite appears to be true for unpleasant emotions (e.g., Larsen, 2000). These assumptions have dominated the field of emotion regulation, leading to the impression that any further study of emotion values and emotion regulatory goals is quite unnecessary. But is that, in fact, the case?

As noted earlier, immediate pleasure is one source of value, but it is not the only source. For instance, value may be derived from adhering to cultural norms or satisfying important needs. To the extent that emotions vary in the extent to which they are consistent with norms or in their implications for need satisfaction, there may be sources other than pleasure that contribute to the value of emotions. In the following sections, we examine how immediate pleasure, cultural norms, and need satisfaction can contribute to the value of emotions.

### *3.3.1 Hedonic Experiences Contribute to Emotion Values and to Emotion Regulation Goals*

Immediate pleasure and pain are prominent sources of value, with pleasure increasing value and pain decreasing it (e.g., Bentham, 1781/1988). Because emotions are hedonic states, their degree of pleasure should contribute to their value. Pleasant emotions should be valued more, whereas unpleasant emotions should be valued less. Consistent with this proposition, Rusting and Larsen (1995) asked participants to rate the desirability of different emotions. Not surprisingly, they found that pleasant emotions were viewed as highly desirable, whereas unpleasant emotions were viewed as undesirable. Replicating such findings, Tsai, Knutson, and Fung (2006) demonstrated that pleasure contributes to the value of emotions across cultures. They asked participants from different cultures to rate how much they would *ideally* like to feel different emotional states. Across cultures, participants rated pleasant emotions more highly than unpleasant emotions. In general, people across the world view pleasant emotions as valuable (Diener, 2000).

Such values, in turn, should shape the goals people pursue as they regulate their emotions. Indeed, people are generally motivated to feel pleasant emotions and avoid unpleasant ones (Vastfjall, Garling, & Kleiner, 2001). As typically assumed in emotion regulation research, immediate pleasure is a critical source of emotion value and emotion regulation goals. However, is it the only source?

### *3.3.2 Cultural Norms Contribute to Emotion Values and to Emotion Regulation Goals*

Values are typically acquired within a social context (Hochschild, 1979; Merton, 1957). There is evidence for cultural differences in the value assigned to emotional experiences. In collectivistic cultures, for instance, guilt is valued more than in individualistic cultures, whereas the opposite is true for pride (Eid & Diener, 2001). In addition, in collectivistic cultures low arousal pleasant emotions, such as calmness, are valued more than in individualistic cultures, whereas the opposite is true for high arousal pleasant emotions, such as excitement (Tsai et al., 2006).

As these examples suggest, cross-cultural differences in emotional values are linked to core cultural principles. Collectivistic cultures emphasize social harmony, whereas individualistic cultures emphasize personal achievement. Because guilt promotes social engagement it should be more valuable in collectivistic cultures, and because pride promotes social dominance (Williams & DeSteno, 2009) it should be more valuable in individualistic cultures (Kitayama, Mesquita, & Karasawa, 2006).

Collectivistic cultures tend to emphasize social harmony and adjustment to others, whereas individualistic cultures emphasize personal achievement and influence on others (Morling, Kitayama, & Miyamoto, 2002). To the extent that low arousal pleasant feelings promote adjustment to others, one might expect them to be more valuable in collectivistic cultures and to the extent that high arousal pleasant emotions promote influencing others, one might expect them to be more valuable in individualistic cultures (Tsai, Miao, Seppala, Fung, & Yeung, 2007). Tsai and colleagues provided evidence in support of these hypotheses, showing that within and across cultures the value of high and low arousal pleasant emotions varied as a function of the importance of influencing versus adjusting to others.

Cultures may differ not only in the appropriateness of different types of emotional experiences, but also in the appropriateness of the intensity with which they are experienced. In a recent study that tested this idea, we measured individuals' values regarding emotion control in a sample of American college students from European and Asian backgrounds (Mauss et al., 2010). European-American participants reported valuing emotions to a greater extent than Asian-American participants. These differences in values, in turn, mediated cultural differences in emotional responses to a standardized laboratory anger provocation, as measured by self-reported anger and by observers' coding of facial and verbal behaviors. These results support the idea that cultures differ in emotional values, and that these values are associated with emotional experiences.

Consistent with the idea that people should be motivated to experience emotions they think are valuable, people who tried to adjust (vs. influence) others were more likely to try to increase low (vs. high) arousal pleasant emotions. Moreover, people who reported valuing emotion control experienced less intense anger in response to a laboratory provocation. Such findings clearly demonstrate that the value of emotions may vary as a function of culture and, furthermore, that it can shape the goals people pursue as they regulate their emotions.

### 3.3.3 *Need Satisfaction Contributes to Emotion Values and to Emotion Regulation Goals*

Value can also be derived from the usefulness of an experience for satisfying needs. For instance, a wool sweater is likely to be more valuable when a person is cold than when she is hot. Emotions, in turn, differ in the extent to which they help satisfy important needs (e.g., Frijda, 1986). Therefore, emotions may differ in value depending on the needs that are prominent in a given context. For instance, excitement promotes successful approach of rewards, whereas fear promotes successful avoidance of threats (e.g., Carver, 2001). From this perspective, people should value excitement relatively more when they need to find a potential mate, but they should value fear more when they need to escape from imminent danger. According to this approach, people may actually value an unpleasant emotion (e.g., fear) more than a pleasant one (e.g., excitement), when it can help satisfy a critical need. Recent evidence is consistent with this proposition.

We found that people tended to value excitement when they needed to obtain rewards (e.g., trying to win a big contest), but they tended to value fear when they needed to avoid threats (e.g., avoid a car accident) (Tamir, Chiu, & Gross, 2007). Furthermore, the more people valued fear as a useful avoidance strategy, the more likely they were to try to increase their fear before a potentially threatening task, as indicated by explicit preferences for fear-inducing activities. These findings demonstrate that the value of emotions can vary as a function of their usefulness, regardless of their hedonic tone. These findings also demonstrate that the value of emotions in a given context can influence what people want to feel in that context.

The idea that people want to feel emotions that are useful, regardless of whether they are pleasant or not, forms the basis for the instrumental approach to emotion regulation (Tamir, 2009a; Tamir, 2005; Tamir, Mitchell, & Gross, 2008). This approach gives rise to at least two empirical predictions. First, because the usefulness of emotions depends on the context in which they are experienced, the emotions people want to feel should differ by context. People may be motivated to experience even unpleasant emotions, when such emotions are useful. Second, because what is useful for one person may not be useful for another, people may differ in the emotions they want to experience.

A series of recent studies from our laboratory provide support for these hypotheses (for a review, see Tamir, 2009a). We demonstrated that people want to feel even unpleasant emotions when such emotions are useful to them. Building on the idea that fear promotes successful avoidance and excitement promotes successful approach, we found that people were motivated to increase their level of fear when they needed to avoid threats, but that they were motivated to increase their level of excitement when they needed to approach rewards (Tamir & Ford, 2009). Similarly, building on the idea that anger promotes successful confrontation, we found that people were motivated to increase their level of anger when they needed to confront others (Tamir et al., 2008). Indeed, increasing their level of anger made them more successful at playing a confrontational computer game, as measured by the number of virtual enemies killed. Thus, people appear to be motivated to experience emotions that are useful, even when they are unpleasant.

As demonstrated above, the value of emotions can vary from one situation to the next. In addition, needs vary from one person to the next. For instance, neuroticism appears to be linked to avoidance motivation (Elliot & Thrash, 2002), such that the need to avoid threats is more prominent among individuals high (vs. low) in neuroticism. Given that emotions such as worry and fear promote successful avoidance, they may be more useful for individuals high (vs. low) in neuroticism, when they are confronted with potential threats. If usefulness is a source of value, that implies that emotions such as fear or worry may be more valuable to individuals high (vs. low) in neuroticism in certain contexts, motivating them to experience such emotions. Indeed, we found that individuals higher in neuroticism were more motivated than those lower in neuroticism to increase their level of worry when preparing for demanding tasks (Tamir, 2005).

Conversely, extraversion appears to be linked to approach motivation (Elliot & Thrash, 2002), such that the need to approach rewards is more prominent among individuals high (vs. low) in extraversion. Given that emotions such as happiness and excitement promote successful approach, they may be more useful for individuals high (vs. low) in extraversion, when they are confronted with potential rewards. That implies that emotions such as happiness may be more valuable to individuals high (vs. low) in extraversion in certain contexts, motivating them to experience such emotions. Supporting this prediction, we found that individuals high (vs. low) in extraversion were more motivated to increase their level of happiness when preparing for demanding tasks (Tamir, 2009b).

These studies suggest that the value of an emotion is not synonymous with its hedonic tone. People may value and, as a result, be motivated to experience either pleasant or unpleasant emotions. Furthermore, emotion values and the goals they give rise to may vary as a function of the situation as well as the individual.

### 3.3.4 Emotion Values as Causal Agents

Most of the studies described above examined existing emotion values. These studies have shown that emotion values are associated with the goals people pursue as they regulate their emotions. To the extent that people are able to regulate their emotions successfully, one might expect emotion values to be associated with emotion experiences. Some of the evidence is consistent with this expectation. For instance, culturally valued emotions are experienced more frequently and more intensely than less valued ones (Eid & Diener, 2001; Mauss et al., 2010; Tsai et al., 2006).

The assumption in such studies is that emotion values determine the goals people pursue as they regulate their emotions, which in turn, help shape emotional experiences. The existing findings are encouraging, yet there is a possibility that the causal arrow is reversed. In other words, instead of emotion values determining emotional experiences, emotional experiences may determine emotion values. To test the causal role of emotion values in determining emotion regulatory goals and emotion experiences, emotion values should be experimentally manipulated and their implications for emotional experiences should be assessed. We recently undertook this challenge.

In a recent study, we manipulated the value of happiness, by having participants read one of two bogus summaries of scientific research (Mauss, Tamir, Anderson, & Savino, in press). In one condition, participants learned that happiness is very beneficial for people's lives. In the control condition, participants learned that making accurate judgments is very beneficial for people's lives. In both conditions, participants were unaware of the nature of the manipulation. Participants then watched film clips selected to evoke either happiness or sadness. As we predicted, compared to participants in the control condition, those who were led to value happiness were more likely to actively try to increase their happiness as they watched the films. These results provide preliminary support for the idea that values influence what people want to feel, which in turn, can influence how they actually feel.

### 3.3.5 *Values and Goals in Emotion Regulation: Implications for Well-Being*

There is relatively little research that directly examines the impact of values and goals in emotion regulation on well-being. Therefore, in this section, we outline several predictions and review research that speaks to them, when it is available. Our predictions reflect two general arguments. First, we argue that the implications of values and goals in emotion regulation for well-being should depend on how useful emotions are in the long-term. Values and goals that lead people to increase emotions that are useful in the long term should enhance well-being, whereas values and goals that lead people to increase emotions that prove harmful in the long-term, are unlikely to enhance well-being.

Second, building on research on conflicting goals and well-being (e.g., Emmons, 1987; Sheldon & Elliot, 1999), we argue that conflicting sources of value in emotion and the goals they give rise to should impair well-being, whereas concordance should enhance it. This is likely the case when any two or more sources of value conflict, but it may be particularly true when one of the sources involves hedonics (i.e., pleasure and pain). We expand on this idea below.

#### 3.3.5.1 Non-Conflicting Hedonic and Nonhedonic Sources of Emotion Value

People may be motivated to experience pleasant emotions to maximize pleasure, to conform to social norms, or to satisfy important needs. For instance, a person may seek to increase pride to feel good or to promote social dominance in an individualistic society (i.e., to adhere to cultural norms). In other words, hedonic and nonhedonic sources can make congruent, yet independent contributions to the value of pleasant emotions. In such cases, we believe that the value of emotions and the goals they give rise to are likely to promote well-being.

First, because they contribute to greater pleasure, values that arise from nonconflicting sources are generally likely to contribute to hedonic well-being. Second, the value of an emotion is likely greater when more than one source contributes to it. People are likely to exert more effort when seeking such emotions. Greater effort in emotion regulation is likely to increase the probability of successful emotion regulation, resulting in greater well-being. In general, therefore, we expect emotion values that arise from nonconflicting hedonic and nonhedonic sources to promote well-being.

Consistent with this prediction, the experience of culturally valued pleasant emotions appears to be a stronger predictor of well-being within a given culture than the experience of equally pleasant emotions that are not culturally valued. For instance, well-being in a collectivistic culture was more closely associated with the experience of friendly feelings than with the experience of pride, whereas well-being in an individualistic culture was more closely associated with the experience of pride than friendly feelings (Kitayama et al., 2006). Similarly, lower levels of depression in collectivistic cultures were associated with calmness, but not excitement, whereas lower levels of depression in individualistic cultures were associated with excitement, but not calmness (Tsai et al., 2006).

In summary, people who value and pursue pleasant emotions not only because they are pleasant (e.g., but also because they are culturally appropriate), are likely to experience greater well-being. Whether the effects of such emotion values on well-being are mediated by successful emotion regulation remains to be tested.

#### 3.3.5.2 Conflicting Hedonic and Nonhedonic Sources of Emotion Value

Hedonic sources increase the value of pleasant emotions and decrease the value of unpleasant emotions. In contrast, nonhedonic sources (e.g., cultural norms, need satisfaction) can increase the value of both pleasant and unpleasant emotions. This implies that unpleasant emotions can actually be valuable at times. In such cases, hedonic and nonhedonic sources of value conflict with each other.

What are the implications of emotion values that are based on conflicting hedonic and nonhedonic sources for well-being? One possible prediction is that pursuing goals that target the decrease of pleasant emotions or increase of unpleasant emotions should always impair well-being. Although this possibility remains to be tested, we do not think it is plausible. Rather, it appears that pursuing goals that target the decrease of pleasant emotions or increase of unpleasant emotions can sometimes promote well-being. Two pieces of evidence support this prediction. First, some degree of unpleasant emotional experiences may actually be necessary for well-being (e.g., Oishi, Diener, & Lucas, 2007; Ryff, 1989). Second, our research has shown that increasing unpleasant emotions can sometimes promote goal attainment, which may promote well-being (e.g., Tamir, 2005; Tamir et al., 2008).

We propose, therefore, that in certain cases emotion values that are based on conflicting sources may promote well-being. For example, increasing momentary anger may lead a person to gain the upper hand in a negotiation (Tamir & Ford, 2010). If the value gained by the successful negotiation is greater than the value lost by experiencing anger, the motivation to increase anger should promote well-being. These ideas are consistent with other cases of self regulation that involve foregoing immediate pleasure to obtain long-term benefits (Mischel, Shoda, & Rodriguez, 1989).

Although there may be times when increasing unpleasant emotions or decreasing pleasant emotions might carry positive implications for well-being, it is important to highlight several caveats. First, any conflict in self regulation can carry some harmful implications for well-being (e.g., Emmons, 1987; Emmons & King, 1988). To the extent that people experience some degree of conflict in emotion regulation when emotion values are based on conflicting hedonic and nonhedonic sources, such conflict may carry negative consequences for well-being, depending on its magnitude and duration.

Second, any goal can be adaptive only to the extent that it is pursued with flexibility (Bonanno, Papa, Lalande, Westphal, & Coifman, 2004). Emotion values and the goals they give rise to should be dynamically evaluated in light of their actual outcomes and abandoned when appropriate (Mischel et al., 1996). Such flexibility, we believe, may be critical when people are motivated to increase unpleasant or decrease pleasant emotions. For example, a person who increases her anger before interacting with a disobedient subordinate may benefit from doing so. However, a person who increases her anger in every situation, even when she interacts with superordinates and significant others is unlikely to benefit from doing so.

Identifying the proper contexts in which increasing unpleasant emotions or decreasing pleasant emotions is actually beneficial requires flexibility and insight. It is no wonder, therefore, that the ability to use pleasant and unpleasant emotions adaptively to attain desirable outcomes is a core component of emotional intelligence (Mayer & Salovey, 1997; Salovey, Hsee, & Mayer, 1993; Salovey & Mayer, 1990). Therefore, we cautiously propose that emotion values that are based on conflicting hedonic and nonhedonic sources and the goals they give rise to may contribute to well-being to the extent that they lead to at least some beneficial outcomes and that they are maintained and pursued with flexibility.

#### 3.3.5.3 Summary

In this section, we highlighted several factors that influence the implications of emotion values and emotion regulatory goals for well-being. First, when emotion values are based on nonconflicting hedonic and nonhedonic sources, they are likely to promote well-being. For instance, the pursuit of pleasant emotions that are valued by one's culture is likely to be particularly beneficial for well-being. Second, when emotion values are based on conflicting hedonic and nonhedonic sources, the implications for well-being are more complex. If such values lead to long-term benefits, they are likely to promote well-being. For instance, increasing one's anxiety before driving on an icy road may promote well-being to the extent that it results in the benefit of avoiding a likely accident at a temporary hedonic cost. However, if such values do not lead to long-term benefits, they are likely to impair well-being. For instance, increasing one's anxiety every time a person enters a car is likely to impair well-being to the extent that it leads to little benefit at a permanent hedonic cost. Future research has the challenging yet exciting task of better understanding how values and goals shape emotion regulation, emotional experiences, and well-being.

## 3.4 Summary and Future Directions

What determines the nature of emotion regulation and its consequences? The past few decades have given rise to an impressive body of research on emotion regulation. Such research has distinguished between various strategies in emotion regulation and delineated their consequences (e.g., antecedent-focused vs. response-focused; Gross, 1998). Such research also identified core skills and competencies that contribute to emotion regulation (e.g., executive functioning; Zelazo & Cunningham, 2007). Clearly, emotion regulation strategies and related competencies shape the process of emotion regulation.

In this chapter, we add to this growing literature, by proposing two other factors that may contribute to the nature and adaptive consequences of emotion regulation. Building on social cognitive approaches to self regulation (e.g., Mischel et al., 1996), we suggested that beliefs about the controllability of emotion may determine whether emotion regulation is initiated, and that emotion values and the goals they give rise to determine the target of emotion regulation. We then discussed the nature of such factors and their potential implications for well-being.

Research on beliefs about the controllability of emotions and research on values and goals in emotion regulation are still in their infancy. Many of the ideas and predictions discussed in this chapter have not yet been tested empirically. For instance, to what extent do the proposed psychological predictors play a causal role in emotion regulation? What are sorely needed are empirical studies that manipulate beliefs about the controllability of emotions and emotion values and goals to examine their implications for emotion regulation and experience.

Another important question involves the origins and development of the social-cognitive factors highlighted in this chapter. For instance, what leads some people to believe that emotions can be controlled and others to believe that they cannot be controlled? Why is it that some people value anger whereas others do not? Finally, little is known about the long-term consequences of such factors. How do they influence emotion regulation, emotion experiences, and well-being over time? As researchers begin to tackle these questions, our understanding of emotion regulation and the role it plays in well-being will become increasingly more sophisticated.

**Acknowledgement** The authors acknowledge support from a National Science Foundation grant SES 0920918 (Tamir), and a National Institutes of Health grant AG031967 (Mauss).

## References

Aspinwall, L. G., & Taylor, S. E. (1992) Modeling cognitive adaptation: A longitudinal investigation of the impact of individual differences and coping on college adjustment and performance. *Journal of Personality and Social Psychology, 63*, 989–1003.

Bandura, A. (1977) Self-efficacy: Toward a unifying theory of behavioral change. *Psychological Review, 84*, 191–215.

Baumeister, R. F., Braslavsky, E., Muraven, M., & Tice, D. M. (1998) Ego depletion: Is the active self a limited resource? *Journal of Personality and Social Psychology, 74*, 1252–1265.

Bentham, J. (1781/1988) *The Principles of Morals and Legislation*. Amherst: Prometheus.

Bonanno, G. A., Papa, A., Lalande, K., Westphal, M., & Coifman, K. (2004) The importance of being flexible: The ability to both enhance and suppress emotional expression predicts long-term adjustment. *Psychological Science, 15*, 482–487.

Catanzaro, S. J., & Mearns, J. (1990) Measuring generalized expectancies for negative mood regulation: Initial scale development and implications. *Journal of Personality Assessment, 54*, 546–563.

Carver, C. S. (2001) Affect and the functional bases of behavior: On the dimensional structure of affective experience. *Personality and Social Psychology Review, 5*, 345–356.

Diener, E. (1984) Subjective well-being. *Psychological Bulletin, 95*, 542–575.

Diener, E. (2000) The science of happiness and a proposal for a National Index. *American Psychologist, 55*, 34–43.

Dweck, C. S. (1999) *Self-Theories: Their Role in Motivation, Personality, and Development.* New York: Psychology Press.

Dweck, C. S., Chiu, C. Y., & Hong, Y. Y. (1995) Implicit theories and their role injudgments and reactions: A world from two perspectives. *Psychological Inquiry, 6*, 267–285.

Eid, M., & Diener, E. (2001) Norms for experiencing emotions in different cultures: Inter- and intranational differences. *Journal of Personality and Social Psychology, 81*, 869–885.

Elliot, A. J., & Thrash, T. M. (2002) Approach-avoidance motivation in personality: Approach and avoidance temperaments and goals. *Journal of Personality and Social Psychology, 82*, 804–818.

Emmons, R. A. (1987) Personal strivings: An approach to personality and subjective well-being. *Journal of Personality and Social Psychology, 51*, 1058–1068.

Emmons, R. A., & King, L. A. (1988) Conflict among personal strivings: Immediate and long-term implications for psychological and physical well-being. *Journal of Personality and Social Psychology, 54*, 1040–1048.

Frijda, N. (1986) *The Emotions*. London: Cambridge University Press.

Gollwitzer, P. M., Fujita, K., & Oettingen, G. (2004) Planning and the implementation of goals. In R. F. Baumeister & K. D. Vohs (Eds.), *Handbook of Self-Regulation: Research, Theory, and Applications* (pp. 211–228). New York: Guilford.

Gollwitzer, P. M., & Moskowitz, G. B. (1996) Goal effects on action and cognition. In E. T. Higgins & A. W. Kruglanski (Eds.), *Social Psychology: Handbook of Basic Principles*. New York: Guilford.

Gross, J. J. (2007) *Handbook of Emotion Regulation*. New York: Guilford.

Gross, J. J. (1998) The emerging field of emotion regulation: An integrative review. *Review of General Psychology*, 2, 271–299.

Gross, J. J., & Muñoz, R. F. (1995) Emotion regulation and mental health. *Clinical Psychology: Science and Practice*, 2, 151–164.

Higgins, E. T. (2006) Value from hedonic experience and engagement. *Psychological Review, 113*, 439–460.

Higgins, E. T. (2007) Value. In A. W. Kruglanski & E. T. Higgins (Eds.), *Social Psychology: Handbook of Basic Principles* (2nd ed., pp. 454–472). New York: Guilford.
Kitayama, S., Mesquita, B., & Karasawa, M. (2006) Cultural affordances and emotional experience: Socially engaging and disengaging emotions in Japan and the United States. *Journal of Personality and Social Psychology, 91*, 890–903.
Hochschild, A. R. (1979) Emotion work, feeling rules, and social structure. *American Journal of Sociology, 85*, 551–575.
Kokkonen, M., & Kinnunen, M. L. (2006) Emotion regulation and well-being. In L. Pulkkinen, J. Kaprio, & R. J. Rose (Eds.), *Socioemotional Development and Health from Adolescence to Adulthood. Cambridge Studies on Child and Adolescent Health* (pp. 197–208). New York: Cambridge University Press.
Kuhl, J. (1984) Volitional aspects of achievement motivation and learned helplessness: Toward a comprehensive theory of action control. In B. A. Maher (Ed.), *Progress in Experimental Personality Research* (Vol. 13, pp. 99–171). New York: Academic.
Larsen, R. J. (2000) Toward a science of mood regulation. *Psychological Inquiry, 11*, 129–141.
Mauss, I. B., Tamir, M., Anderson, C. L., & Savino, N. S. (in press). *Can seeking happiness make people unhappy? Paradoxical effects of valuing happiness*. Emotion.
Mauss, I. B., Butler, E.A., Roberts, N. A., & Chu, A. (2010). Emotion control values and responding to an anger provocation in Asian-American and European-American individuals. *Cognition and Emotion. 24*, 1026–1043.
Mayer, J. D., & Salovey, P. (1997) What is emotional intelligence? In P. Salovey & D. J. Sluyter (Eds.), *Emotional Development and Emotional Intelligence: Educational Implications* (pp. 3–34). New York: Basic.
Merton, R. K. (1957) *Social Theory and Social Structure*. Glencoe: The Free Press.
Mischel, W., Cantor, N., & Feldman, S. (1996) Principles of self-regulation: The nature of willpower and self-control. In E. T. Higgins & A. W. Kruglanski (Eds.), *Social Psychology: Handbook of Basic Principles* (pp. 329–360). New York: Guilford.
Mischel, W., & Shoda, Y. (1995) A cognitive-affective system theory of personality: Reconceptualizing situations, dispositions, dynamics, and invariance in personality structure. *Psychological Review, 102*, 246–268.
Mischel, W., Shoda, Y., & Rodriguez, M. L. (1989) Delay of gratification in children. *Science, 244*, 933–938.
Morling, B., Kitayama, S., & Miyamoto, Y. (2002) Cultural practices emphasize influence in the United States and adjustment in Japan. *Personality and Social Psychology Bulletin, 28*, 311–323.
Oishi, S., Diener, E., & Lucas, R. E. (2007) The optimum level of well-being: Can people be too happy? *Perspectives on Psychological Science, 2*, 346–360.
Povey, R., Conner, M., Sparks, P., James, R., & Sheperd, R. (2000) Application of the Theory of Planned Behaviour to two dietary behaviours: Roles of perceived control and self-efficacy. *British Journal of Health Psychology, 5*, 121–139.
Rimal, R. N. (2000) Closing the knowledge-behavior goal in health promotion: The mediating role of self-efficacy. *Health Communication, 12*, 219–237.
Rottenberg, J., & Gross, J. J. (2007) Emotion and emotion regulation: A map for psychotherapy researchers. *Clinical Psychology: Science and Practice, 14*, 323–328.
Rusting, C. L., & Larsen, R. J. (1995) Moods as sources of stimulation: Relationships between personality and desired mood states. *Personality and Individual Differences, 18*, 321–329.
Ryan, R. M., & Deci, E. L. (2000) On happiness and human potentials: A review of research on hedonic and eudaimonic well-being. *Annual Review of Psychology, 52*, 141–166.
Ryff, C. D. (1989) Happiness is everything, or is it? Explorations on the meaning of psychological well-being. *Journal of Personality and Social Psychology, 57*, 1069–1081.
Salovey, P., Hsee, C. K., & Mayer, J. D. (1993) Emotional intelligence and the self-regulation of affect. In D. Wegner & J. W. Pennebaker (Eds.), *Handbook of Mental Control* (pp. 258–277). New York: Prentice Hall.
Salovey, P., & Mayer, J. D. (1990) Emotional intelligence. Imagination, Cognition and Personality, *9*, 185–211.

Seligman, M. E. P. (1975) *Helplessness: On Depression, Development, and Death.* San Francisco: Freeman.

Sheldon, K. M., & Elliot, A. J. (1999) Goal striving, need satisfaction, and longitudinal well-being: The self-concordance model. *Journal of Personality and Social Psychology*, *76*, 482–497.

Tamir, M. (2009a) What do people want to feel and why? Pleasure and utility in emotion regulation. *Current Directions in Psychological Science. 18*, 101–105.

Tamir, M. (2009b) Differential preferences for happiness: Extraversion and trait-consistent emotion regulation. *Journal of Personality. 77*, 447–470.

Tamir, M. (2005) Don't worry, be happy? Neuroticism, trait-consistent affect regulation, and performance. *Journal of Personality and Social Psychology*, *89*, 449–461.

Tamir, M., Chiu, C.Y., & Gross, J.J. (2007) Business or pleasure? Utilitarian versus hedonic consideration in emotion regulation. *Emotion*, *7*, 546–554.

Tamir, M., & Ford, B. Q. (2009) Choosing to be afraid: Preferences for fear as a function of goal pursuit. *Emotion. 9*, 488–497.

Tamir, M., & Ford, B. Q. (2010). Instrumental emotion regulation in negotiations: Goals and the expected usefulness of emotions. Paper under review.

Tamir, M., John, O. P., Srivastava, S., & Gross, J. J. (2007) Implicit theories of emotion: Affective and social outcomes across a major life transition. *Journal of Personality and Social Psychology*, *92*, 731–744.

Tamir, M., Mitchell, C., & Gross, J. J. (2008) Hedonic and instrumental motives in anger regulation. *Psychological Science*, *19*, 324–328.

Tsai, J. L., Knutson, B., & Fung, H. H. (2006) Cultural variation in affect valuation. *Journal of Personality and Social Psychology*, *90*, 288–307.

Tsai, J. L., Miao, F. F., Seppala, E., Fung, H. H., & Yeung, D. Y. (2007) Influence and adjustment goals: Sources of cultural differences in ideal affect. *Journal of Personality and Social Psychology*, *92*, 1102–1117.

Teasdale, J. D., (1988) Cognitive vulnerability to persistent depression. *Cognition & Emotion*, *2*, 247–274.

Vastfjall, D., Garling, T., & Kleiner, M. (2001) Does it make you happy feeling this way? A core affect account of preferences for current mood. Journal *of Happiness Studies*, *2*, 337–354.

Vingerhoets, A., Nyklíček, I., & Denollet, J. (2008) *Emotion Regulation: Conceptual and Clinical Issues*. New York: Springer Science.

Williams, L. A., & DeSteno, D. (2009) Pride: Adaptive social emotion or seventh sin? *Psychological Science. 20*, 284–288.

Zelazo, P. D., & Cunningham, W. A. (2007) Executive function: Mechanisms underlying emotion regulation. In J. J. Gross (Ed.), *Handbook of Emotion Regulation* (pp. 135–158). New York: Guilford.

# Chapter 4
# Retracted Chapter: From (Unconscious) Perception to Emotion: A Global-to-Specific Unfolding View of Emotional Responding

**Kirsten I. Ruys, Diederik A. Stapel, and Henk Aarts**

## 4.1 Introduction

Emotions are driven by people's perceptions. Seeing the picture of a loved one elicits happiness, smelling a dirty toilet elicits disgust, hearing the voice of an enemy elicits anger, and looking down from a steep cliff elicits fear. The emotions that arise in these cases are not surprising: Happiness arises from positive events, disgust is triggered by health threatening conditions, anger occurs when treated unfairly, and fear is induced when encountering danger. What is less obvious, however, is how these emotions occur, and whether people need to be consciously aware of the emotional event. Do people need to know what caused their emotions before emotional reactions can arise? More generally, what happens between the exposure to an emotional event and the emotional reactions that follow?

The view on emotional responding that we put forward in this chapter is that people's emotional reactions are primarily triggered by what people (unconsciously) perceive (see also Prinz, 2004). We assume that people's interpretations of the sensory input that enters the brain determine the emotions that arise. An important implication of this viewpoint is that emotional reactions may unfold in a way that is similar to the unfolding of perception. Based on Navon's (1977) idea that perception typically unfolds from global to specific, we propose that emotions unfold from global emotional reactions to more specific emotional reactions. First, the gist or essence of an emotional event is perceived, which triggers a global positive–negative reaction. Then, specific details of the event – necessary to trigger more specific emotional responses such as fear, disgust, or anger – are perceived.

The core of our global-to-specific unfolding view of emotional responding is that emotional responses are not static or fixed, but that emotional responses unfold as a function of the emotional information that is perceived (Ruys & Stapel, 2009). This explains why the same emotional stimulus can elicit different responses. For example, an old picture of your grandfather may sometimes elicit general positive

K.I. Ruys (✉)
Utrecht University, Psychology Department, P.O. Box 80140, 3508 TC Utrecht, Netherlands
e-mail: k.i.ruys@uu.nl

I. Nyklíček et al. (eds.), *Emotion Regulation and Well-Being*,
DOI 10.1007/978-1-4419-6953-8_4, © Springer Science+Business Media, LLC 2011

feelings because the picture activates the knowledge that your grandfather was such a wonderful person and at other times may elicit sadness when the picture also activates more specific memories of the last years of his life when he suffered from Alzheimer's disease. The emotional response to an emotional event or stimulus depends on the specificity of the information that is perceived or activated in memory at the time the emotional response is triggered.

Another core assumption of our global-to-specific unfolding view on emotional responding is that people can experience emotions and their associated emotional reactions without knowing the cause of these emotions. Although our intuition rules out the idea of experiencing a specific emotion like fear or disgust without knowing why, there are important theoretical and empirical reasons to assume that emotional reactions may occur without conscious awareness of the emotion-eliciting stimulus.

We start this chapter by clarifying and providing evidence for our global-to-specific unfolding view of emotional responding. After discussing research showing that initial emotional responses are mostly global and later emotional responses are more specific, we explain in detail why we think that emotional reactions unfold similar to perception, how this link between perception and emotion relates to unconscious emotions, and how our view differs from appraisal theories of emotion. Then, we discuss research involving the interaction between global and more specific emotional reactions, and speculate about how global and specific emotional reactions interact with further emotional processing such as recognition and simulation of facial emotional expressions.

## 4.2 Global-to-Specific Unfolding of Perception

A global-to-specific unfolding view on emotional responding assumes that emotional responses parallel the perception of emotional stimuli. The question is then, how do people perceive emotional events? The ideas of the Gestalt psychologists – and Navon (1977) in particular – suggest that visual perception unfolds from global to more specific processing (see also, Derryberry & Tucker, 1994; Kimchi, 1992; Rosenthal, 2004; Werner, 1956). First, people typically extract the gist or essence of a visual scene as a result from global processing. Then, if necessary, people fill in the details of a visual scene by processing it in a more specific, fine-grained way. Thus, global processing primarily activates the big picture from a relatively distant perspective, whereas specific processing activates the details from a nearby, zoomed-in perspective (see Avramova & Stapel, 2008). For example, when you walk into a busy train station and notice the swarm of people going in and out of the station, you are unlikely to specifically perceive the individual persons passing by. What you see is a crowd while trying to find your way to the train. Suddenly, a familiar (and therefore positive) face triggers your attention, you "zoom in" and recognize the face of a colleague who is trying to catch the same train.

The idea that people initially process a visual scene in a global, holistic way, followed by more specific, detailed processing of the visual scene can be illustrated by

Navon's (1977) now classic experiments. In one of these experiments, participants looked at pictures that consisted of a large character made out of small characters, for example, a big capital letter L made up of small capital letters P. The task of the participants was to name the identity of the large character, or the identity of the small characters, as quickly as possible. The results showed that the identity of the small characters did not influence how quickly participants identified the large character, indicating that participants did not process the small characters before identifying the large character. Interestingly however, the identity of the large character did influence how quickly participants identified the small characters, indicating that participants processed the identity of the large character before identifying the small characters. This experiment points out that global perception typically occurs prior to more specific perception.

## 4.3 Global and Specific Emotional Reactions

The question is whether the global-to-specific unfolding that occurs in visual perception also occurs in the emotional reactions that emotional events trigger. We propose that not only seeing and thinking but also feeling unfolds from global to specific. A global way to represent an emotional event is in terms of its positive or negative valence, whereas specific processing is focused on features and details. Therefore, we expect that global processing of an emotional event typically elicits positive–negative emotional reactions such as a positive or negative mood, and that specific processing of an emotional event elicits more fine-grained emotional reactions such as fear, anger, or disgust. Thus, a sudden glimpse of a dangerous, poisonous snake crossing your trail when you are hiking in the woods may elicit a general negative reaction, but may also elicit a more specific fear reaction that takes into account specific characteristics of the snake such as its colors and size. On a concrete action level, a general negative reaction may be the preparation of an *avoidance* response (as opposed to *approach*), whereas a more specific fear reaction may be a *freeze* or *flight* response.

Two experiments directly show that emotional reactions may indeed develop from global to specific. In this research of Ruys and Stapel (2008a), participants were either quickly or super quickly subliminally exposed to fearful pictures (e.g., a growling, mad dog, a pointed gun), disgusting pictures (e.g., a dirty, non-flushed toilet, a moldy cooking pot), or neutral pictures (e.g., a horse, a chair) in a parafoveal vigilance task (see also Bargh & Chartrand, 2000; Stapel, Koomen, & Ruys, 2002). The hypothesis was that *super quick* subliminal exposure to these emotional stimuli would merely allow for global processing of the emotional stimuli and therefore that super quick exposures to these emotional stimuli would trigger global emotional reactions. Thus, participants who were super quickly exposed to fearful or disgusting pictures would show a general, negative emotional response compared to participants who were exposed to neutral pictures in the parafoveal vigilance task. A second hypothesis was that *quick* subliminal exposure to these emotional stimuli would also allow for more specific processing of the emotional stimuli and therefore that quick exposures to these stimuli would trigger specific emotional reactions. Participants who were quickly exposed to fearful or disgusting pictures would thus show a fear or disgust response, respectively, compared to participants who were exposed to neutral pictures.

These hypotheses were examined by assessing participants' global and specific emotional responses with cognitive, feeling, and behavioral measures (see Ruys & Stapel, 2008a). Results on the cognitive measures – a word-completion task and a scenario measure – showed that super quick exposures to either disgusting or fearful pictures increased the cognitive accessibility of general negative concepts (i.e., bad, stupid), whereas quick exposures to disgusting pictures increased the cognitive accessibility of concepts related to disgust (e.g., vomit, sick) specifically and quick exposures to the fearful pictures increased accessibility of the concept of fear (e.g., worry, panic). The feeling measures showed a similar pattern of results. Super quick exposures to either disgusting or fearful pictures resulted in more negative mood reports than exposures to neutral pictures, whereas quick exposures to disgusting pictures resulted in specific feelings of disgust and quick exposures to fearful pictures resulted in specific feelings of fear. As a measure of behavior, participants were asked to choose between seeing scary movies or sampling exotic, potentially disgusting food. We expected that fearful participants would choose the strange-food test to avoid more fear-eliciting materials, whereas disgusted participants would choose the scary-movie test to avoid exposure to exotic, potentially disgusting food. The results indeed showed that participants were more likely to choose the scary movies over the exotic food after quick exposures to disgusting compared to fearful pictures. The behavioral results are especially important because semantic activation of the concepts of disgust and fear would produce the opposite pattern of findings. The behavioral results thus support the idea that the subliminally presented emotional pictures triggered genuine emotional responses.

The research of Ruys and Stapel (2008a) illustrates how an emotional response unfolds over time from a global mood to a specific, meaning-based emotion like fear or disgust. Importantly, a global-to-specific unfolding of emotional responses was revealed on various emotion measures, in line with a multicomponent perspective on emotion (Frijda, 1988; Scherer, 1984). When little time was available to process the emotional pictures, suggesting that participants only perceived global evaluative information, this elicited a global negative mood and activated general negative cognitions. However, when relatively plenty of time was available to process the emotional pictures, suggesting that participants also perceived specific fine-grained information, this triggered specific emotions. Thus, emotional stimuli may on the one hand elicit global emotional responses such as a positive or negative mood and accessibility of general positive or negative concepts, and on the other hand elicit specific emotional responses such as feelings of disgust or fear, accessibility of specific emotion concepts, and the inclination to make a specific choice. These various emotional reactions can occur directly in response to the emotional event and together form the emotional experience.

To obtain more evidence for a global-to-specific unfolding of emotional responding, Ruys and Stapel performed two additional studies that examined participants' global and specific emotional responses to facial emotional expressions (Ruys & Stapel, 2008c). In this research, participants were either super quickly or quickly subliminally exposed to disgusted, fearful, angry, or neutral faces in a parafoveal vigilance task. After the exposure phase, participants completed global and specific measures of feeling and cognition, similar to the ones used in Ruys and Stapel (2008a). In line with global-to-specific unfolding, the results showed that super quick exposures to disgusted, fearful, or angry faces primarily activated a global, negative evaluative response that was reflected in participants' moods and an increased accessibility of general negative cognitions. Interestingly however, quick subliminal exposures to disgusted, fearful, or angry faces resulted in the activation of specific emotion knowledge, without influencing people's global and specific feelings.

These results indicate that people's responses to facial emotional expressions differ from responses to other more direct emotion elicitors (Hariri, Tessitore, Mattay, Fera, & Weinberger, 2002; Ruys & Stapel, 2008a, 2008c). Initially, facial emotional expressions and other emotion elicitors like poisonous snakes or favorite desserts elicited similar positive–negative responses, whereas later, more specific, fine-grained responses differed such that more direct emotion elicitors elicited a corresponding specific emotion (e.g., disgust or fear) and facial emotional expressions merely activated emotion knowledge (e.g., increased accessibility of emotion-related words). This makes perfect sense because automatically taking over other people's emotions can be quite dysfunctional. It does not seem functional to always feel angry when other people feel angry, or to feel scared when other people feel scared. It does seem functional, however, to immediately know about other people's feelings of anger or fear, as to determine your own optimal course of action.

## 4.4 Unconscious Perception Triggers Emotional Responses

Besides showing a global-to-specific unfolding of emotional responses, the research of Ruys and Stapel (2008a) illustrates another important aspect of our unfolding view, namely that emotional responses may occur *without being consciously aware* of their cause: Participants felt scared without knowing about the frightening pictures that caused their fear and participants felt disgusted without knowing about the sickening pictures that caused their disgust (Ruys & Stapel, 2008a). Thus, people actually experienced specific emotional feelings and showed emotional behavior after being unconsciously exposed to emotion-eliciting stimuli. To our knowledge, this research was the first to show the unconscious nature of specific emotions without using facial emotional expressions as emotional stimuli (Ruys & Stapel, 2008a). Because facial emotional expressions are principally *reactions* to emotional stimuli (see Ruys & Stapel, 2008c), it was important to show the unconscious elicitation of specific emotions like fear and disgust by subliminally exposing people to regular emotional stimuli like growling mad dogs and dirty non-flushed toilets.

As we also point out in the title of this chapter, the influence of perception on emotional responding is thus not restricted to conscious perception. We should acknowledge, however, that the likelihood that perceivers consciously perceive an emotional stimulus during specific, fine-grained processing may be greater than during global, positive—negative processing because specific processing starts later and takes more time to complete than global processing. However, there are several important reasons why we assume that both global and specific emotional information processing do not need awareness to occur.

An important theoretical reason for our assumption that emotional responding emerges without awareness of its cause is the survival value of emotions and emotional reactions. According to an evolutionary perspective on emotions, quick emotional reactions such as immediate flight or withdrawal increase people's chances of survival (Cacioppo & Gardner, 1999; Ekman, 1984; Frijda, 1994; Keltner & Gross, 1999; Öhman, 1992; Scherer, 1984). Fear, for example elicited by a big truck that is quickly approaching, may reduce risk-taking behavior (Lerner & Keltner, 2001) and may elicit a freeze response before crossing the street. Considering that the speed of emotional responding increases when instigated before an emotional event reaches awareness, it seems likely that emotional responses indeed occur unconsciously. An evolutionary perspective also entails that not only humans but also non-human animals display specific emotional reactions (e.g., Darwin, 1872; Frijda, 1986; Panksepp, 1998). However, most non-human animals are not widely assumed to be consciously aware of their actions, let alone being aware of the reasons behind their actions.

For adequate responding, our emotional system should be able to automatically detect the valence of the stimulus as well as its specific meaning. Specific body posture cues may, for example, reveal whether one should fear or aggress a potential attacker (Parkinson & Manstead, 1992). The idea that awareness is not necessary for the emergence of both global and specific information processing has also received empirical support. In addition to the research of Ruys and Stapel (2008a, 2008c), neuroimaging techniques have shown that unconscious exposure to disgusted, fearful, sad, angry, and happy facial emotional expressions led to differential levels of amygdala and anterior cingulate activity (e.g., Killgore & Yurgelun-Todd, 2004; Morris, de Gelder, Weiskrantz, & Dolan, 2001; Palermo & Rhodes, 2007; Phillips et al., 2004). Furthermore, physiological techniques have demonstrated that unconscious exposures to happy and angry facial emotional expressions evoke distinctive facial electromyographic (EMG) reactions in emotion-relevant facial muscles (Dimberg, Thunberg, & Elmehed, 2000).

Thus, research provides strong support for the idea that emotions can occur without conscious awareness of their cause. However, does this mean that emotions can be unconscious altogether? To answer this question, we need to define more closely what we mean by unconscious emotions. We can distinguish between being unconscious of the emotional event, being unconscious of the link between the emotional event and the experienced emotion, and being unconscious of the emotion or emotional reactions itself. Thus, the emotion elicitor can be unconscious, the link between emotion and elicitor can be unconscious, and the elicited response can be unconscious (Prinz, 2004).

We think the first case – being unconscious of the emotional event – is most interesting, because it allows us to study relatively "pure" emotional reactions. We say "pure" because these emotional reactions are less contaminated with folk ideas on the causes of emotions and the appropriate emotional reactions. When emotions are elicited unconsciously, people need more time to consciously control their emotional responses and expressions than when they are conscious of the emotion induction because the emotion has already kicked in. When people are unconscious of the link between a specific emotional event and the experienced emotion, for example when multiple possible causes are present, people are likely to regulate their emotional reactions, despite the fact that they are unaware of the actual cause of the emotional reaction. Regarding the last case, being unconscious of the emotional reactions, one may question what it means if people are unconscious of the emotion itself. As we have argued previously, when people do not become aware of their emotional reactions following an emotional event, this could mean that these emotional reactions are not very intense (see also, Ruys & Stapel, 2008a). When an emotional event is meaningful, the event is likely to trigger an intense emotional reaction and reach awareness. This reasoning is in line with Rolls (2008), who proposed that people become aware of their emotional state because emotions often arise in situations where higher order behavior planning is necessary to deal with an emotional event.

## 4.5 The Perception–Emotion Link and Appraisal Theories

A global-to-specific unfolding view on emotional responding entails that emotional responses may arise without conscious awareness of their cause. Initial global processing of an emotional event results in global positive–negative reactions and later, more specific processing results in specific, fine-grained emotional reactions. An important question to address is whether this prediction is unique or whether this prediction can also be derived from other theories of emotion, such as appraisal theories. We primarily relate our unfolding view to appraisal theories of emotion to illustrate the assumptions underlying our global-to-specific unfolding view on emotional responding in more detail.

Whereas our global-to-specific unfolding view can be distinguished from other theories of emotion by its emphasis on emotional responses, appraisal theories of emotion can be distinguished by their emphasis on cognition. A core assumption of appraisal theories is that estimates of the situation (i.e., appraisals) generate specific emotions (e.g., Arnold, 1960; Frijda & Zeelenberg, 2001; Lazarus, 1968). Specifically, a detailed set of appraisal criteria predicts which particular configuration of appraisals will produce a specific emotion in an individual (Frijda, 1988; Lazarus, 1991; Scherer, 1984; Manstead & Fischer, 2001; Zeelenberg, van den Bos, van Dijk, & Pieters, 2002). One could argue that appraisal theories also distinguish between global and specific processing of emotional events. The component process model of Scherer (1984, 1999), for example, postulates a fixed number of predefined stimulus evaluation checks (i.e., appraisals of novelty, intrinsic pleasantness, goal/need conduciveness, coping potential, and compatibility with standards) that determine whether people experience an emotion and what kind of emotion people experience. These stimulus evaluation checks, which are hypothesized to occur sequentially, can be seen as increasingly specific (Grandjean & Scherer, 2008).

A crucial difference between our global-to-specific unfolding view on emotional responding and appraisal theories is that appraisal theories invoke a limited set of cognitive computations (i.e., appraisals) to arrive at emotional reactions, whereas we assume that emotional reactions are directly related to what people perceive. An important example of research showing the relation between perception and emotion is the work of LeDoux (1989), who demonstrated a subcortical pathway between the retinae of our eyes and the amygdala via the thalamus, through which fear responses could be elicited. The thalamus can distinguish coarse visual features that are sufficiently specific to elicit emotional reactions. This work strongly suggests that emotional responding can occur without mediation of the neocortex and thus without cognitive appraisals. Of course, the fact that emotions occur without cognitive processing does not mean that emotional reactions always occur without cognitive processing. We refer to this work (and we are not the first) only to show that appraisals need not be a prerequisite for emotional responding.

The question is how perception "translates" to emotional reactions without intermediate appraisal processes. In keeping with an embodiment perspective (Niedenthal, Barsalou, Winkielman, Krauth-Gruber, & Ric, 2005), we assume that emotional reactions are associated to specific emotional events or stimulus configurations, just like other physical reactions can be associated to concepts. First, people learn to associate certain stimulus configurations with particular positive or negative consequences and their physical, emotional responses to these consequences. Then, the activation of these stimulus configurations may trigger the associated emotional reactions even before the positive or negative consequences have yet occurred through an automatic pattern completion mechanism. For example, when the brain "recognizes" a stimulus configuration that was associated to a dangerous situation in the past, the system automatically reproduces the associated fear response that accompanied the previous dangerous situation. Consequently, the more specific the information that is available, the more specific the emotional reactions that occur.

The idea that the specificity of the information that is available determines the specificity of the emotional reaction can more easily explain individual differences in emotional responding than the assumption that each emotional event is always appraised on a specific set of universal appraisal dimensions. It also solves the debate between appraisal theorists on which specific, universal appraisals are necessary to distinguish between different emotions. According to some theorists, emotional events are primarily appraised in terms of personal significance followed by secondary coping appraisals (e.g., Lazarus, 1991; Weiner, 1985), whereas other appraisal theorists argue that emotional events need to be differentiated along a relatively larger number of appraisal dimensions (e.g., Evers, Fischer, Mosquera, & Manstead, 2005; Manstead & Fischer, 2001; Parkinson & Manstead, 1992; Scherer, 1984, 1999). Our global-to-specific unfolding perspective on emotional responding predicts that the stimulus configurations that trigger emotional reactions vary between persons, not because different people make different appraisals, but because different people have different prior experiences and have acquired different associations between emotional events and emotional reactions. For example, for people who witnessed the assault on the Dutch queen that was committed by a person driving a black Suzuki Swift, the confrontation with a black Suzuki Swift is likely to trigger fear, despite the realization that other black Suzuki Swifts (and their drivers) are unlikely to be dangerous. For people who did not witness the assault, exposure to a black Suzuki Swift is unlikely to trigger fear.

Our global-to-specific unfolding view of emotional responding also assumes that people can be flexible in how they process information. In contrast to, for example, the component process model (Scherer, 1984, 1999), we argue that global and specific emotional reactions do not have to occur sequentially. Sometimes people extract specific, detailed knowledge before global evaluative meaning (see Stapel & Koomen, 2006). Often it makes sense to immediately extract global positive–negative information, for example to see whether an animal is cute or threatening. However, sometimes it more useful to know whether an animal is a wasp or a mosquito by extracting detailed information. Specifically, immediate specific processing occurs when the emotional event is processed *top-down*. This means that people are already attuned to a specific kind of information, for instance due to the activation of a particular goal or when specific features are diagnostic for a task (Storbeck & Robinson, 2004; Corbetta & Shulman, 2002). However, when information processing is stimulus-driven or *bottom-up*, we assume that a global-to-specific unfolding of emotional responding occurs. Thus, when people are confronted with an unexpected emotion elicitor (e.g., a favorite dessert, a poisonous snake, a smiling face) global positive–negative reactions typically occur prior to specific, detailed emotional reactions.

Appraisal theories of emotion and our global-to-specific unfolding view on emotional responding also differ in that our view emphasizes emotional *reactions* rather than the cognitions that may precede emotions. In contrast to most appraisal theories of emotion, our global-to-specific unfolding view on emotional responding provides more detail on emotional reactions that develop in response to an emotional event. At present, it remains relatively unclear how people react in response to the generation of appraisals. We propose that which specific emotion is produced after exposure to an emotion-eliciting stimulus depends on the information that is cognitively activated during such exposure and on prior emotional experiences. The accessibility of global positive–negative feelings, cognitions, and behaviors is increased after global processing of the emotional event, which may result in a positive or negative mood. Accessibility of specific, fine-grained emotional responses is increased after specific processing of the emotional event, which may result in a specific emotion like fear, anger, happiness, disgust, surprise, or sadness. Thus, moods can be characterized by the activation of global, diffuse evaluative information, whereas emotions are characterized by the activation of specific, fine-grained information.

At first sight, our global-to-specific unfolding view on emotional responding might seem similar to appraisal theories of emotion. However, as we made clear, the assumptions underlying both viewpoints show profound differences. Most important is our assumption that emotions unfold in a way that is similar to the unfolding of perception because emotions arise as a result of prior associations with these perceptions. We also assume that emotional responding is flexible in the instigation of global and specific processing and emphasize people's emotional reactions in terms of feelings, cognitions, and behaviors.

## 4.6 Interaction of Global and Specific Processing

In the previous sections of this chapter, we have emphasized the idea that emotional events can be processed globally and more specifically resulting in global and specific emotional responses. A natural question is whether the systems that are responsible for these two modes of processing operate independently, or whether these systems interact. We argue for the latter option and assume that initial diffuse evaluative reactions (resulting from global processing) may influence the kind of specific fine-grained reactions that occur (resulting from specific processing). For example, the initial positive or negative reaction to a friend's proposal to go on a skiing trip to Austria might influence whether you focus on the positive aspects of the skiing trip (e.g., snow guaranteed) or the negative aspects of this trip (e.g., long drive). Thus, an intriguing possibility is that initial evaluative reactions resulting from global coarse information processing may determine the details that receive attention during specific information processing.

This possibility that initial evaluative reactions influence later detailed, specific reactions is supported by neurological evidence. Neurological research indicates that global and specific processing depend on different systems in the brain (Adolphs, 2003; Derryberry & Tucker, 1994; Fink, Halligan, Marshall, Frith, Frackowiak, & Dolan, 1996; LeDoux, 1989; Tucker & Williamson, 1984; Zajonc, 2000). Adolphs (2003) for example suggested that coarse perceptual processing is initiated at the superior colliculus and feeds into the amygdala, striatum, and orbitofrontal cortex, whereas detailed perceptual processing takes place at the higher order sensory cortices, including the fusiform gyrus and the superior temporal gyrus. Importantly, the coarse processing system responsible for global evaluative reactions to stimulus events has numerous physical interactions with the fine-grained processing system responsible for specific, descriptive processing (Adolphs, 2003). Thus, if we consider that global evaluative processing of a stimulus ends before specific descriptive processing is complete, it seems likely that through the interactions between the two systems, early positive–negative reactions may serve as input for specific, descriptive processing.

A psychological phenomenon that illustrates how global evaluative processing interacts with specific descriptive processing is the formation of impressions. When positive impressions are important, many people refer to the following famous expression: "you never get a *second* chance to make a good *first* impression." This folk wisdom suggests that initial first impressions have a strong impact on the remainder of the person perception process. Thus, a positive first impression of a job candidate makes it easier to see the positive aspects of this person than a negative first impression. The idea that first impressions influence later, more secondary impression formation processes is in line with our global-to-specific unfolding view on emotional responding. Global-to-specific unfolding predicts that perceivers initially experience global positive–negative reactions to a target person, which are followed by more specific fine-grained emotional reactions (Ruys & Stapel, 2008a, 2008b, 2008c; Stapel et al., 2002). An interesting additional hypothesis is that global processing *interacts* with specific processing. Because global evaluative reactions typically occur prior to more specific detailed reactions, it seems highly plausible that global reactions indeed influence the content of more specific reactions.

The idea that global evaluative reactions to a person influence later specific processing is supported by a study of Niedenthal and Cantor (1986). They showed that people are more likely to apply a given description to a target person when this description and the first impression of the target person have the same valence (i.e., are evaluatively congruent). Participants judged it, for instance, more likely that a target person was a "recreational sportsman" (a positive description) than a "scheming politician" (a negative description) when this target person displayed dilated pupils that typically cause a positive first impression, rather than constricted pupils that typically cause a negative first impression (Niedenthal & Cantor, 1986). Thus, people's initial global impressions of a target person determined to what extent people were willing to apply specific detailed information to this target person.

A next question is whether global evaluative reactions to a target person also spontaneously influence later specific fine-grained processing of features that are inherent to the target person. Is it, for instance, the case that global evaluative reactions facilitate the spontaneous activation of evaluatively congruent descriptive features? If global evaluative processing indeed interacts with specific descriptive processing, this could mean that perceivers are likely to focus on those specific features (e.g., gender, race, dress) that are evaluatively congruent with the perceivers' first impression. For example, when exposure to a very unattractive cigarette-smoking woman initially elicits a global negative reaction, it seems more likely that this negative reaction facilitates the activation of "smoking" (an evaluatively congruent, negative feature), rather than the activation of "woman" (an evaluatively incongruent, positive feature).

Ruys, Dijksterhuis, and Corneille (2008) tested the hypothesis that initial, global evaluative reactions spontaneously facilitate the activation of evaluatively congruent specific information. In two speeded dichotomous categorization experiments, participants were instructed to indicate (as quickly as possible) the social category of the target person that appeared on the screen, choosing between a positive and a negative social category. Ruys et al. (2008) expected that *attractive* target persons would elicit a global *positive* reaction that would lead to faster and more accurate responses when the remaining specific features of the target person were also positive (e.g., "fellow-citizen," "bride"), compared to when these features were negative (e.g., "foreign," "prostitute"). They also expected that *unattractive* target persons would elicit a global *negative* reaction that would lead to faster and more accurate responses when the remaining specific features of the target person were also negative, compared to when these features were positive. Participants should thus respond more quickly and more accurately when global evaluative reactions to a target person evaluatively match the specific features of the person, because these global evaluative reactions facilitate the activation of evaluatively congruent specific features (Ruys et al., 2008).

In one study, Ruys et al. (2008) tested this hypothesis by having participants categorize target persons either as "foreign" or as "fellow-citizen," features that were pretested as negative and positive, respectively. To remove the intergroup confound, they also conducted a second study where participants categorized target persons either as "prostitute" or as "bride." Both studies show that categorization was more rapid and more accurate when the attractiveness of the person evaluatively matched the remaining specific features (e.g., with "unattractive foreigners," "unattractive prostitutes," "attractive fellow-citizens," and "attractive brides") than when the attractiveness of the person evaluatively mismatched the remaining specific features (e.g., with "attractive foreigners," "attractive prostitutes," "unattractive fellow-citizens," and "unattractive brides"). These findings indicate that initial global evaluative reactions may indeed facilitate the activation of remaining specific information when this information is evaluatively congruent (Ruys et al., 2008). On a more general level, these studies provide evidence for the hypothesis that global and specific processing interact.

Interestingly, these recent findings (Ruys et al., 2008) and our global-to-specific unfolding view contradict the common view that the activation of stereotypes guides initial impressions of people (Allport, 1954; Brewer, 1988; Kawakami, Dion, & Dovidio, 1998; Macrae, Milne, & Bodenhausen, 1994). According to this view, when perceivers form an impression, they categorize people as Black, female, or skinhead, and this categorization process results in the activation of specific knowledge associated with that category (i.e., the stereotype). The activated specific knowledge, in turn, further guides the impression formation process. We call into question whether the activation and application of stereotypes is indeed the first thing social perceivers do upon encountering a person, and suggest that stereotype activation is better characterized as a "downstream" process that follows from earlier processes. As predicted by global-to-specific unfolding and demonstrated empirically, most stimuli initially elicit global evaluative reactions ("Barney is nice") prior to more specific detailed reactions like the activation of stereotypical information ("Barney is a priest").

## 4.7 Recognition and Simulation of Facial Emotional Expressions

Besides examining the interactions between global and specific emotional reactions, another interesting angle is to examine how global and specific emotional reactions interact with further emotional processing such as recognition and simulation of facial emotional expressions. We speculate that global and specific emotional reactions have a differential impact on these processes.

Based on affective priming research in general (e.g., Fazio, 2001) and research regarding the interaction of global and specific processing of emotional information in particular (Niedenthal & Cantor, 1986; Ruys et al., 2008), we expect that global emotional reactions (i.e., positive or negative moods) facilitate the recognition of affectively congruent facial emotional expressions and delay the recognition of affectively incongruent facial emotional expressions. Thus, people detect and recognize a happy facial expression more readily than a fearful or angry facial expression when they feel good compared to when they feel bad.

Specific emotional reactions might impact the recognition of facial emotional expressions in a different way. Researchers have proposed that covert or overt simulation of a facial emotional expression facilitates the recognition of that facial emotional expression (Enticott, Johnston, Herring, Hoy, & Fitzgerald, 2008; Gallese, 2006; Goldman & Sripada, 2005; Hess & Blairy, 2001; Niedenthal, Brauer, Halberstad, & Innes-Ker, 2001; Oberman, Winkielman, & Ramachandran, 2007). For example, recognition of a joyful expression is facilitated when the joyful expression also activates the same joyful expression in the perceiver.

This assumption – that simulation facilitates recognition – suggests that impeding simulation of a particular facial emotional expression also impedes recognition of that facial emotional expression in someone else. We think that the experience of a specific emotion might be a situation wherein simulation of the associated emotional expression is impeded. When people experience a specific emotion such as fear, this involves the (micro) activation of a fearful facial emotional expression. In particular, experiencing a specific emotion activates the motor program that is responsible for contracting or relaxing of the facial muscles that produce the associated facial expression. The occupation this motor program and activation of the associated facial musculature could impede imitation of a similar facial emotional expression. Thus, the experience of fear might render recognition of fearful facial expressions more difficult.

The idea that the experience of a specific emotion hinders recognition of the facial emotional expression associated to that emotion has received some empirical support (Niedenthal et al., 2001). In this research, participants indicated, after the induction of happiness or sadness, the offset of a happy (or sad) facial expression that changed into a sad (or happy) facial expression. The results showed that participants more quickly detected the offset of a congruent facial emotional expression than the offset of an incongruent facial emotional expression. Another interpretation of these results is that participants more quickly detected the *onset* of an incongruent facial emotional expression than the *onset* of a congruent facial emotional expression. The experience of happiness or sadness thus seemed to delay recognition of the corresponding facial emotional expression. This is in line with our idea that experiencing a specific emotion hinders recognition of the associated facial expression in others. However, to conclude that the experience of a specific emotion hinders recognition of the facial emotional expression associated to that emotion requires more evidence.

A final note we need to make is that the impact of simulation on the recognition of a facial emotional expression is minimal when recognition of the expression is fairly easy. Simulation of facial emotional expressions plays a more profound role in recognition when facial emotional expressions are more difficult to distinguish. Consequently, we assume that the influence of experiencing a specific emotion on the recognition of the associated facial emotional expression increases when the facial emotional expression becomes harder to decipher. However, these claims remain to be tested empirically.

## 4.8 Conclusion

In this chapter, we presented a global-to-specific unfolding view on emotional responding. This view entails that emotional responses follow the unfolding of perception and processing of emotional events. In keeping with the contention that perception typically unfolds form global to specific (Navon, 1977), we showed that emotional responding develops from global positive-negative emotional reactions (e.g., moods) to more specific fine-grained emotional reactions (e.g., anger, fear, disgust). We also demonstrated that both global and specific emotional reactions occur without knowing the cause of these emotional reactions. Thus, both moods and emotions can be triggered unconsciously.

We discussed the assumptions that underlie our global-to-specific unfolding view on emotional responding in more detail by contrasting our view with appraisal theories of emotion. One assumption is that the two systems responsible for global and specific processing are highly intertwined. We discussed research suggesting that global and specific processing do not operate independently but may interact. We ended this chapter by speculating about the differential impact of global and specific emotional responding on recognition of facial emotional expressions. Looking into the consequences of global and specific emotional responding on further emotional processing seems a promising avenue for future research.

## References

Adolphs, R. (2003) Cognitive neuroscience of human social behavior. *Nature Reviews Neuroscience*, *4*,165–178.

Allport, G. W. (1954) *The nature of prejudice*. Reading, MA: Addison-Wesley.

Arnold, M. B. (1960) *Emotion and personality*. New York, NY: Columbia University Press.

Avramova, Y. R., & Stapel, D. A. (2008) Moods as spotlights: The influence of mood on accessibility effects. *Journal of Personality and Social Psychology*, *95*, 542–554.

Bargh, J. A., & Chartrand, T. L. (2000) The mind in the middle. A practical guide to priming and automaticity research. In H. T. Reis & C. M. Judd (Eds.), *Handbook of Research Methods in Social and Personality Psychology* (pp. 253–285). New York: Cambridge University Press.

Brewer, M. B. (1988) A dual process model of impression formation. In T. K. Srull & R. S. Wyer (Eds.), *Advances in Social Cognition: Vol. 1. A Dual Process Model of Impression Formation* (pp. 1–36). Hillsdale, NJ: Erlbaum.

Cacioppo, J. T., & Gardner, W. L. (1999) Emotion. *Annual Review of Psychology, 50*, 191–214.

Corbetta, M., & Shulman, G. L. (2002) Control of goal-directed and stimulus-driven attention in the brain. *Nature Reviews Neuroscience, 31*, 201–215.

Darwin, C. (1872) *The expression of the emotions in man and animals*. London: John Murray.

Derryberry, D., & Tucker, D. M. (1994) Motivating the focus of attention. In P. M. Niedenthal & S. Kitayama (Eds.), *The Heart's Eye: Emotional Influences in Perception and Attention* (pp. 167–196). San Diego: Academic Press.

Dimberg, U., Thunberg, M., & Elmehed, K. (2000) Unconscious facial reactions to emotional facial expressions. *Psychological Science, 11*, 86–89.

Ekman, P. (1984) Expression and the nature of emotion. In K. R. Scherer & P. Ekman (Eds.), *Approaches to Emotion* (pp. 319–343). Hillsdale, NJ: Erlbaum.

Enticott, P. G., Johnston, P. J., Herring, S., Hoy, K. E., & Fitzgerald, P. B. (2008) Mirror neuron activation is associated with facial emotion processing. *Neuropsychologia, 46*, 2851–2854.

Evers, C., Fischer, A. H., Mosquera, P. M. R., & Manstead, A. S. R. (2005) Anger and social appraisal: A "spicy" sex difference? *Emotion, 5*, 258–266.

Fazio, R. H. (2001) On the automatic activation of associated evaluations: An overview. *Cognition and Emotion, 15*, 115–141.

Fink, G. R., Halligan, P. W., Marshall, J. C., Frith, C. D., Frackowiack, R. S. J., & Dolan, R. J. (1996) Where in the brain does visual attention select the forest and the trees? *Nature, 382*, 626–628.

Frijda, N. H. (1986) *The emotions*. Cambridge: Cambridge University Press.

Frijda, N. H. (1988) The laws of emotion. *American Psychologist, 43*, 349–358.

Frijda, N. H. (1994) Emotions are functional, most of the time. In P. Ekman & R. J. Davidson (Eds.), *The Nature of Emotion. Fundamental Questions*. New York: Oxford University Press.

Frijda, N. H., & Zeelenberg, M. (2001) Appraisal. What is the dependent? In K. R. Scherer, A. Schorr, & T. Johnstone (Eds.), *Appraisal Processes in Emotion: Theory, Methods, Research* (pp. 141–155). New York: Oxford University Press.

Gallese, V. (2006) Intentional attunement: A neurophysiological perspective on social cognition and its disruption in autism. *Brain Research, 1079*, 15–24.

Goldman, A. I., & Sripada, C. S. (2005) Simulationist models of face-based emotion recognition. *Cognition, 94*, 193–213.

Grandjean, D., & Scherer, K. R. (2008) Unpacking the cognitive architecture of emotion processes. *Emotion, 8*, 341–351.

Hariri, A. R., Tessitore, A., Mattay, V. S., Fera, F., & Weinberger, D. R. (2002) The amygdala response to emotional stimuli: A comparison of faces and scenes. *NeuroImage, 17*, 317–323.

Hess, U., & Blairy, S. (2001) Facial mimicry and emotional contagion to dynamic emotional facial expressions and their influence on decoding accuracy. *International Journal of Psychophysiology, 40*, 129–141.

Kawakami, K., Dion, K. L., & Dovidio, J. F. (1998) Racial prejudice and stereotype activation. *Personality and Social Psychology Bulletin, 24*, 407–416.

Keltner, D., & Gross, J. J. (1999) Functional accounts of emotions. *Cognition and Emotion, 13*, 467–480.

Killgore, W. D. S., & Yurgelun-Todd, D. A. (2004) Activation of the amygdala and anterior cingulate during nonconscious processing of sad versus happy faces. *NeuroImage, 21*, 1215–1223.

Kimchi, R. (1992) Primacy of wholistic processing and global/local paradigm: A critical review. *Psychological Bulletin, 112*, 24–38.

Lazarus, R. S. (1968) Emotions and adaptation. In W. J. Arnold (Ed.), *Nebraska Symposium on Motivation* (pp. 175–266). Lincoln: University of Nebraska Press.

Lazarus, R. S. (1991) Progress on a cognitive-motivational-relational theory of emotion. *American Psychologist, 46*, 819–834.

LeDoux, J. E. (1989) Cognitive-emotional interactions of the brain. *Cognition and Emotion, 3*, 267–289.

Lerner, J. S., & Keltner, D. (2001) Fear, anger, and risk. *Journal of Personality & Social Psychology, 81*, 146–159.

Macrae, C. N., Milne, A. B., & Bodenhausen, G. V. (1994) Stereotypes as energy-saving devices: A peek inside the cognitive toolbox. *Journal of Personality and Social Psychology*, *66*, 37–47.
Manstead, A. S. R., & Fischer, A. H. (2001) Social appraisal: The social world as object of and influence on appraisal processes. In K. R. Scherer, A. Schorr, & T. Johnstone (Eds.), *Appraisal Processes in Emotion* (pp. 221–232). New York: Oxford University Press.
Morris, J. S., de Gelder, B., Weiskrantz, L., & Dolan, R. J. (2001) Differential extrageniculostriate and amygdala responses to presentation of emotional faces in a cortically blind field. *Brain*, *124*, 1241–1252.
Navon, D. (1977) Forest before trees: The precedence of global features in visual perception. *Cognitive Psychology*, *9*, 353–383.
Niedenthal, P. M., Barsalou, L. W., Winkielman, P., Krauth-Gruber, S., & Ric, F. (2005) Embodiment in attitudes, social perception, and emotion. *Personality and Social Psychology Review*, *9*, 184–211.
Niedenthal, P. M., Brauer, M., Halberstadt, J. B., & Innes-Ker, A. H. (2001) When did her smile drop? Facial mimicry and the influences of emotional state on the detection of change in emotional expression. *Cognition and Emotion*, *15*, 853–864.
Niedenthal, P. M., & Cantor, N. (1986) Affective responses as guides to category-based inferences. *Motivation and Emotion*, *10*, 217–232.
Oberman, L., Winkielman, P., & Ramachandran, V. S. (2007) Face to face: Blocking facial mimicry can selectively impair recognition of emotional expressions. *Social Neuroscience*, *2*, 167–178.
Öhman, A. (1992) The psychophysiology of emotion: Evolutionary and non-conscious origins. In G. d'Ydewalle, P. Eelen, & P. Bertelson (Eds.), *International Perspectives on Psychological Science; Volume 2: The State of the Art* (Vol. 2, pp. 197–227). Hillsdale, NJ: Lawrence Erlbaum.
Palermo, R., & Rhodes, G. (2007) Are you always on my mind? A review of how face perception and attention interact. *Neuropsychologia*, *45*, 75–92.
Panksepp, J. (1998) *Affective neuroscience: The foundations of human and animal emotions*. New York: Oxford University Press.
Parkinson, B., & Manstead, A. S. R. (1992) Appraisal as a cause of emotion. In M. S. Clark (Ed.), *Emotion, Review of Personality and Social psychology*. Newbury Park, CA: Sage Publishers.
Phillips, M. L., Williams, L. M., Heining, M., Herba, C. M., Russell, T., Andrew, C., et al. (2004) Differential neural responses to overt and covert presentations of facial expressions of fear and disgust. *NeuroImage*, *21*, 1484–1496.
Prinz, J. (2004) *Gut reactions: A perceptual theory of emotion*. New York: Oxford University Press.
Rolls, E. T. (2008) Emotion, higher order syntactic thoughts, and consciousness. In L. Weiskrantz & M. K. Davies (Eds.), *Frontiers of Consciousness* (pp. 131–167). Oxford: Oxford University Press.
Rosenthal, V. (2004) Microgenesis, immediate experience and visual processes in reading. In A. Carsetti (Ed.), *Seeing, Thinking and Knowing: Meaning and Self-Organisation in Visual Cognition and Thought* (pp. 221–243). Dordrecht, Netherlands: Kluwer Academic Publishers.
Ruys, K. I., Dijksterhuis, A., & Corneille, O. (2008) On the (mis)categorization of unattractive brides and attractive prostitutes: Extending evaluative congruency effects to social category activation. *Experimental Psychology*, *55*, 182–188.
Ruys, K. I., & Stapel, D. A. (2008a) The secret life of emotions. *Psychological Science*, *19*, 385–391.
Ruys, K. I., & Stapel, D. A. (2008b) How to heat up from the cold: Examining the preconditions for (unconscious) mood effects. *Journal of Personality and Social Psychology*, *94*, 777–791.
Ruys, K. I., & Stapel, D. A. (2008c) Emotion elicitor or emotion-messenger? Subliminal exposure to two faces of facial expressions. *Psychological Science*, *19*, 593–600.
Ruys, K. I., & Stapel, D. A. (2009) *The unconscious unfolding of emotions*. European Review of Social Psychology, 20, 232–271.
Scherer, K. R. (1984) On the nature and function of emotion: A component process approach. In K. R. Scherer & P. Ekman (Eds.), *Approaches to Emotion* (pp. 293–318). Hillsdale, NJ: Erlbaum.
Scherer, K. R. (1999) On the sequential nature of appraisal processes: Indirect evidence from a recognition task. *Cognition and Emotion*, *13*, 763–793.

Stapel, D. A., & Koomen, W. (2006) The flexible unconscious: Investigating the judgmental impact of varieties of unaware perception. *Journal of Experimental Social Psychology*, *42*, 112–119.

Stapel, D. A., Koomen, W., & Ruys, K. I. (2002) The effects of diffuse and distinct affect. *Journal of Personality and Social Psychology*, *83*, 60–74.

Storbeck, J., & Robinson, M. D. (2004) Preferences and inferences in encoding visual objects: A semantic comparison of semantic and affective priming. *Personality and Social Psychology Bulletin*, *30*, 81–93.

Tucker, D. M., & Williamson, P. A. (1984) Asymmetric neural control systems in human self-regulation. *Psychological Review*, *91*, 185–215.

Weiner, B. (1985) An attributional theory of achievement motivation and emotion. *Psychological Review*, *92*, 548–573.

Werner, H. (1956) Microgenesis and aphasia. *Journal of Abnormal Social Psychology*, *52*, 347–353.

Zajonc, R. B. (2000) Feeling and thinking. Closing the debate over the independence of affect. In J. Forgas (Ed.), *Feeling and Thinking: The Role of Affect in Social Cognition* (pp. 31–58). Cambridge: Cambridge University Press.

Zeelenberg, M., van den Bos, K., van Dijk, E., & Pieters, R. (2002) The inaction effect in the psychology of regret. *Journal of Personality and Social Psychology*, *82*, 314–327.

# Chapter 5
# Self-Regulatory Interplay Between Negative and Positive Emotions: The Case of Loneliness and Nostalgia

**Tim Wildschut, Constantine Sedikides, and Filippo Cordaro**

## 5.1 Introduction

The past 20 years have seen a surge in psychological research on emotions. Most of this attention has been devoted to negative affective states such as shame (Tangney, 2003), guilt (Baumeister, Stillwell, & Heatherton, 1994), embarrassment (Keltner & Buswell, 1996), regret (Gilovich & Medvec, 1995), social anxiety (Leary & Kowalski, 1995), and loneliness (Cacioppo et al., 2006). Historically, the study of positive emotions has lagged behind, but in recent years there has been a welcome increase in research on positive affective states such as gratitude (Emmons & McCullough, 2003), pride (Tracy & Robins, 2007), joy (Fredrickson, 2001), self-compassion (Neff, 2003), inspiration (Thrash & Elliot, 2003), passion (Vallerand et al., 2003), and nostalgia (Sedikides, Wildschut, Arndt, & Routledge, 2008).

Much of the impetus for the burgeoning interest in positive emotions was provided by the influential idea that these emotions play a vital role in the regulation of psychological distress and the maintenance of psychological and physiological homeostasis (Aspinwall, 1998; Folkman & Moskowitz, 2000). This view was expressed succinctly, for instance, in Levenson's (1988) *undoing hypothesis*. Levenson proposed that: "the evolutionary meaning of positive emotions such as happiness might be to function as efficient 'undoers' of states of ANS (autonomic nervous system) arousal produced by certain negative emotions" (p. 25). Building on this hypothesis, Fredrickson and Levenson (1998) suggested that:

> If negative emotions promote the activation of a limited number of well-rehearsed, time-tested, adaptive actions along with their attendant physiological support, certain positive emotions can be seen as assuming a complementary role, efficiently restoring equilibrium to the organism both in terms of returning physiological activation to prior levels, and restoring psychological openness to a wide range of action possibilities (p. 215).

The objective of this chapter is to review empirical research that highlights the complementary relation between loneliness (a negative emotional state) and

T. Wildschut (✉)
School of Psychology, University of Southampton, Southampton, SO17 1BJ, England, UK
e-mail: timw@soton.ac.uk

I. Nyklíček et al. (eds.), *Emotion Regulation and Well-Being*,
DOI 10.1007/978-1-4419-6953-8_5, © Springer Science+Business Media, LLC 2011

nostalgia (a positive emotional state). Specifically, we propose that the psychological significance of nostalgia resides in part in its capacity to regulate feelings of loneliness by increasing perceived social connectedness. We review findings showing that loneliness increases nostalgia and that, in turn, nostalgia increases perceived social connectedness. We then examine evidence for the vital implication that, whereas the direct effect of loneliness is to reduce perceived social connectedness, its indirect effect is to increase perceived social connectedness via nostalgia. Finally, we examine how the relation between loneliness and nostalgia is shaped by individual differences that play a governing role in emotion regulation: resilience (Block & Kremen, 1996; Bonanno, 2005) and the attachment-related dimensions of avoidance and anxiety (Mikulincer & Shaver, 2003).

### *5.1.1 Loneliness*

Loneliness is a complex emotion marked by negative feelings and cognitions, including unhappiness, pessimism, self-blame, and depression (Cacioppo & Hawkley, 2005). Loneliness is also characterized by perceived lack of social support (Cacioppo et al., 2006) and by having fewer and less satisfying relationships than desired (Archibald, Bartholomew, & Marx, 1995). Furthermore, loneliness is a universal experience, as documented by studies with diverse cultural samples including Chinese Canadians (Goodwin, Cook, & Yung, 2001), Turks and Argentines (Rokach & Bacanli, 2001), Americans and Canadians (Rokach & Neto, 2000), Portuguese (Neto & Barrios, 2001), and British Asians (Shams, 2001). Broadly defined, loneliness may comprise negative affective states such as hurt feelings (Leary, Springer, Negel, Ansell, & Evans, 1998) and unrequited love (Baumeister, Wotman, & Stillwell, 1993). Hurt feelings arise from relational devaluation: that is, the feeling that close others do not value one's relationship with them. Betrayal, criticism, disassociation, and being unappreciated are important precursors to hurt feelings, and hurt feelings are strongly correlated with a sense of social exclusion (Leary et al., 1998). Unrequited love occurs when romantic attraction is not reciprocated, and involves a particularly poignant form of relational devaluation (Baumeister et al., 1993).

### *5.1.2 Nostalgia*

The term "nostalgia" derives from the Greek words nostos (*return*) and algos (*pain*). It was coined by the Swiss physician Johannes Hofer (1688/1934) to describe the adverse symptoms displayed by Swiss mercenaries fighting in the service of European monarchs. Hofer conceptualized nostalgia as "a cerebral disease" (p. 387), and his view of nostalgia as a neurological affliction persisted throughout the seventeenth and the eighteenth century. By the early nineteenth century, nostalgia came to be regarded as a form of melancholia or depression, and it remained relegated to the realm of psychological disorders for much of the twentieth century. In part, this disconsolate perspective was due to the equation of nostalgia with homesickness. Only in the latter part of the twentieth century did nostalgia acquire a separate conceptual status (Davis, 1979; Sedikides, Wildschut, & Baden, 2004). Current dictionary definitions of homesickness and nostalgia reflect this distinctness. *The New Oxford Dictionary of English* (1998) defines "homesick" as "experiencing a longing for one's home during a period of absence from it" and "nostalgia" as "a sentimental longing for the past" (p. 1266). Whereas there is now a sizeable literature on homesickness (Van Tilburg & Vingerhoets, 2005; Watt & Badger, 2009), empirical research on nostalgia remains scarce and, until recently, confined mainly to the field of marketing and consumer preferences (Holbrook, 1993). Focused on accounting for the market success of certain consumer goods, this research has demonstrated how product styles (e.g., of music) that were popular during one's youth influence one's lifelong preferences. Although these findings are important, we have attempted to lay the foundation for a broader perspective in order to understand more fully the psychological significance of nostalgia (Sedikides et al., 2008; Sedikides, Wildschut, Arndt, & Routledge, 2006).

Nostalgia is a self-relevant and social emotion: The self almost invariably figures as the protagonist in nostalgic memories and is almost always surrounded by close others. Along with close others (family members, friends, romantic partners), the most common objects of nostalgia are momentous events (birthdays, anniversaries, vacations; Wildschut, Sedikides, Arndt, & Routledge, 2006, Studies 1–2). Although nostalgia is characterized by some affective ambivalence, it is a predominantly positive emotion. On the one hand, the simultaneous expression of happiness and sadness is more commonly found in recollections of nostalgic events, compared with ordinary events, and the co-activation of happiness and sadness occurs more frequently as a result of reflection about nostalgic events than as a result of reflection about ordinary or positive events (Wildschut, Stephan, Sedikides, Routledge, & Arndt, 2008). On the other hand, recollections of nostalgic events include more frequent expressions of happiness than of sadness, and nostalgic reflection generates more positive affect (but not more negative affect) than reflection about ordinary events (Wildschut et al., 2006, 2008; Zhou et al., 2008). Moreover, in nostalgic narratives, positive and negative elements are often juxtaposed in a redemption sequence – a narrative pattern that progresses from a bleak to a triumphant life scene (McAdams, 2001).

### 5.1.3 Interplay Between Loneliness and Nostalgia

Loneliness can be combated in more than one way. Deficiencies in social connectedness elicit a range of compensatory mechanisms geared toward replenishing social connectedness (Maner, DeWall, Baumeister, & Schaller, 2007). For instance, Williams and Sommer (1997) found that women responded to rejection from a group by working harder on a subsequent collective task. Support from social networks alleviates loneliness (Asher & Paquette, 2003) and individuals form social bonds with relative ease (Festinger, Schachter, & Back, 1950). Furthermore, once formed, individuals attempt tenaciously to maintain social bonds (Vaughan, 1986). Yet, frequently, the formation and maintenance of social networks is impeded or interrupted by situational or individual factors. For instance, the deterioration or even dissolution of valued social bonds that often accompanies life transitions (e.g., transition to college, relocation, migration) can make individuals feel adrift and lonely (Sedikides, Wildschut, Routledge, Arndt, & Zhou, 2009; Van Tilburg & Vingerhoets, 2005). Social networks can also be disrupted by interpersonal rejections (Williams, 1997), and personality dispositions (e.g., shyness, social anxiety) can frustrate the maintenance and formation of social networks (Leary & Kowalski, 1995).

An alternative strategy for coping with loneliness is to strengthen subjective perceptions of social connectedness and support by drawing on nostalgic memories. In nostalgic reverie, "the mind is 'peopled'" (Hertz, 1990, p. 195). By rekindling meaningful relationships, nostalgia bolsters social bonds and renders accessible positive relational knowledge structures (Baldwin, Keelan, Fehr, Enns, & Koh-Rangarajoo, 1996). Important figures from one's past are brought to life and become part of one's present (Davis, 1979).

## 5.2 The Relationship Between Nostalgia and Loneliness

### *5.2.1 Does Loneliness Increase Nostalgia?*

There is compelling empirical evidence that lonely individuals seek refuge in nostalgic reverie. Initial results indicating a link between loneliness and nostalgia came from a study in which British undergraduate participants were asked simply to write about the circumstances under which they become nostalgic (Wildschut et al., 2006, Study 2). Analysis of these narrative descriptions revealed that negative affect was the most frequently mentioned trigger of nostalgia (e.g., "Generally I think about nostalgic experiences when things are not going very well – lonely or depressed"). Specifically, 38% of participants listed negative affect as a trigger of nostalgia. The next most frequent trigger (24%) was social interaction (e.g., "Meeting up with people who were there and discussing what happened and laughing/crying about it"). Considering the prominence of negative affect as a trigger of nostalgia, Wildschut et al. examined more closely descriptions coded into this category. They made a distinction between discrete negative affective states (e.g., lonely, scared) and generalized affective states often referred to as negative mood (e.g., sad, depressed). In contrast to more discrete affective states, which "arise from appraisals of specific actual or contemplated states of the world" (Bodenhausen, Sheppard, & Kramer, 1994, p. 46), generalized affective states often lack a clearly delineated referent or antecedent. Some participants mentioned both discrete and generalized negative affective states (e.g., "If I ever feel lonely or sad, I tend to think of my friends or family whom I haven't seen for a long time") and therefore the two categories were not mutually exclusive. Of those who listed negative affect as a trigger of nostalgia, 78% referred to negative mood, and 58% referred to discrete negative affective states. Within the latter category, 59% of participants referred to loneliness, making it the most frequently mentioned discrete affective state by far.

In a follow-up study, Wildschut et al. (2006, Study 4) investigated directly the causal impact of loneliness on nostalgia. Does experimentally induced loneliness increase in-the-moment feelings of nostalgia? Wildschut et al. manipulated loneliness by giving British undergraduates false questionnaire feedback. Participants completed a questionnaire labeled "Southampton Loneliness Scale," which comprised 15 statements drawn from the UCLA Loneliness Scale (Russell, 1996). In the high loneliness condition, participants completed items that were designed to elicit agreement by prefacing them with the words "I sometimes" (e.g., "I sometimes feel isolated from others"). In the low loneliness condition, participants completed items that were designed to elicit disagreement by prefacing them with the words "I always" (e.g., "I always feel isolated from others"). As intended, participants in the high loneliness (compared to low loneliness) condition agreed with a greater number of statements. Next, participants in the high loneliness condition were told that they fell in the 62nd percentile of the loneliness distribution and therefore were "above average on loneliness," whereas participants in the low loneliness condition were told that they fell in the 12th percentile and therefore were "very low on loneliness." Participants then completed a manipulation check and Batcho's (1995) Nostalgia Inventory (NI). On this questionnaire, participants rated how much they miss 18 aspects of their past (e.g., "my family," "not having to worry," "music," "having someone to depend on," "holidays I went on," "my family house"). Results revealed that participants in the high loneliness (compared to low loneliness) condition felt more lonely and experienced stronger in-the-moment feelings of nostalgia.

### *5.2.2 Does Nostalgia Increase Social Connectedness?*

The documented effect of loneliness on nostalgia is consistent with the possibility that nostalgia serves to regulate deficiencies in social connectedness. To further examine this idea, Wildschut et al. (2006, Studies 5–7) tested whether nostalgia strengthens social connectedness. They randomly assigned participants to a nostalgia or control condition. In the nostalgia condition, participants were instructed to recall a nostalgic event from their lives, and to reflect upon the event and how it made them feel. In the control condition, participants were instructed to recall an ordinary event from their lives, and to reflect upon the event and how it made them feel. Following a manipulation check, social connectedness was assessed with either (1) the items "loved" and "protected," (2) the Revised Experiences in Close Relationships Scale (ECR-R; Fraley, Waller, & Brennan, 2000) which measures attachment-related anxiety and avoidance, and (3) the Interpersonal Competence Questionnaire (Buhrmester, Furman, Wittenberg, & Reis, 1988) which taps perceived competence in initiating social interactions, self-disclosing, and providing emotional support. Nostalgic (compared to control) participants manifested stronger feelings of nostalgia (as assessed by the manipulation check) and stronger social connectedness: they felt more loved and protected, evinced reduced attachment-related anxiety and avoidance, and reported greater interpersonal competence. In a subsequent study with Chinese undergraduates, Zhou, Sedikides, Wildschut, and Gao (2008, Study 3) further found that nostalgic (compared to control) participants scored higher on perceived social support, as assessed by the Multidimensional Scale of Perceived Social Support (MSPSS; Zimet, Dahlem, Zimet, & Farley, 1988), and estimated that they had a greater number of friends who would help them to earn research credits.

### *5.2.3 Does Loneliness Increase Social Connectedness Via Nostalgia?*

So far, we have reviewed evidence that loneliness increases nostalgia and that nostalgia, in turn, increases social connectedness. This evidence raises the possibility that loneliness affects social connectedness in two distinct ways. The direct effect of loneliness is to reduce social connectedness: The lonelier one feels, the fewer social connections one perceives. However, loneliness may also have an indirect positive effect by increasing social connectedness via nostalgia: The lonelier one feels, the more nostalgic one becomes, and the more social connectedness one may then experience. This pattern of relations would give rise to a situation of "statistical suppression." Such situations can be described in terms of an implicit causal model involving an initial predictor (e.g., loneliness), an intervening variable (e.g., nostalgia), and an outcome (e.g., perceived social connectedness). Suppression occurs when the direct effect of the initial predictor is directionally opposite to its indirect effect via the intervening variable. When the intervening variable is controlled, the direct effect of the initial predictor is strengthened (Paulhus, Robins, Trzesniewski, & Tracy, 2004).

In a series of studies with Chinese participants, Zhou et al. (2008) examined the possibility that nostalgia counteracts reductions in perceived social support caused by loneliness. In one study, 758 Chinese children who had migrated with their parents from rural to urban areas completed measures of loneliness, nostalgia (Southampton Nostalgia Scale [SNS]; Routledge, Arndt, Sedikides, & Wildschut, 2008), and perceived social support. The results of this study are presented in Fig. 5.1 (top panel). Zero-order correlations revealed that (1) loneliness was negatively associated with perceived social support, (2) loneliness was positively associated with nostalgia, and (3) nostalgia was positively associated with perceived social support. These results showed that, whereas the direct effect of loneliness is to decrease perceived social support, the indirect effect of loneliness is to increase perceived social support via nostalgia. Indeed, when Zhou et al. regressed perceived social support onto both loneliness and nostalgia, they found a unique negative association between loneliness and perceived social support, and a unique positive association between nostalgia and perceived social support. Importantly, the negative

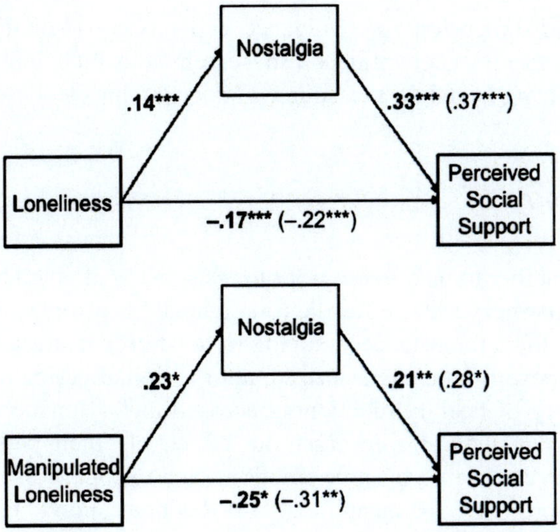


**Fig. 5.1** Associations among loneliness, nostalgia, and perceived social support in Study 1 (*top*; $N = 758$) and Study 2 (*bottom*; $N = 84$). Shown are zero-order correlations (in **boldface**) and standardized regression coefficients (in *parentheses*); $^{*}p < 0.05$; $^{**}p < 0.01$; $^{***}p < 0.001$

association between loneliness and perceived social support became significantly more negative after the palliative effect of nostalgia was controlled. In sum, lonely migrant children perceived little social support but were also the most nostalgic. This high level of nostalgia, in turn, increased their perceptions of social support.

A subsequent experiment by Zhou et al. (2008) involved Chinese university students who were randomly assigned to either a high loneliness or a low loneliness condition. Loneliness was manipulated by giving participants false feedback regarding questionnaire scores (Wildschut et al., 2006, Study 4). Following this manipulation, participants completed state measures of nostalgia and perceived social support. Results revealed that loneliness reduced social support but increased nostalgia, and that nostalgia was positively associated with social support. Importantly, whereas the direct effect of loneliness was to reduce social support, its indirect effect was to increase social support via nostalgia (Fig. 5.1, bottom panel). Participants in the high loneliness (compared to low loneliness) condition perceived less social support, but they also felt more nostalgic. In turn, this nostalgic reverie boosted their perceptions of social support.

## 5.3 The Role of Individual Differences

The evidence reviewed so far is consistent with the idea that nostalgia facilitates the regulation of loneliness by strengthening social connectedness. We now focus on individual differences that have been shown to affect self-regulation in a broad range of domains. These are resilience (Block & Kremen, 1996; Bonanno, 2005) and the attachment-related dimensions of avoidance and anxiety (Mikulincer & Shaver, 2003). Do these factors also influence the extent to which individuals regulate loneliness by utilizing nostalgia as a source of social connectedness and support?

### 5.3.1 *Resilience*

Resilience is the ability to recover from (or to resist being affected by) shock, insult, or disturbance (Garmezy, 1991). Resilient individuals confronted with challenging or even traumatic life circumstances (ranging from a terrorist attack to divorce, death of a spouse, and poverty) are characterized, after an initial period of adjustment, by a "stable trajectory of healthy functioning across time" (Bonanno, 2005, p. 136). Such individuals are then able to carry out effectively their personal and social responsibilities, to experience positive emotions, and to engage in creative activities (Block & Kremen, 1996; Bonanno, 2005). Resilient individuals capitalize on available personal and social resources to self-regulate effectively in the face of adversity (Tugade & Fredrickson, 2004).

A study by Zhou et al. (2008, Study 4) revealed that resilience plays an important role in shaping the association between loneliness and nostalgia. These researchers assessed resilience (Resilience Scale; Wagnild & Young, 1993), loneliness, nostalgia, and perceived social support in a sample of Chinese factory workers. Results again showed that, whereas the direct effect of loneliness is to reduce perceived social support, its indirect effect is to increase perceived social support via nostalgia. More importantly, the positive association between loneliness and nostalgia was significantly stronger among participants who were high (compared to low) in resilience. Thus, it is highly resilient individuals who are most likely to recruit nostalgia in response to loneliness. Resilience did not qualify the strength of the association between nostalgia and perceived social support. In all, the Zhou et al. findings showed that both resilient and non-resilient people derive social support from nostalgia, but that highly resilient people are more likely to recruit nostalgia when lonely.

### 5.3.2 *Attachment-Related Individual Differences*

Attachment-related individual differences, like individual differences in resilience, are known to play a critical role in the regulation of emotional distress (Mikulincer & Shaver, 2003). In a series of studies, Wildschut, Sedikides, Routledge, Arndt, & Cordaro (2010) examined how individual differences in attachment-related avoidance (avoidance) and attachment-related anxiety (anxiety) shape the dynamic relation between loneliness and nostalgia. According to attachment theory (Bowlby, 1982; Brennan, Clark, & Shaver, 1998; Mikulincer & Shaver, 2003), individual differences in reactions to distress are a manifestation of two underlying dimensions: anxiety and avoidance. The former reflects the extent to which the self is seen as worthy of love and support, whereas the latter reflects the extent to which others are seen as responsive to one's distress. These internal working models of self and others begin to develop early in life in response to experiences with attachment figures (Ainsworth, Blehar, Waters, & Wall, 1978) and are thought to remain relatively stable across time (Sharfe & Bartholomew, 1994).

There is strong empirical evidence that avoidance in particular is negatively associated with support-seeking behavior (Feeney, 2006). Such evidence is consistent with the idea that highly avoidant individuals view others as unavailable or unresponsive and, hence, do not rely on social bonds to regulate distress. Importantly, research has also revealed that avoidance interacts with emotional distress to shape support-seeking behavior (Fraley & Shaver, 2000). That is, the positive association between emotional distress and support-seeking is stronger when others are seen as responsive (i.e., when avoidance is low) than when others are seen as unresponsive (i.e., when avoidance is high).

#### 5.3.2.1 Is the Effect of Loneliness on Nostalgia Shaped by Attachment-Related Individual Differences?

To the extent that nostalgia serves as a source of social connectedness and support, one would expect the positive association between loneliness and nostalgia to be stronger when avoidance is low rather than high. Wildschut et al. (2010, Study 1) tested this idea by assessing avoidance and anxiety, and then asking participants to write about the circumstances under which they become nostalgic. Afterwards, participants' responses were coded for instances in which loneliness was identified as trigger of nostalgia. Low-avoidance (compared to high-avoidance) participants more frequently stated that they become nostalgic in response to loneliness.

To achieve a more detailed understanding of the association between loneliness and nostalgia, Wildschut et al. (2010, Study 2) conducted a follow-up study that distinguished among three facets of loneliness connectedness (Hawkley, Browne, & Cacioppo, 2005): isolation (reflecting feelings of aloneness, anonymity, and withdrawal), relational connectedness (corresponding to familiarity, intimacy, and emotional support), and collective connectedness (dealing with feelings of group cohesion and similarity). Wildschut et al. measured how often participants felt lonely (differentiating between different facets of loneliness as assessed by the UCLA Loneliness Scale, see Hawkley et al.) and how frequently participants experienced nostalgia. They then tested whether the strength of the association between loneliness facets and nostalgia varied as a function of attachment-related individual differences. Results revealed that deficiencies in relational connectedness were the strongest predictor of increased nostalgia, and that this association between relational connectedness and nostalgia was present only for low-avoidance participants. That is, for low-avoidance (but not high-avoidance) participants, a perceived lack of emotional support and intimacy was linked with increased nostalgia.

Building on these findings, Wildschut et al. (2010, Study 3) sought to corroborate the postulated causal impact of deficiencies in relational connectedness on increased nostalgia among low-avoidance (compared to high-avoidance) persons.

They examined the impact of a validated social exclusion manipulation (Twenge, Baumeister, Tice, & Stucke, 2001) on in-the-moment feelings of nostalgia. In the *future alone* condition, participants were given false personality feedback suggesting that they would not enjoy lasting friendships or marriages. In the *future belonging* condition, participants were given false personality feedback suggesting that they would enjoy a stable marriage and rewarding friendships throughout life. This manipulation thus targets specifically (anticipated) deficiencies in relational connectedness. After participants received the false personality feedback, they reported on their in-the-moment feelings of nostalgia. Results revealed that social exclusion (compared to social inclusion) increased nostalgia among low-avoidance participants, but not among high-avoidance participants. These findings provided further convergent evidence for the idea that the psychological significance of nostalgia resides partly in its capacity to strengthen social connectedness, and that low-avoidance (compared to high-avoidance) persons are more apt to regulate deficiencies in relational connectedness by recruiting nostalgia.

#### 5.3.2.2 Is the Effect of Nostalgia on Social Connectedness Shaped by Attachment-Related Individual Differences?

An important remaining question is whether deficiencies in relational connectedness elicit nostalgia more strongly among low-avoidance (compared to high-avoidance) persons, given that low-avoidance persons are more capable of deriving from nostalgia precisely the feelings of intimacy and emotional support that are optimally suited to redress deficiencies in relational connectedness (Cutrona & Russell, 1990). There are, of course, alternative explanations. Perhaps low-avoidance (compared to high-avoidance) persons are more likely to turn to nostalgia, not because they derive from it more social connectedness, but because nostalgia has other desirable effects, such as augmenting positive affect and boosting self-esteem (Wildschut et al., 2006).

To address this question, Wildschut et al. (2010, Study 4) assessed attachment-related individual differences and then randomly assigned participants to a nostalgia or control condition. Participants in the nostalgia condition were instructed to recall a nostalgic event, whereas participants in the control condition were instructed to recall an ordinary event from their past. Following this manipulation (and a successful manipulation check), participants completed brief state-level measures of positive affect ("Thinking about this event makes me feel happy," "… makes me feel in a good mood"), positive self-esteem ("… makes me feel I have many positive qualities," "… makes me value myself more"), and social connectedness ("… makes me feel loved," "… makes me feel connected to loved ones"). Results revealed that, whereas manipulated nostalgia increased positive affect and positive self-esteem irrespective of attachment-related individual differences, manipulated nostalgia strengthened social connectedness only among low-avoidance participants. These findings suggest that low-avoidance (compared to high-avoidance) persons are more apt to derive social connectedness (but not positive affect or self-esteem) from nostalgia.

## 5.4 Concluding Remarks and Future Directions

Whereas negative emotions have long been the focus of attention for emotion research, recent years have witnessed a marked shift toward increased interest in positive emotions. Research on positive emotions has highlighted their vital role in many aspects of daily experience and their involvement in the regulation of, and adjustment to, negative affective states. In this chapter, we reviewed recent studies that have examined the question of whether nostalgia – a predominantly positive self-relevant emotion – plays a role in the regulation of, and adjustment to, loneliness. These studies provided evidence for the idea that the psychological significance of nostalgia resides in part in its capacity to diminish loneliness by increasing perceived social connectedness.

### *5.4.1 Summary of Evidence*

The first question we examined was whether loneliness increases nostalgia. The evidence on this point showed that British university students often spontaneously identified loneliness as a trigger of nostalgia, and that they showed increased levels of state nostalgia following an experimental loneliness induction. The second question we examined was whether nostalgia increases perceived social connectedness. The evidence on this point revealed that both British and Chinese university students who recalled a nostalgic (compared to ordinary) event from their lives scored higher on various measures of social connectedness. Third, we addressed the issue of whether loneliness could increase perceived social connectedness via nostalgia. A series of studies with different Chinese samples found that, whereas the direct effect of loneliness is to reduce perceived social support, the indirect effect of loneliness is to increase perceived social support via nostalgia. Finally, we considered the role of individual differences in resilience and the attachment-related dimensions of avoidance and anxiety. Here, the evidence indicated that the association between loneliness and nostalgia (but not the association between nostalgia and perceived social support) was stronger among highly resilient individuals. It would appear that resilient (compared to non-resilient) individuals are more inclined to recruit nostalgia in response to loneliness. Studies on the role of attachment-related avoidance and anxiety revealed an important role for avoidance (but not for anxiety). These studies underscored the particular importance of deficits in relational connectedness as an antecedent to nostalgia among low-avoidance (but not high-avoidance) individuals. Furthermore, evidence revealed that, for low-avoidance (but not high-avoidance) individuals, nostalgia provided precisely the feelings of intimacy and emotional support that are optimally suited to redress deficiencies in relational connectedness.

### 5.4.2 Limitations and Further Research Directions

One must keep in mind that the research reviewed here was conducted predominantly (although not exclusively) with samples of college-age, British female subjects. The question whether age-related changes in motivation have a bearing on nostalgia presents one suitable avenue for future research. The interaction between gender and culture in shaping nostalgia is another issue that deserves careful scrutiny.

According to socio-emotional selectivity theory (Carstensen, Isaacowitz, & Charles, 1999), with advancing age people come to view their life-span as limited and shift attention from future-oriented, knowledge-related goals toward a desire to find purpose and meaning in life, to enjoy intimate friendships, and to be embedded in a social network. This raises two important issues pertaining to nostalgia. First, are such age-related changes in motivation reflected in the frequency and content of nostalgia? We would expect older (as compared to younger) adults to be more prone to nostalgia and more likely to give center stage to close others in their nostalgic reverie. The second issue is whether nostalgia acquires greater significance in old age. Although the problem of loneliness is not specific to old age, bereavements and declines in health status may render older adults particularly vulnerable to social isolation (Victor, Scambler, Bowling, & Bond, 2005), thus impairing the formation of intimate friendships and social networks they so highly value. Under these circumstances, nostalgia may play a vital role in reestablishing at least a symbolic connection with significant others.

Relevant to the role of gender, it seems plausible that British college students do not identify strongly with narrowly prescribed gender roles, and that gender differences in this population are therefore attenuated. In cultural contexts that place a stronger emphasis on traditional gender roles, however, strong differences between women and men may well arise. In general, gender differences are shaped by culture (Hyde, 2003) and so it would be unwarranted to generalize possible gender differences in a British college sample across different cultural settings.

Many other issues await empirical investigation. For instance, the extant literature does not inform the important question of whether, by virtue of its capacity to strengthen social connectedness, nostalgia can increase psychological and physical well-being. With respect to psychological well-being, there is a wealth of evidence that strong social bonds are associated with increased happiness (Sarason, Sarason, & Gurung, 1997). Concerning physical well-being, Berkman (1995) reviewed eight prospective epidemiological studies and concluded that mortality rates are lower among individuals with strong social bonds. Based on this evidence, we expect nostalgia to be positively associated with indices of both psychological and physical well-being. Could it be that these beneficial effects of nostalgia may accrue particularly to low-avoidance individuals because they are more likely than high-avoidance individuals to derive social connectedness from nostalgia?

Equally as important, the psychological significance of nostalgia may extend beyond its capacity to regulate loneliness by increasing social connectedness. For instance, nostalgia may also serve to imbue life with meaning, which could facilitate coping with existential fears. One of the primary human challenges is carving out a meaningful existence. Yet, awareness of inevitable mortality presents a major obstacle on the path to psychological equanimity. According to terror management theory (Pyszczynski, Greenberg, Solomon, Arndt, & Schimel, 2004), one can mitigate existential anxiety through shared beliefs about the nature of reality that imbue life with meaning. Nostalgia can contribute an overall sense of enduring meaning to one's life. In recent studies, we have explored this line of inquiry. For instance, in several studies testing American undergraduates, Routledge et al. (2008) examined this existential function of nostalgia. After being reminded of their mortality (relative to an aversive dental procedure), the more nostalgic the participants felt, the more meaningful they perceived their life to be. Also, after reminders of mortality (relative to a dental procedure or failing an important exam), participants who were more prone to nostalgia (e.g., had reported frequent engagement in nostalgia), or who had received a nostalgia induction, actually had fewer death-related thoughts. Nostalgia boosted perceptions of life as meaningful and assuaged existential threat.

Another interesting question is whether nostalgia can facilitate continuity between past and present selves. Nostalgia may facilitate use of positive perceptions about the past to bolster a sense of continuity and meaning in one's life (Sedikides, Wildschut, Gaertner, Routledge, & Arndt, 2008). An additional function of nostalgia may be its motivating potential. Nostalgia may boost optimism, spark inspiration, and foster creativity (Stephan, Wildschut, Sedikides, Routledge, & Arndt, 2008). Recent research provides initial evidence for both of these possibilities.

Nostalgia is emerging as a fundamental human strength. It is part of the fabric of everyday life and plays a versatile role in maintaining psychological equanimity. By so doing, nostalgia can help people navigate successfully the vicissitudes of life.

## References

Ainsworth, M. D. S., Blehar, M. C., Waters, E., & Wall, S. (1978) *Patterns of attachment: A psychological study of the strange situation*. Hillsdale, NJ: Erlbaum.

Archibald, F. S., Bartholomew, K., & Marx, R. (1995) Loneliness in early adolescence: A test of the cognitive discrepancy model of loneliness. *Personality and Social Psychology Bulletin*, *21*, 296–301.

Asher, S. R., & Paquette, J. A. (2003) Loneliness and peer relations in childhood. *Current Directions in Psychological Science*, *12*, 75–78.

Aspinwall, L. G. (1998) Rethinking the role of positive affect in self-regulation. *Motivation and Emotion*, *22*, 1–32.

Baldwin, M. W., Keelan, J. P. R., Fehr, B., Enns, V., & Koh-Rangarajoo, E. (1996) Social-cognitive conceptualization of attachment working models: Availability and accessibility effects. *Journal of Personality and Social Psychology*, *71*, 94–109.

Batcho, K. I. (1995) Nostalgia: A psychological perspective. *Perceptual and Motor Skills*, *80*, 131–143.

Baumeister, R. F., Stillwell, A. M., & Heatherton, T. F. (1994) Guilt: An interpersonal approach. *Psychological Bulletin*, *115*, 243–267.

Baumeister, R. F., Wotman, S. R., & Stillwell, A. M. (1993) Unrequited love: On heartbreak, anger, guilt, scriptlessness, and humiliation. *Journal of Personality and Social Psychology 64*, 377–394.

Berkman, L. F. (1995) The role of social relations in health promotion. *Psychosomatic Medicine*, *57*, 245–254.

Block, J.,& Kremen, A. (1996) IQ and Ego-resiliency: Clarifying their conceptual and empirical linkage and separateness. *Journal of Personality and Social Psychology*, *70*, 349–361.

Bodenhausen, G. V.,Sheppard, L. A.,& Kramer,G. P. (1994) Negative affect and social judgment: The differential impact of anger and sadness.*European Journal of Social Psychology*, *24*, 45–62.

Bonanno, G. A. (2005) Resilience in the face of potential trauma. *Current Directions in Psychological Science*, *4*, 135–138.

Bowlby, J. (1982) *Attachment and loss: Vol. 1. Attachment*. New York: Basic Books.

Brennan, K. A., Clark, C. L., & Shaver, P. R. (1998) Self-report measurement of adult attachment. An integrative overview. In J. A. Simpson & W. S. Rholes (Eds.), *Attachment theory and close relationships* (pp. 46–76). New York, NY: Guilford.

Buhrmester, D., Furman, W., Wittenberg, M. T., & Reis, H. T. (1988) Five domains of interpersonal competence in peer relationships. *Journal of Personality and Social Psychology*, *55*, 991–1108.

Cacioppo, J. T., & Hawkley, L. C. (2005) People thinking about people: The vicious cycle of being a social outcast in one's own mind. In K. D. Williams, J. P. Forgas, & W. von Hippel (Eds.), *The social outcast: Ostracism, social exclusion, rejection, and bullying* (pp. 91–108). New York, NY: Psychology Press.

Cacioppo, J. T., Hawkley, L. C., Ernst, J. M., Burleson, M., Berntson, G. G., Nouriani, B., & Spiegel, D. (2006) Loneliness within a nomological net: An evolutionary perspective. *Journal of Research in Personality*, *40*, 1054–1085.

Carstensen, L. L., Isaacowitz, D. M., & Charles, S. T. (1999) Taking time seriously. A theory of socioemotional selectivity. *American Psychologist*, *54*, 165–181.

Cutrona, C. E., & Russell, D. (1990) Type of social support and specific stress: Toward a theory of optimal matching. In I. G. Sarason, B. R. Sarason, & G. R. Pierce (Eds.), *Social support: An interactional view* (pp. 319–366). New York, NY: Wiley.

Davis, F. (1979) *Yearning for yesterday: A sociology of nostalgia*. New York: Free Press.

Emmons, R. A., & McCullough, M. E. (2003) Counting blessings versus burdens: An experimental investigation of gratitude and subjective well-being in daily life. *Journal of Personality and Social Psychology*, *84*,377–389.

Feeney, B. C. (2006) An attachment theory perspective on the interplay between intrapersonal and interpersonal processes. In K. D. Vohs & E. J. Finkel (Eds.), *Self and relationships: Connecting intrapersonal and interpersonal processes* (pp. 133–159). New York, NY: Guilford.

Festinger, L., Schachter, S., & Back, K. (1950) *Social pressures in informal groups: A study of a housing community*. Palo Alto, CA: Stanford University Press.

Folkman, S., & Moskowitz, J. T. (2000) Positive affect and the other side of coping. *American Psychologist*, *55*, 647–654.

Fraley, R. C., & Shaver, P. R. (2000) Adult romantic attachment: Theoretical developments, emerging controversies, and unanswered questions. *Review of General Psychology*, *4*, 132–154.

Fraley, R. C., Waller, N. G., & Brennan, K. A. (2000) An item response theory analysis of self-report measures of adult attachment. *Journal of Personality and Social Psychology*, *78*, 350–365.

Fredrickson, B. L. (2001) The role of positive emotions in positive psychology: The broaden-and-build theory of positive emotions. *American Psychologist*, *56*, 218–226.

Fredrickson, B. L., & Levenson, R. W. (1998) Positive emotions speed recovery from the cardiovascular sequelae of negative emotions. *Cognition and Emotion*, *12*, 191–220.

Garmezy, N. (1991) Resilience and vulnerability to adverse developmental outcomes associated with poverty. *American Behavioral Scientist*, *34*, 416–430.

Gilovich, T., & Medvec, V. H. (1995) The experience of regret: What, when, and why. *Psychological Review*, *102*, 379–395.

Goodwin, R., Cook, O., & Yung, Y. (2001) Loneliness and life satisfaction among three cultural groups. *Personal Relationships*, *8*, 225–230.

Hawkley, L. C., Browne, M. W., & Cacioppo, J. T. (2005) How can I connect with thee? Let me count the ways. *Psychological Science, 16*, 798–804.

Hertz, D. G. (1990) Trauma and nostalgia: New aspects of the coping of aging holocaust survivors. *Israeli Journal of Psychiatry and Related Sciences, 27*, 189–198.

Hofer, J. (1934) Medical dissertation on nostalgia (C. K. Anspach, Trans.). *Bulletin of the History of Medicine, 2*, 376–391. (Original work published 1688.)

Holbrook, M. B. (1993) Nostalgia and consumption preferences: Some emerging patterns of consumer tastes. *Journal of Consumer Research, 20*, 245–256.

Hyde, J. S. (2003) *Half the human experience: The psychology of women*. Boston, MA: Houghton-Mifflin.

Keltner, D., & Buswell, B. N. (1996) Evidence for the distinctness of embarrassment, shame, and guilt: A study of recalled antecedents and facial expressions of emotion. *Cognition and Emotion, 10*, 155–171.

Leary, M. R., & Kowalski, R. M. (1995) *Social anxiety*. New York, NY: Guilford Press.

Leary, M. R., Springer, C., Negel, L., Ansell, E., & Evens, K. (1998) The causes, phenomenology, and consequences of hurt feelings. *Journal of Personality and Social Psychology, 74*, 1225–1237.

Levenson, R. W. (1988) Emotion and the autonomic nervous system: A prospectus for research on autonomic specificity. In H. L. Wagner (Ed.), *Social psychophysiology and emotion: Theory and clinical applications* (pp. 17–42). London: Wiley.

Maner, J. K., DeWall, C. N., Baumeister, R. F., & Schaller, M. (2007) Does social exclusion motivate interpersonal reconnection? Resolving the "porcupine problem." *Journal of Personality and Social Psychology, 92*, 42–55.

McAdams, D. P. (2001) The psychology of life stories. *Review of General Psychology, 5*, 100–122.

Mikulincer, M., & Shaver, P. R. (2003) The attachment behavioral system in adulthood: Activation, psychodynamics, and interpersonal processes. In M. P. Zanna (Ed.), *Advances in experimental social psychology* (Vol. 35, pp. 53–152). New York, NY: Academic Press.

Neff, K. (2003) The development and validation of a scale to measure self-compassion. *Self and Identity, 2*, 223–250.

Neto, F., & Barrios, J. (2001) Predictors of loneliness among adolescents from Portuguese immigrant families in Switzerland. *Social Behavior and Personality, 28*, 193–206.

Paulhus, D., Robins, R., Trzesniewski, K., & Tracy, J. (2004) Two replicable suppressor situations in personality research. *Multivariate Behavioral Research, 39*, 301–326.

Pyszczynski, T., Greenberg, J., Solomon, S., Arndt, J., & Schimel, J. (2004) Why do people need self-esteem? A theoretical and empirical review. *Psychological Bulletin, 130*, 435–468.

Rokach, A., & Bacanli, H. (2001) Perceived causes of loneliness: A cross-cultural comparison. *Social Behavior and Personality, 29*, 169–182.

Rokach, A., & Neto, F. (2000) Coping with loneliness in adolescence: A cross-cultural study. *Social Behavior and Personality, 28*, 329–342.

Routledge, C., Arndt, J., Sedikides, C., & Wildschut, T. (2008) A blast from the past: The terror management function of nostalgia. *Journal of Experimental Social Psychology, 44*, 132–140.

Russell, D. (1996) The UCLA loneliness scale (Version 3): Reliability, validity, and factor structure. *Journal of Personality Assessment, 66*, 20–40.

Sarason, B. R., Sarason, I. G., & Gurung, R. A. R. (1997) Close personal relationships and health outcomes: A key to the role of social support. In S. Duck (Ed.), Handbook of personal relationships (pp. 547–573). New York, NY: Wiley.

Sedikides, C., Wildschut, T., Arndt, J., & Routledge, C. (2008) Nostalgia: Past, present, and future. *Current Directions in Psychological Science, 17*, 304–307.

Sedikides, C., Wildschut, T., Arndt, J., & Routledge, C. D. (2006) Affect and the self. In J. P. Forgas (Ed.), *Affect in social thinking and behavior: Frontiers in social psychology* (pp. 197–215). New York, NY: Psychology Press.

Sedikides, C., Wildschut, T., & Baden, D. (2004) Nostalgia: Conceptual issues and existential functions. In J. Greenberg, S. Koole, & T. Pyszczynski (Eds.), *Handbook of experimental existential psychology* (pp. 200–214). New York, NY: Guilford Press.

Sedikides, C., Wildschut, T., Gaertner, L., Routledge, C., & Arndt, J. (2008) Nostalgia as enabler of self-continuity. *Self-continuity: Individual and collective perspectives* (pp. 227–239). New York, NY: Psychology Press.

Sedikides, C., Wildschut, T., Routledge, C., Arndt, J., & Zhou, X. (2009) Buffering acculturative stress and facilitating cultural adaptation: Nostalgias as a psychological resource. In R. S. Wyer, Jr., C.-Y. Chiu, & Y.-Y. Hong (Eds.), *Understanding culture: Theory, research and application* (pp. 351–368). New York, NY: Psychology Press.

Shams, M. (2001) Social support, loneliness and friendship preference among British Asian and non-Asian adolescents. *Social Behavior and Personality, 29*, 399–404.

Sharfe, E., & Bartholomew, K. (1994) Reliability and stability of adult attachment patterns. *Personal Relationships, 1*, 23–44.

Stephan, E., Wildschut, T., Sedikides, C., Routledge, C. R., & Arndt, J. (2008) *The magic of the past: Nostalgia inspires*. Unpublished manuscript, University of Southampton.

Tangney, J. P. (2003) Self-relevant emotions. In M. R. Leary & J. P. Tangney (Eds.), *Handbook of self and identity* (pp. 384–400). New York, NY: Guilford Press.

*The New Oxford Dictionary of English*. (1998) Oxford: Oxford University Press.

Thrash, T. M., & Elliot, A. J. (2003) Inspiration as a psychological construct. *Journal of Personality and Social Psychology, 84*, 871–889.

Tracy, J. L., & Robins, R. W. (2007) The psychological structure of pride: A tale of two facets. *Journal of Personality and Social Psychology, 92*, 506–525.

Tugade, M. M., & Fredrickson, B. L. (2004) Resilient individuals use positive emotions to bounce back from negative emotional experiences. *Journal of Personality and Social Psychology, 86*, 320–333.

Twenge, J. M., Baumeister, R. F., Tice, D. M., & Stucke, T. S. (2001) If you can't join them, beat them: Effects of social exclusion on aggressive behavior. *Journal of Personality and Social Psychology, 81*, 1058–1069.

Vallerand, R. J., Blanchard, C., Mageau, G. A., Koestner, R., Ratelle, C., Léonard, M., & Gagné, M. (2003) Les passions de l'âme: On obsessive and harmonious passion. *Journal of Personality and Social Psychology, 85*, 756–767.

Van Tilburg, M. A. L., & Vingerhoets, A. J. J. M. (Eds.). (2005) *Psychological aspects of geographical moves: Homesickness and acculturation stress* (2nd ed). Amsterdam, The Netherlands: Amsterdam University Press.

Vaughan, D. (1986) *Uncoupling*. New York, NY: Oxford University Press.

Victor, C. A., Scambler, S. J., Bowling, A., & Bond, J. (2005) The prevalence of, and risk factors for, loneliness in later life: a survey of older people in Great Britain. *Ageing & Society, 25*, 357–375.

Wagnild, G. M., & Young, H. M. (1993) Development and psychometric evaluation of the resilience scale. *Journal of Nursing Measurement, 1*, 165–178.

Watt, S. E., & Badger, A. J. (2009) Effects of social belonging on homesickness: An application of the belongingness hypothesis. *Personality and Social Psychology Bulletin, 35*, 516–530.

Wildschut, T., Sedikides, C., Arndt, J., & Routledge, C. (2006) Nostalgia: Content, triggers, functions. *Journal of Personality and Social Psychology, 91*, 975–993.

Wildschut, T., Sedikides, C., Routledge, C., Arndt, J., & Cordaro, F. (2009) *Nostalgia as a repository of social connectedness: The role of attachment-related avoidance.* Journal of Personality and Social Psychology, 98, 573–586.

Wildschut, T., Stephan, E., Sedikides, C., Routledge, C., & Arndt, J. (2008) *Feeling happy and sad at the same time: Nostalgia informs theories of affect.* Paper presented at the 9th Annual Meeting of the Society for Personality and Social Psychology, Albuquerque, NM.

Williams, K. D. (1997) Social ostracism. In R. M. Kowalski (Ed.), *Aversive interpersonal behaviors* (pp. 133–170). New York, NY: Plenum Press.

Williams, K. D., & Sommer, K. L. (1997) Social ostracism by one's coworkers: Does rejection lead to loafing or compensation? *Personality and Social Psychology Bulletin*, *23*, 693–706.

Zhou, X., Sedikides, C., Wildschut, T., & Gao, D.-G. (2008) Counteracting loneliness: On the restorative function of nostalgia. *Psychological Science*, *19*, 1023–1029.

Zimet, G. D., Dahlem, N. W., Zimet, S. G., & Farley, G. K. (1988) The multidimensional scale of perceived social support. *Journal of Personality Assessment*, *52*, 30–41.

# Chapter 6
# Perseverative Cognition, Psychopathology, and Somatic Health

**Bart Verkuil, Jos F. Brosschot, Winifred A. Gebhardt, and Julian F. Thayer**

## 6.1 General Introduction: The Perseverative Cognition Hypothesis

A long tradition of research into the effects of stressful events has demonstrated that such events can lead to mental (Hammen, 2005) as well as somatic health problems (Cohen & Williamson, 1991; Rozanski, Blumenthal, & Kaplan, 1999). It has also been well documented that the way people perceive and appraise events codetermines whether a situation or event is experienced as stressful and that stressful appraisals, in turn, initiate and activate the physiological stress reaction (Lazarus, 1991). Thus, "stress" can make us sick and that is in part due to what we think about stressful events. Yet, stress researchers have confined their attention mainly to what we think *during* these events and how that leads to enhanced physiological stress reactions *during* a stressful situation. Little attention has been paid to how these thoughts, when they persevere after (or before, in anticipation of) stressful events, can prolong the stress response. As we will argue in this chapter, it is the prolongation of stress responses, and not so much acute stress responses that forms a crucial link between stressors and later mental (McEwen, 2003; Thayer & Lane, 2000) and somatic problems (Selye, 1951; Ursin & Eriksen, 2004; Linden, Earle, Gerin, & Christenfeld, 1997; Brosschot, Pieper, & Thayer, 2005; Brosschot, Gerin, & Thayer, 2006). As yet, scientists have hardly addressed the important issue of *when*, *how often*, and *how long* we think about stressful events and how "perseverative thinking" about stressors might prolong the stress response. In psychopathology research though, during the past decade perseverative cognitive processes have received increasing attention, and have been recognized as core etiological factors in the maintenance of several mental disorders, such as mood and anxiety disorders. We have recently hypothesized perseverative cognition (PC) as the mediator of the effects of stressors on not only mental but also somatic

B. Verkuil (✉)
Leiden University, Institute of Psychology, Clinical, Health and Neuropsychology Unit, P.O. Box 9555, 2300 RB Leiden, Netherlands
e-mail: bverkuil@fsw.leidenuniv.nl

I. Nyklíček et al. (eds.), *Emotion Regulation and Well-Being*,
DOI 10.1007/978-1-4419-6953-8_6, © Springer Science+Business Media, LLC 2011

illness, because it prolongs not only psychological but also physiological responses to stressors. Brosschot et al. (2006) have stated that stress can only lead to disease when physiological stress responses are prolonged by PC. PC refers to mental representations of the stressful events, such as worrisome anticipation before or ruminative thinking after the stressful events. Just as stressful cognitions during stressful events shape the concomitant physiological and emotional stress reaction, perseveration of these representations is hypothesized to prolong this physiological and emotional activity, thereby adding to the total time that stressors can have an impact on our mental and somatic well-being. This focus on the temporal aspects of the stress response beyond the presence of stressful events, we suggest, is important for a better understanding of how "stress" affects our health.

In this chapter, we will review recent evidence for the PC hypothesis, including its effects on mental as well as somatic health. Furthermore, we will argue that PC is in fact the default response to stressful situations, a response which is successfully inhibited by most healthy people. We will illustrate how goal directed cognition can lead to pathological PC as seen in mood and anxiety disorders. But first, the concept of PC itself will be introduced.

## 6.2 The Concept of Perseverative Cognition

PC is defined as "the repeated or chronic activation of the cognitive representation of one or more psychological stressors" (Brosschot et al., 2006). A stressor is defined as a situation involving potential harm, without or with low perceived control, that is, a *threat* to the psychobiological integrity of oneself or to the attainment of one's higher order goals. The term "perseverative" implies that the pathological ingredient of mentally representing stressors is their *perseveration*, that is, the *duration of exposure* of the organism to the (cognitive representation of) the stressor (threat). As mentioned above, we suggest that the duration of the stress response is its toxic element, for mental as well as for somatic health. Only persistent emotional or physiological responses can lead to problems in either mental or somatic health.

The term PC encompasses concepts involving conscious perseverative thinking that have been studied traditionally within the context of psychopathology, such as worry (anxious thoughts about the future) and depressive rumination (sad thoughts about ones current mood). The definition of PC as a "cognitive representation of psychological stressors" also allows for the inclusions of prolonged *automatic* or unconscious processing of stressor related information, as reflected in for example attentional hypervigilance or enhanced memory retrieval of stress related information (e.g., Rothermund, 2003). The PC hypothesis is therefore not strictly limited to conscious thinking about stressors, but also accommodates automatic, or unconscious, stress related cognition, that may have substantial health relevant effects. Since the greater part of any cognitive processing appears to operate without awareness (Bargh & Ferguson, 2000), a considerable part of PC is likely to be unconscious as well. Even minor stressful events cause people to persistently scan the environment for threat and this attentional hypervigilance is only possible when a mental representation, or "cognition" concerning threat is still present (Wells & Matthews, 1996). This very basic representation of threat is fundamental for survival, and it occurs automatically and without conscious awareness (LeDoux, 2000).

## 6.3 Perseverative Cognition, Psychopathology and Somatic Health Problems

Below we provide an overview of the mental and somatic problems that have been associated with PC.

### *6.3.1 Psychopathology*

Research into the mental health effects of worry started in the early 1980s with the finding that frequent nighttime worrying is a predictor of the onset and maintenance of insomnia (Borkovec, 1982). Nowadays, perseverative thoughts like worry and rumination are recognized as fundamental characteristics of several psychopathological conditions (Watkins, 2008). For example, worry is a central feature of generalized anxiety disorder (GAD; Borkovec, Ray, & Stöber, 1998; Wells & Matthews, 1996) and depressive rumination is recognized as a central feature of depression (Nolen-Hoeksema, 1991). Moreover, PC is found in hypochondriasis (Looper & Kirmayer, 2001), social phobia (Abbott & Rapee, 2004), and post traumatic stress disorder (Holeva, Tarrier, & Wells, 2001).

PC is not just a symptom or epiphenomenon of these pathological conditions. Experimental studies show that PC is causally related to negative mood. In addition, in prospective studies it has been observed that perseverative thoughts predict the onset and maintenance of anxious and depressed mood (for a review see Watkins, 2008). Yet, it is unclear at what levels of intensity, that is, at which frequency and duration, PC can be regarded as pathological.

Automatic, unconscious or other "low-level" threat related cognitive processes have been associated with mental health in a plethora of studies during the past 30 years (Williams, Watts, MacLeod, & Mathews, 1997; Mineka, 1992). Attentional hypervigilance, for example operationalized as selective attention for threatening stimuli, as well as memory biases, for example operationalized as enhanced memory for threatening stimuli, have been amply documented to play a role in mental health problems. Yet, very few of these studies have actually sought evidence that these forms of PC preceded or caused the disorder. A thrilling recent development in experimental psychopathology is that researchers are now attempting to address these automatic processes in order to develop new therapeutic tools. Evidence is now growing that reversing cognitive biases by "attentional retraining" procedures can reduce symptoms of mood and anxiety disorders.

This suggests that these biases may have a causal role in the onset and maintenance of such disorders (MacLeod, Rutherford, Campbell, Ebsworthy, & Holker, 2002; Hazen, Vasey, & Schmidt, 2009; Wilson, MacLeod, Mathews, & Rutherford, 2006).

### *6.3.2 Somatic Health*

Importantly, for *somatic* outcomes, the PC hypothesis is not restricted to *pathological* worry. It is likely that somatic problems can be caused by much less intense levels of worry, if only maintained long enough. One of the earliest findings suggesting that PC plays an important role in the link between stress and somatic disease was that among elderly men who had a myocardial infarction, those who frequently worried were at heightened risk for experiencing a second myocardial infarction (Kubzansky et al., 1997). In addition, it has been observed that during experimentally induced worry as well as during worry in daily life cardiovascular activity is increased (Lyonfields, Borkovec, & Thayer, 1995; Thayer, Friedman, & Borkovec, 1996; Verkuil, Brosschot, Borkovec, & Thayer, 2009; Pieper, Brosschot, Van der Leeden, & Thayer, 2007). Furthermore, a recent review concluded that PC is associated with enhanced activation in endocrine and immune systems (see Brosschot et al., 2006). Finally, more recently worry appeared to be associated with lowered levels of antibody titers in caregivers (Segerstrom et al., 2008) and ruminating after emotional events has been linked to enhanced levels of cortisol, in daily life (McCullough, Orsulak, Brandon, & Akers, 2007), as well as in the laboratory (Zoccola, Dickerson, & Zaldivar, 2008).

These findings are in line with the PC hypothesis (Brosschot et al., 2006), stating that PC prolongs physiological activity which, in turn, leads to a pathogenic state in which one is more vulnerable to developing a somatic disease. However, the discussed studies have mainly focused on physiological activity, and not so much on disease outcomes. Few studies have suggested that PC can indeed lead to somatic disease. Recently, a study by Holman et al. (2008) showed that in US citizens suffering from acute stress after the 9/11 attacks, ongoing worries about terrorism predicted cardiovascular health problems up to 3 years after the attacks. More indirect evidence for the impact of PC on somatic disease is provided by the fact that risk for cardiovascular problems is heightened in people suffering from anxiety disorders and depression (e.g., Wulsin, Vaillant, & Wells, 1999), which are characterized by high PC. In addition, studies focusing on work stress have found that experiencing problems in recovering or "unwinding" after work is predictive of cardiovascular mortality (Van Amelsvoort, Kant, Bultmann, & Swaen, 2003; Kivimaki et al., 2006). Furthermore, at least two studies among patients suffering from somatic health problems have suggested that PC might be an important mediator of the effects of some somatic treatments. In one study it was found that in patients awaiting surgery for their hernia, greater worry about the surgery predicted lower levels of immune cells at the wound site, greater pain, poorer self-rated recovery and a longer recovery time (Broadbent, Petrie, Alley, & Booth, 2003). Furthermore, heightened levels of trait worry in psoriasis patients were predictive of a slowed recovery from photochemotherapy (Fortune et al., 2003). Still more evidence is needed to test the PC hypothesis with respect to disease outcomes. An important venture for future research is to conduct more prospective studies examining whether PC is indeed the pathogenic link between stressful events and the onset and maintenance of somatic disease.

It is a highly exciting notion that automatic or unconscious PC can cause prolonged stress related physiological activity, and in the long term even somatic disease. To date, the possibility that automatic vigilance or other forms of unconscious PC have physiological effects has hardly been investigated. Some exceptions are studies showing relatively subtle effects of subliminal emotional stimulation on brain activity (Morris, Öhman, & Dolan, 1999), startle reflex (Ruiz-Padial & Vila, 2007) and skin conductance (Öhman & Mineka, 2001). Moreover, two of our own recent studies have yielded some indirect evidence for the somatic effects of unconscious PC. Firstly, in an ambulatory study we found – quite unexpectedly – that worry episodes were not only associated with enhanced heart activity, but that the worry episodes *themselves* also had prolonged cardiac effects, until up to 2h *after* the worry episode had ended (Pieper et al., 2007). This effect was independent of ongoing worry, emotions, health behaviors and physical activity, and therefore we concluded that it must have been due to some unconscious, or at least not verbally reportable form of worry. Secondly, in another ambulatory study we found that conscious daytime worrying predicted heightened heart rate during the subsequent night (Brosschot, Van Dijk, & Thayer, 2007). During sleep people obviously do not worry consciously, but the hypervigilance that is evoked by stressful events might be prolonged into the night. Although a lot has to be discovered on what exactly happens cognitively during sleep, studies with rats and humans have shown that daytime neuronal activity seems to be repeated or "replayed" just before or during sleep (Skaggs & McNaughton, 1996; Stickgold, Malia, Maguire, Roddenberry, & O'Connor, 2000). Furthermore, sleep promotes the consolidation of memories, especially negative ones (Walker & Stickgold, 2004). It may, therefore, be likely that daytime stressful events are mentally represented during sleep in one way or another and that this interferes with physiological recovery during sleep. It is obvious that this will prolong the total amount of physiological "wear and tear" that stressful events have on the human body, since sleep covers about one third of our lives. Future studies are warranted to investigate to what extent and how stressful events and hypervigilance influence physiological activity during sleep.

### *6.3.3 Subjective Somatic Health*

Ambulatory studies by our group have shown that in several nonclinical populations (students, high school teachers) nonclinical levels of worry were positively and prospectively associated with subjective health complaints like fatigue, headache and lower back pain (Brosschot & Van Der Doef, 2006). A simple worry intervention, consisting of postponing worry to a daily 30-min worry period, reduced the duration of worry episodes, which, in turn, predicted the reduction of health complaints. The effects of the intervention were not restricted to certain types of complaints, but pertained to a range of different complaints (e.g., cough, palpitations, neck pain). Further evidence for the effects of PC on subjective health comes from another ambulatory study. In this study, it was found that people who ruminated a lot about conflicting goals reported heightened levels of somatic complaints (Emmons & King, 1988).

Health worry or illness worry, that is, PC concerning health problems, seems to be important for the occurrence of somatic health complaints. Somatic health problems – often severe stressors themselves – usually give rise to worries. For example, chronic pain patients have been found to worry about pain for 20min/day on average, compared to 17min for non-pain related topics (Eccleston, Crombez, Aldrich, & Stannard, 2001). Next to having physiological effects just as other types of worries, these health worries may also affect subjective somatic health through an alternative pathway: Enhanced worrisome thinking about somatic signals might promote complaining about them. Indeed, health worry and the related construct of catastrophizing predict the occurrence of health complaints (Kaptein et al., 2005; Petrie et al., 2005; Devoulyte & Sullivan, 2003) and are associated with increases in pain (Turner, Mancl, & Aaron, 2004). Furthermore, health worry has been associated with increased doctor consulting (Hay, Buckley, & Ostroff, 2005) and with intensive health care utilization (Looper & Kirmayer, 2001). One mechanism that may underlie these effects is that in people who worry excessively about illness bodily sensations are more likely to trigger illness related cognitive networks which promote selective attention to and misinterpretations of bodily sensations as symptoms of illness (Brosschot, 2002; Brown, 2004). In turn, such worries might lower the threshold for actually complaining about these presumed symptoms of illness. Indeed, we recently found that the association between illness related cognitive bias (increased recall of illness information) and health complaints was mediated by illness worry (Verkuil, Brosschot, & Thayer, 2007).

In short, PC, even at nonclinical levels, might influence somatic health either via prolonged activity in endocrine, immune and cardiovascular systems or, in the case of specific health worry, via enhanced processing of illness related information.

## 6.4 A Self Regulation Perspective on Perseverative Cognition

The stress response, and its prolongation via PC, can both basically be understood as the (default) response to threats to the attainment of a person's goals. The detection of potential threats to one's goals and of signs of failure in attaining these goals is a continuous process. Environmental stimuli are first quickly and briefly – and largely automatically – scanned for their threat value (i.e., "fast route, " LeDoux, 2000). Once something has been detected that could be a possible threat to one's goals, it immediately leads to a rapid and indiscriminate defensive response, even if it eventually turns out to be only a novel or ambiguous (nonthreatening) stimulus (LeDoux, 2000; Thayer & Lane, 2000). This defensive response, or motivational state, consists of changes on several levels in the organism: Cognitive changes (attentional hypervigilance and conscious PC), physiological changes (e.g., increased autonomic nervous activity and release of stress hormones) and behavioral changes (avoidance or approach behavior; Lang, 1995). The duration of the defensive response depends on how quickly the system ascertains the safety of the situation. This shutting down of the response because of safety is dependent on a more deliberate cortical processing ("slow route"; LeDoux, 2000) of the potential threat. Thus, the *default* response to any potential threat is this immediate defensive response, served by subcortical networks in the brain, which under normal circumstances is under chronic inhibitory control by the prefrontal cortex (Amat et al., 2005). From an evolutionary perspective it makes sense that this defense system initially "errs on the side of caution" by often responding initially to novel or ambiguous neutral information as if it was threatening, and subsequently either continues or stops after a more deliberate appraisal process has taken place. When no safety signals can be provided however, the stress response is prolonged. This seems to be the case in conditions such as anxiety disorders and during chronically stressful situations. There is some evidence that at least in some people, especially high worriers, that is, people suffering from GAD, this is due to a failure to recognize these safety signals. We will return to this possible explanation later in the chapter. For more information about the neurobiological underpinnings of PC the reader is referred to Thayer and Brosschot (2005) and Thayer and Lane (2000, 2007).

In the remainder of this chapter, the concept of PC will be regarded from a self-regulation perspective.

### 6.4.1 *Why People Perseverate: Perseverative Cognition as the Default Response to Potential Threat to Goal Attainment*

The essence of PC is to keep attention directed towards one's goals, to anticipate threats to goal attainment and, in the case of rumination, to protect oneself from the recurrence of mistakes made in the past (for related theoretical accounts see Wells & Matthews, 1996; Martin & Tesser, 1996). It has been consistently shown that intensive engagement in the pursuit of a goal has effects on information processing (Johnson, Chang, & Lord, 2006). Goal engagement leads to alterations in pre-attentive processes and the content of thoughts and dreams, and it enhances the perception and processing of goal related stimuli (Klinger, 1975).

In terms of self-regulation, a psychological stress response arises when people experience a discrepancy between an expected state and the actual state that they are in (Ursin & Eriksen, 2004). Expected states can either be desired states in the present ("standards, " such as being healthy or having enough money to buy food) as well as desired states that lie in the future ("goals, " such as becoming a successful employee, Boldero & Francis, 2002). In daily life, one's actual state is continuously monitored, occurring mostly automatically, and compared to these desired states, or, reference values. People can be confronted with discrepancies between one's current state and one's standards or between one's current state and the desired speed with which one is making progress towards one's goals. Information concerning these discrepancies then tends to stay activated in the brain, whereas when goals are attained information about goal discrepancies is inhibited. Again, this suggests that the default response to perceiving a goal discrepancy is cognitive *perseveration*, in the sense that this response is simply maintained as long as the discrepancy is present. This was first shown by Zeigarnik more than 80 years ago, who showed that memory for interrupted tasks is better than for completed tasks (Zeigarnik, 1927). Perseveration of goal directed cognition has been found in several other studies (Marsh, Hicks, & Bink, 1998; Goschke & Kuhl, 1993; Rothermund, 2003; Koole, Smeets, Van Knippenberg, & Dijksterhuis, 1999). For example, Rothermund (2003) found that failure on a cognitive task was associated with slowed responses in a dual tasking experiment when participants were presented with failure related words, indicative of hypervigilance after failure. In line with these findings on hypervigilance, conscious PC has also been found to be associated with experiencing discrepancy, for example, between one's actual self and one's ideal self (Roelofs et al., 2007; Jones, Papadakis, Hogan, & Strauman, 2009).

Most studies have taken place in laboratory settings and have measured this perseveration of stressor related cognition immediately after the goal frustration (e.g., Rothermund, 2003) or after a brief period (e.g., 6min; Koole et al., 1999). Thus, it remains to be established how long this initial perseveration of stressor related cognition lasts.

### *6.4.2 Psychological Moderators of Perseverative Cognition Duration*

In the next sections we will discuss how PC can get enhanced, thereby foremost discussing studies that have been conducted with chronic (trait) worriers, that is, people suffering from GAD.

#### 6.4.2.1 Goal Commitment

Most anxiety and mood disorders are characterized by extreme hypervigilance and perseverative thinking. What determines difficulties to stop perseverating, or – to the same end – stimulates its continuation, to the extent that it starts to have health consequences?

The initial duration of PC after one has encountered a threat to goal attainment depends on how strong one is committed to attaining the goal, which differs between individuals and between situations. According to several authors (Shah & Higgins, 1997;

Feather, 1963) the strength of goal commitment is a function of the interaction between (a) the importance or value that people attach to their goals and (b) the expectancy that one can either cope or not cope with the goal discrepancy and is either still able to attain the goal or not any more: both expectancies appear to influence PC. Here, we will review evidence that shows that high trait worriers are likely to be more committed to their goals when confronted with threats to attainment.

Several studies have found that the duration of hypervigilance is a function of *higher level goals*. For example, Koole et al. (1999) showed that hypervigilance persisted longer after failure on a task when people thought that completing this task successfully was very important for one of their higher order goals, for example, obtaining a good job later in life. In contrast, when people had the opportunity to scale down the importance of this task by focusing on other goals hypervigilance was reduced. In addition, several other studies have shown that goal commitment (Gebhardt, Van der Doef, Massey, Verhoeven, & Verkuil, 2010), the tendency to link the (non) attainment of lower level goals to the (non)attainment of higher level goals (Mcintosh, Harlow, & Martin, 1995), spending much energy in the pursuit of one single goal (Magee, MacLeod, Tata, & Regan, 2003) and perfectionism, are all associated with high levels of rumination.

A second important factor that influences the initial duration of goal directed cognition is the expectancy of the outcome of the stressful event, or goal discrepancy. As PC is the default response to stress, it will arise when people hold negative or no outcome expectancies. Indeed, worry was found to be associated with doubts concerning ones problem-solving skills and the tendency to be pessimistic about the outcome (Robichaud & Dugas, 2005). Likewise, people with low self-esteem are more prone to ruminate (Wood & Dodgson, 1996).

#### 6.4.2.2 Reinforcement of Perseverative Cognition: Coping

Although people who frequently worry or ruminate might lack confidence in general coping skills, they paradoxically report to be very motivated to use PC as a strategy to cope with goal discrepancies. For example, Szábo and Lovibond (2002) asked students to keep a log of their worries for a week and they found that almost 50% of the reported worries consisted of problem solving attempts. Furthermore, cross-sectional studies have shown that people who frequently worry think that "worrying helps solving problems" (Roelofs et al., 2007; Papageorgiou & Wells, 2001). In addition, high trait worriers report that worry serves as a distraction from more emotionally laden topics (Borkovec & Roemer, 1995), suggesting that in some people worry might serve to cognitively avoid intense negative emotions. Both the motivated use of PC as a problem solving strategy and the use of PC as a cognitive avoidance strategy have been proposed to be reinforcing PC.

Despite many worriers' beliefs that worrying is helpful in solving one's problems, research has shown that worry and rumination are ineffective strategies to cope with stressful situations, yielding only more PC as a result. First, worry and rumination are characterized by an abstract way of thinking about problems, and "abstract models are unlikely to lead to concrete actions" (cited from Borkovec et al., 1998, p. 566). For example, in the case of rumination, Watkins and Baracaia (2002) found that depressed patients who were led to ask themselves abstract, ruminative problem solving questions (e.g., "why do I feel this way?") in a problem solving task came up with less relevant solutions than depressed patients who were led to ask themselves concrete, process focused questions (e.g., "how am I deciding what to do next?"). Second, even if worrying leads to concrete solutions, high trait worriers are not highly likely to come into action and implement their solutions. High trait worriers, compared to low trait worriers, have less confidence in their problem solving skills (Davey, 1994), have elevated needs for evidence that a given solution will work (Tallis, Eysenck, & Mathews, 1991) and try to come up with as many solutions as possible before trying out these solutions (Startup & Davey, 2003; Davey, 2006). Behaviorally implementing a solution is also difficult when the problems that people are worrying about have already happened or might happen in the future.

In sum, although worry itself might be appraised by the individual as helpful, negative outcome expectancies will likely persist as no concrete action will be taken to reduce or remove the current or future threat. This will lead to a vicious cycle in which threatening events are coped with by worrying. Furthermore, although the discussed studies have mainly focused on the outcome expectancies associated with *conscious* PC, unconscious PC (threat related hypervigilance or cognitive bias) is suggested to be part of a worrisome coping style (Wells & Matthews, 1996) and is likely to be subject to the same reinforcing factors.

Another way in which PC is reinforced has been forwarded by Borkovec et al. (1998). In studies with nonclinical as well as clinical populations he demonstrated that worry might be a cognitive avoidance response to threat. High trait worriers are thought to have learned to use worry as an emotion regulation strategy because worry suppresses somatic anxiety, due to the abstract verbal nature of worrying (Borkovec, Lyonfields, Wiser, & Deihl, 1993; Borkovec & Hu, 1990). Indeed, threatening thoughts yield smaller cardiovascular responses than threatening images about the same material (Vrana, Cuthbert, & Lang, 1986). Correspondingly, abstract anticipatory thoughts yield smaller increases in heart rate than concrete thoughts (Kindt, Brosschot, & Boiten, 1999). In addition, worry, in contrast to relaxation, has been associated with blunted cardiovascular responses to threatening imagery (Borkovec & Hu, 1990). Furthermore, worry is likely to bias information processing away from threatening images. Several studies have shown that verbally memorizing information impairs the retrieval of the visual memory of this material, called "verbal overshadowing" (Schooler & Engstler-School, 1990). Importantly, "verbal overshadowing" result in a reduction of the total time that people are exposed to aversive, possibly traumatic, images and this is thought to reinforce the use of worry as an emotion regulation strategy. Although this might be adaptive in the short term, persistently avoiding threatening information and its associated somatic arousal, by relying on worrisome thought, interferes with the integration and extinction of threatening material in memory (Foa & Kozak, 1986). It increases the risk that threatening information is repetitively retrieved from memory (for example, in the form of intrusive thoughts; Holmes, Brewin, & Hennessy, 2004) and warrants further use of worry.

Although most studies have focused on the avoidance function of worry, it is likely that rumination has the same function, which is also a verbal and abstract thinking style. Furthermore, it is unknown whether this avoidance function also pertains to unconscious PC, and to date it is unclear to what extent unconscious mental representations consist of verbal parts or images.

In short, there are several reasons why worrying might become associated with positive outcome expectancies, and as a result might be prolonged and difficult to unlearn (disengage from). Since worry seldom actually helps to solve problems, these positive reinforcers suggest a vicious circle leading to ever more worry.

#### 6.4.2.3 Not Recognizing Safety Signals

A third important factor that influences the duration of PC is the (in)ability to recognize novel and ambiguous stimuli as safe. As mentioned above, the default cognitive response to stressful events will cease once a safety signal is recognized that implies that no goal is currently threatened. In line with this idea, Woody and Rachman (1994, p. 745) stated that: "Safety signals de-limit the range and duration of threat and, hence, of fear. In the presence of an established safety signal the animal/person is assured of safety from threat in that place at that time. Having attained a safety signal, the person/animal can rest and reduce vigilance for a time." As mentioned earlier, high trait worriers are strongly engaged in the pursuit of their goals. They require a lot of evidence before they dare to implement a solution to try solve the problem or to disengage from it. A consequence of this might be that at least pathological worriers do not easily recognize novel and ambiguous situations as safe. Recent evidence supports this idea. GAD patients show subcortical brain activity to neutral information as if it was threatening (Hoehn-Saric, Schlund, & Wong, 2004; Nitschke et al., 2009). In addition, whereas the cardiac responses of healthy people to neutral words show habituation to the repeated presentation of these neutral words, GAD patients show no habituation to neutral words (cf. Thayer, Friedman, Borkovec, Johnsen, & Molina, 2000). Thus, high worriers seem to indiscriminately keep on responding to threatening as well as neutral stimuli, and thereby do not recognize safety signals. By not recognizing safety, the fear response and PC are therefore prolonged.

## 6.5 Conclusions

In this chapter, we have provided an overview of the role that PC plays in the onset and maintenance of stress related mental and somatic health problems. PC is a common reaction to stressful events in everyday life, and it can account for stress related physiological activity that is prolonged beyond the presence of actual real life stressors. This prolonged physiological activity is proposed to be the missing link in the relationship between psychosocial factors and the chronic pathogenic state in which one is more prone to develop mental and somatic problems. Furthermore, we have discussed that PC forms part of the default response to threat, novelty and ambiguity, which basically is an adaptive self-regulatory response. We also outlined which psychological factors enhance this default response: excessive commitment to one's goals, the motivated but exaggerated use of PC as a strategy to cope with possible threats to goal attainment and the inability to recognize signals of safety. These factors were forwarded as pathogenic psychological processes that lead to a vicious cycle where one worry episode enhances the likelihood of the occurrence of another episode. This increases the total amount of time that stressful events have a prolonged "wear and tear" effect on the human body.

Although the pivotal (causal) role of unconscious PC in psychopathology has been acknowledged for a long time, its effects on somatic health have remained largely unexplored. However, while evidence is accumulating, numerous studies have already supported the PC hypothesis. We have speculated on a role of unconscious PC that may be as important as that of conscious PC. By focusing on conscious PC alone we may have been only touching the tip of the iceberg of stress related causes of mental and somatic problems.

**Acknowledgment** This writing of this chapter was financially supported by grants from The Ohio State University, Department of Psychology.

## References

Abbott, M. J., & Rapee, R. M. (2004) Post-event rumination and negative self-appraisal in social phobia before and after treatment. *Journal of Abnormal Psychology*, *113*, 136–144.

Amat, J., Baratta, M. V., Paul, E., Bland, S. T., Watkins, L. R., & Maier, S. F. (2005) Medial prefrontal cortex determines how stressor controllability affects behavior and dorsal raphe nucleus. *Nature Neuroscience*, *8*, 365–371.

Bargh, J. A., & Ferguson, M. J. (2000) Beyond behaviorism: On the automaticity of higher mental processes. *Psychological Bulletin*, *126*, 925–945.

Boldero, J., & Francis, J. (2002) Goals, standards, and the self: Reference values serving different functions. *Personality and Social Psychology Review*, *6*, 232.

Borkovec, T. (1982) Insomnia. *Journal of Consulting and Clinical Psychology*, *50*, 880–896.

Borkovec, T. D., & Hu, S. (1990) The effect of worry on cardiovascular response to phobic imagery. *Behaviour Research and Therapy*, *28*, 69–73.

Borkovec, T. D., Lyonfields, J. D., Wiser, S. L., & Deihl, L. (1993) The role of worrisome thinking in the suppression of cardiovascular response to phobic imagery. *Behaviour Research and Therapy*, *31*, 321–324.

Borkovec, T. D., Ray, W. J., & Stöber, J. (1998) Worry: A cognitive phenomenon intimately linked to affective, physiological, and interpersonal behavioral processes. *Cognitive Therapy and Research*, *22*, 561–576.

Borkovec, T. D., & Roemer, L. (1995) Perceived functions of worry among generalized anxiety disorder subjects: Distraction from more emotionally distressing topics? *Journal of Behavior Therapy and Experimental Psychiatry*, *26*, 25–30.

Broadbent, E., Petrie, K. J., Alley, P. G., & Booth, R. J. (2003) Psychological stress impairs early wound repair following surgery. *Psychosomatic Medicine*, *65*, 865–869.

Brosschot, J. F. (2002) Cognitive-emotional sensitization and somatic health complaints. *Scandinavian Journal of Psychology*, *43*, 113–121.

Brosschot, J. F., Gerin, W., & Thayer, J. F. (2006) The perseverative cognition hypothesis: A review of worry, prolonged stress-related physiological activation, and health. *Journal of Psychosomatic Research*, *60*, 113–124.

Brosschot, J. F., Pieper, S., & Thayer, J. F. (2005) Expanding stress theory: prolonged activation and PC. *Psychoneuroendocrinology*, *30*, 1043–1049.

Brosschot, J. F., & Van Der Doef, M. (2006) Daily worrying and somatic health complaints: Testing the effectiveness of a simple worry reduction intervention. *Psychology and Health*, *21*, 19–31.

Brosschot, J. F., Van Dijk, E., & Thayer, J. F. (2007) Daily worry is related to low heart rate variability during waking and the subsequent nocturnal sleep period. *International Journal of Psychophysiology*, *63*, 39–47.

Brown, R. J. (2004) Psychological mechanisms of medically unexplained symptoms: An integrative conceptual model. *Psychological Bulletin*, *130*, 793–812.

Cohen, S., & Williamson, G. M. (1991) Stress and infectious disease in humans. *Psychological Bulletin*, *109*, 5–24.

Davey, G. C. L. (1994) Worrying, social problem-solving abilities, and social problem-solving confidence. *Behaviour Research and Therapy*, *32*, 327–330.

Davey, G. C. L. (2006) A mood-as-input account of perseverative worrying. In G. C. L. Davey & A. Wells (Eds.), *Worry and its psychological disorders: Theory, assessment and treatment* (pp. 217–237). Chicester: Wiley.

Devoulyte, K. B. A., & Sullivan, M. J. L. P. (2003) Pain catastrophizing and symptom severity during upper respiratory tract illness. *Clinical Journal of Pain*, *19*, 125–133.

Eccleston, C., Crombez, G., Aldrich, S., & Stannard, C. (2001) Worry and chronic pain patients: A description and analysis of individual differences. *European Journal of Pain*, *5*, 309–318.

Emmons, R. A., & King, L. A. (1988) Conflict among personal strivings: Immediate and long-term implications for psychological and physical well-being. *Journal of Personality and Social Psychology*, *54*, 1040–1048.

Feather, N. T. (1963) Mowrer's revised two-factor theory and the motive-expectancy-value model. *Psychological Review*, *70*, 500.

Foa, E. B., & Kozak, M. J. (1986) Emotional processing of fear: Exposure to corrective information. *Psychological Bulletin*, *99*, 20–35.

Fortune, D. G., Richards, H. L., Kirby, B., McElhone, K., Markham, T., Rogers, S., et al. (2003) Psychological distress impairs clearance of psoriasis in patients treated with photochemotherapy. *Archives of Dermatology*, *139*, 752–756.

Gebhardt, W. A., Van Der Doef, M., Massey, E. K., Verhoeven, C., & Verkuil, B. (2010) Goal commitment to finding a partner and satisfaction with life among female singles: The mediating role of rumination. *Journal of Health Psychology*, *15*, 122–130.

Goschke, T., & Kuhl, J. (1993) Representation of intentions: Persisting activation in memory. *Journal of Experimental Psychology: Learning, Memory, & Cognition*, *19*, 1211–1226.

Hammen, C. (2005) Stress and depression. *Annual Review of Clinical Psychology*, *1*, 293.

Hay, J. L., Buckley, T. R., & Ostroff, J. S. (2005) The role of cancer worry in cancer screening: A theoretical and empirical review of the literature. *Psycho-Oncology*, *14*, 517–534.

Hazen, R. A., Vasey, M. W., & Schmidt, N. B. (2009) Attentional retraining: A randomized clinical trial for pathological worry. *Journal of Psychiatric Research*, *43*, 627–633.

Hoehn-Saric, R., Schlund, M. W., & Wong, S. H. Y. (2004) Effects of citalopram on worry and brain activation in patients with generalized anxiety disorder. *Psychiatry Research: Neuroimaging*, *131*, 11–21.

Holeva, V., Tarrier, N., & Wells, A. (2001) Prevalence and predictors of acute stress disorder and PTSD following road traffic accidents: Thought control strategies and social support. *Behavior Therapy*, *32*, 65–83.

Holman, E. A., Silver, R. C., Poulin, M., Andersen, J., Gil-Rivas, V., & McIntosh, D. N. (2008) Terrorism, acute stress, and cardiovascular health: A 3-year national study following the September 11th attacks. *Archives of General Psychiatry*, *65*, 73.

Holmes, E. A., Brewin, C. R., & Hennessy, R. G. (2004) Trauma films, information processing, and intrusive memory development. *Journal of Experimental Psychology: General*, *133*, 3–22.

Johnson, R. E., Chang, C. H., & Lord, R. G. (2006) Moving from cognition to behavior: What the research says. *Psychological Bulletin*, *132*, 381–415.

Jones, N. P., Papadakis, A. A., Hogan, C. M., & Strauman, T. J. (2009) Over and over again: Rumination, reflection, and promotion goal failure and their interactive effects on depressive symptoms. *Behaviour Research and Therapy*, *47*, 254–259.

Kaptein, A. A., Helder, D. I., Kleijn, W. C., Rief, W., Moss-Morris, R., & Petrie, K. J. (2005) Modern health worries in medical students. *Journal of Psychosomatic Research*, *58*, 453–457.

Kindt, M., Brosschot, J. F., & Boiten, F. (1999) High-level cognition in phobics: Abstract anticipatory memory is associated with the attenuation of physiological reactivity to threat. *Journal of Anxiety Disorders*, *10*, 473–489.

Kivimaki, M., Leino-Arjas, P., Kaila-Kangas, L., Luukkonen, R., Vahtera, J., Elovainio, M., et al. (2006) Is incomplete recovery from work a risk marker of cardiovascular death? Prospective evidence from industrial employees. *Psychosomatic Medicine*, *68*, 402–407.

Klinger, E. (1975) Consequences of commitment to and disengagement from incentives. *Psychological Review*, *82*, 1–25.

Koole, S. L., Smeets, K., Van Knippenberg, A., & Dijksterhuis, A. (1999) The cessation of rumination through self-affirmation. *Journal of Personality and Social Psychology*, *77*, 111–125.

Kubzansky, L. D., Kawachi, I., Spiro, A., III, Weiss, S. T., Vokonas, P. S., & Sparrow, D. (1997) Is worrying bad for your heart?: A prospective study of worry and coronary heart disease in the normative aging study. *Circulation*, *95*, 818–824.

Lang, P. J. (1995) The emotion probe: Studies of motivation and attention. *American Psychologist*, *50*, 372–385.

Lazarus, R. S. (1991) Progress on a cognitive-motivational-relational theory of emotion. *American Psychologist*, *46*, 819–834.

LeDoux, J. E. (2000) Emotion circuits in the brain. *Annual Review of Neuroscience*, *23*, 155–184.

Linden, W., Earle, T. L., Gerin, W., & Christenfeld, N. (1997) Physiological stress reactivity and recovery: Conceptual siblings separated at birth? *Journal of Psychosomatic Research*, *42*, 117–135.

Looper, K. J., & Kirmayer, L. J. (2001) Hypochondriacal concerns in a community population. *Psychological Medicine*, *31*, 577–584.

Lyonfields, J. D., Borkovec, T. D., & Thayer, J. F. (1995) Vagal tone in generalized anxiety disorder and the effects of aversive imagery and worrisome thinking. *Behavior Therapy*, *26*, 457–466.

MacLeod, C., Rutherford, E., Campbell, L., Ebsworthy, G., & Holker, L. (2002) Selective attention and emotional vulnerability: Assessing the causal basis of their association through the experimental manipulation of attentional bias. *Journal of Abnormal Psychology*, *111*, 107–123.

Magee, P. L., MacLeod, A. K., Tata, P., & Regan, L. (2003) Psychological distress in recurrent miscarriage: The role of prospective thinking and role and goal investment. *Journal of Reproductive and Infant Psychology*, *21*, 35–47.

Marsh, R. L., Hicks, J. L., & Bink, M. L. (1998) Activation of completed, uncompleted, and partially completed intentions. *Journal of Experimental Psychology: Learning, Memory, & Cognition*, *24*, 350–361.

Martin, L. L., & Tesser, A. (1996) Some ruminative thoughts. In R. S. Wyer (Ed.), *Ruminative thoughts: Advances in social cognition*, Volume IX (pp. 1–47). Hillsdale, NJ: Lawrence Erlbaum Associates.

McCullough, M. E., Orsulak, P., Brandon, A., & Akers, L. (2007) Rumination, fear, and cortisol: An in vivo study of interpersonal transgressions. *Health Psychology*, *26*, 126–132.
McEwen, B. S. (2003) Mood disorders and allostatic load. *Biological Psychiatry*, *54*, 200–207.
Mcintosh, W. D., Harlow, T. F., & Martin, L. L. (1995) Linkers and nonlinkers – Goal beliefs as a moderator of the effects of everyday hassles on rumination, depression, and physical complaints. *Journal of Applied Social Psychology*, *25*, 1231–1244.
Mineka, S. (1992) Cognitive biases and the emotional disorders. *Psychological Science*, *3*, 65.
Morris, J. S., Öhman, A., & Dolan, R. J. (1999) A subcortical pathway to the right amygdala mediating "unseen" fear. *Proceedings of the National Academy of Sciences of the United States of America, 96*, 1680–1685.
Nitschke, J. B., Sarinopoulos, I., Oathes, D. J., Johnstone, T., Whalen, P. J., Davidson, R. J., et al. (2009) Anticipatory activation in the amygdala and anterior cingulate in generalized anxiety disorder and prediction of treatment response. *American Journal of Psychiatry*, *166*, 302–310.
Nolen-Hoeksema, S. (1991) Responses to depression and their effects on the duration of depressive episodes. *Journal of Abnormal Psychology*, *100*, 569–582.
Öhman, A., & Mineka, S. (2001) Fears, phobias, and preparedness: toward an evolved module of fear and fear learning. *Psychological Review*, *108*, 483–522.
Papageorgiou, C., & Wells, A. (2001) Positive beliefs about depressive rumination: Development and preliminary validation of a self-report scale. *Behavior Therapy*, *32*, 13–26.
Petrie, K. J., Broadbent, E. A., Kley, N., Moss-Morris, R., Horne, R., & Rief, W. (2005) Worries about modernity predict symptom complaints after environmental pesticide spraying. *Psychosomatic Medicine*, *67*, 778–782.
Pieper, S., Brosschot, J. F., Van der Leeden, R., & Thayer, J. F. (2007) Cardiac effects of momentary assessed worry episodes and stressful events. *Psychosomatic Medicine*, *69*, 901–909.
Robichaud, M., & Dugas, M. J. (2005) Negative problem orientation (Part II): construct validity and specificity to worry. *Behaviour Research and Therapy*, *43*, 403–412.
Roelofs, J., Papageorgiou, C., Gerber, R. D., Huibers, M., Peeters, F., & Arntz, A. (2007) On the links between self-discrepancies, rumination, metacognitions, and symptoms of depression in undergraduates. *Behaviour Research and Therapy*, *45*, 1295–1305.
Rothermund, K. (2003) Automatic vigilance for task-related information: Perseverance after failure and inhibition after success. *Memory & Cognition*, *31*, 343–352.
Rozanski, A., Blumenthal, J. A., & Kaplan, J. (1999) Impact of psychological factors on the pathogenesis of cardiovascular disease and implications for therapy. *Circulation*, *99*, 2192–2217.
Ruiz-Padial, E., & Vila, J. (2007) Fearful and sexual pictures not consciously seen modulate the startle reflex in human beings. *Biological Psychiatry*, *61*, 996–1001.
Schooler, J. W., & Engstler-School, T. Y. (1990) Verbal overshadowing of visual memories: Some things are better left unsaid. *Cognitive Psychology*, *22*, 36–71.
Segerstrom, S. C., Schipper, L. J., & Greenberg, R. N. (2008) Caregiving, repetitive thought, and immune response to vaccination in older adults. *Brain, Behavior, and Immunity*, *22*, 744–752.
Selye, H. (1951) The general-adaptation-syndrome. *Annual Review of Medicine*, *2*, 327–342.
Shah, J., & Higgins, E. T. (1997) Expectancy x value effects: Regulatory focus as determinant of magnitude and direction. *Journal of Personality & Social Psychology*, *73*, 447–458.
Skaggs, W. E., & McNaughton, B. L. (1996) Replay of neuronal firing sequences in rat hippocampus during sleep following spatial experience. *Science*, *271*, 1870–1873.
Startup, H. M., & Davey, G. C. L. (2003) Inflated responsibility and the use of stop rules for catastrophic worrying. *Behaviour Research and Therapy*, *41*, 495–503.
Stickgold, R., Malia, A., Maguire, D., Roddenberry, D., & O'Connor, M. (2000) Replaying the game: Hypnagogic images in normals and amnesics. *Science*, *290*, 350–353.
Szábo, M., & Lovibond, P. F. (2002) The cognitive content of naturally occurring worry episodes. *Cognitive Therapy and Research*, *26*, 167–177.
Tallis, F., Eysenck, M., & Mathews, A. (1991) Elevated evidence requirements and worry. *Personality and Individual Differences*, *12*, 21–27.

Thayer, J. F., & Brosschot, J. F. (2005) Psychosomatics and psychopathology: looking up and down from the brain. *Psychoneuroendocrinology, 30*, 1050–1058.
Thayer, J. F., Friedman, B. H., & Borkovec, T. D. (1996) Autonomic characteristics of generalized anxiety disorder and worry. *Biological Psychiatry, 39*, 255–266.
Thayer, J. F., Friedman, B. H., Borkovec, T. D., Johnsen, B. H., & Molina, S. (2000) Phasic heart period reactions to cued threat and nonthreat stimuli in generalized anxiety disorder. *Psychophysiology, 37*, 361.
Thayer, J. F., & Lane, R. D. (2000) A model of neurovisceral integration in emotion regulation and dysregulation. *Journal of Affective Disorders, 61*, 201–216.
Thayer, J. F., & Lane, R. D. (2007) The role of vagal function in the risk for cardiovascular disease and mortality. *Biological Psychology, 74*, 224–242.
Turner, J. A., Mancl, L., & Aaron, L. A. (2004) Pain-related catastrophizing: a daily process study. *Pain, 110*, 103–111.
Ursin, H., & Eriksen, H. R. (2004) The cognitive activation theory of stress. *Psychoneuroendocrinology, 29*, 567–592.
Van Amelsvoort, L. G. P. M., Kant, I. J., Bultmann, U., & Swaen, G. M. H. (2003) Need for recovery after work and the subsequent risk of cardiovascular disease in a working population. *Occupational and Environmental Medicine, 60*, 83–87.
Verkuil, B., Brosschot, J. F., Borkovec, T. D., & Thayer, J. F. (2009) Acute autonomic effects of experimental worry and cognitive problem solving: Why worry about worry? *International Journal of Clinical and Health Psychology, 9*, 439–453.
Verkuil, B., Brosschot, J. F., & Thayer, J. F. (2007) A sensitive body or a sensitive mind? Associations among somatic sensitization, cognitive sensitization, health worry, and subjective health complaints. *Journal of Psychosomatic Research, 63*, 673–681.
Vrana, S. R., Cuthbert, B. N., & Lang, P. J. (1986) Fear imagery and text processing. *Psychophysiology, 23*, 247–253.
Walker, M. P., & Stickgold, R. (2004) Sleep-dependent learning and memory consolidation. *Neuron, 44*, 121.
Watkins, E. R. (2008) Constructive and unconstructive repetitive thought. *Psychological Bulletin, 134*, 163–206.
Watkins, E. R., & Baracaia, S. (2002) Rumination and social problem-solving in depression. *Behaviour Research and Therapy, 40*, 1179–1189.
Wells, A., & Matthews, G. (1996) Modelling cognition in emotional disorder: The S-REF model. *Behaviour Research and Therapy, 34*, 881–888.
Williams, J. M., Watts, F. N., MacLeod, C., & Mathews, A. (1997) *Cognitive psychology and emotional disorders*. New York: Wiley.
Wilson, E. J., MacLeod, C., Mathews, A., & Rutherford, E. M. (2006) The causal role of interpretive bias in anxiety reactivity. *Journal of Abnormal Psychology, 115*, 103–111.
Wood, J. V., & Dodgson, P. G. (1996) When is self-focused attention an adaptive coping response? Rumination and overgeneralization versus compensation. In I. G. Sarason, G. R. Pierce, & B. R. Sarason (Eds.), *Cognitive interference: theories, methods, and findings* (pp. 231–259). Hillsdale, NJ: Erlbaum.
Woody, S., & Rachman, S. (1994) Generalized anxiety disorder (GAD) as an unsuccessful search for safety. *Clinical Psychology Review, 14*, 743–753.
Wulsin, L. R., Vaillant, G. E., & Wells, V. E. (1999) A systematic review of the mortality of depression. *Psychosomatic Medicine, 61*, 6–17.
Zeigarnik, B. (1927) Das Behalten erledigter und unerledigter Handlungen [The memory of completed and uncompleted actions]. *Psychologische Forschung, 9*, 1–85.
Zoccola, P. M., Dickerson, S. S., & Zaldivar, F. P. (2008) Rumination and cortisol responses to laboratory stressors. *Psychosomatic Medicine, 70*, 661–667.

# Chapter 7
# Mindfulness, Emotion Regulation, and Well-Being

**Ivan Nyklíček**

## 7.1 Mindfulness

Mindfulness is a term originally stemming from ancient Asian spiritual traditions, mainly Buddhism (Nhat Hanh, 1976), seeking liberation from human suffering. In their view, human suffering is inevitably based on human desire for things to be different than they are, creating an inner conflict between the present state and an ideal state. This conflict is constructed and maintained by the human nonaccepting and judgmental mind, separating phenomena in "good," which should be strived for and "bad," which should be avoided and fighted against. Mindfulness can be seen as a state of mind opposite to the state just described. This state can be cultivated, mainly by insight (vipassana) meditation, which is also an important aspect of the Mindfulness-Based Stress Reduction (MBSR) intervention, the most frequently applied and researched intervention aimed at stress reduction by cultivating mindfulness, which will be discussed below.

Various definitions of mindfulness have been provided, which mostly agree upon a three component definition, consisting of intention, attention, and attitude (Shapiro, Carlson, Astin, & Freedman, 2006), such as in "paying attention in a particular way: on purpose, in the present moment, and non-judgmentally" (Kabat-Zinn, 1994), and "bringing one's complete attention to the experiences occurring in the present moment, in a nonjudgmental or accepting way" (Baer, Smith, Hopkins, Krietemeyer, & Toney, 2006, p. 27). In these definitions, intention and attention are reflected by the purposeful attention in the present moment and attitude is reflected by the nonjudgmental and accepting quality. A related operational definition has been provided by a group of mindfulness researchers, stating that mindfulness is "a process of regulating attention in order to bring a quality of nonelaborative awareness to current experience and a quality of relating to one's experience within an orientation of curiosity, experiential openness, and acceptance" (Bishop et al., 2004, p. 234).

I. Nyklíček (✉)
Center of Research on Psychology in Somatic disease (CoRPS), Tilburg University,
P.O. Box 90153, 5000 LE Tilburg, Netherlands
e-mail: i.nyklicek@uvt.nl

I. Nyklíček et al. (eds.), *Emotion Regulation and Well-Being*,
DOI 10.1007/978-1-4419-6953-8_7, 

One may wonder whether it is necessary to have such an elaborate definition, making a distinction between a process and a resulting state and even more fundamentally, whether the description of certain qualities of awareness (reflecting the attitude component) is necessary. The old definition of an experienced mindfulness practitioner may do as well: "the clear and single-minded awareness of what actually happens to us and in us at the successive moments of perception" (Thera, 1972). Because this awareness is situated "at the successive moments of perception," it implies a dynamic process of following the ever-changing phenomena occurring from moment to moment. The "clear and single-minded" property implies the perception to be open, accepting and nonjudgmental, otherwise the awareness would be obscured by thoughts narrowing and evaluating or judging the perception (Chambers, Gullone, & Allen, 2009). Also, one may wonder whether the intention aspect is necessary: is it really impossible to be completely mindful, aware of the present-moment experience, without the intention to do that? Of course there is always an intention when one is *practicing* mindfulness (Shapiro et al., 2006), but that does not mean that mindfulness as a *state* of mind is not possible without this intention. Indeed, many practitioners (and "ordinary" nonmeditators alike) report on a state of mindfulness just happening to them at unpredictable moments. In my view, the aspects of intention and attitude are inherent in the practice of mindfulness, but are not necessary to describe the state of mindfulness.

## 7.2 Mindfulness and Well-Being

### *7.2.1 Theory*

From Buddhist theory, the four noble truths are about the causes of human suffering and ways to liberate oneself from this suffering. The main cause of human suffering is claimed to be the judging of phenomena as "good vs. bad," striving for reaching the "good" things, which become attached to, and avoiding the "bad" ones, which become feared, suppressed, and avoided. Not only the feared objects of the mind, but also the attached result in anxiety, as the latter is associated with the fear of losing the things one is attached to. Theoretically, nonjudgmental (and therefore nonattached) mindfulness of what is taking place in the moment resolves the resulting human stress, enhancing psychological well-being.

Modern western psychologists have elaborated on this theory (Ekman, Davidson, Ricard, & Wallace, 2005; Wallace & Shapiro, 2006). Wallace and Shapiro describe the four kinds of mental balance resulting from Buddhist meditation practice: conative, attentional, cognitive, and affective. Mindfulness, as a central component in Buddhist meditation, has been described in operational cognitive-attentional terms in order to facilitate research into the phenomenon (Bishop et al., 2004). In the broadest sense, mindfulness may be viewed with the glasses of self-determination theory, postulating three basic human psychological needs that are necessary for good mental health, these needs being competence, autonomy, and relatedness

(Ryan & Deci, 2000). The latter two factors are important in Buddhist thought as well, but not competence (Nhat Hanh, 1988). Interestingly, a couple of years later, the importance of self-esteem, of which competence is an important component, for mental health has been questioned by one of the self-determination theorists, discussing vulnerability to mental disturbances as a consequence of the preoccupation with ones self-esteem (Ryan & Brown, 2003). Although a fascinating and provoking thought, it goes beyond the frame of the present chapter.

Most theories of mindfulness do not explicitly discuss emotion regulation (ER) strategies as mechanisms by which mindfulness exerts its putatively beneficial effects (Bishop et al., 2004; Brown & Ryan, 2003). The association between mindfulness and ER is discussed below. First, empirical research on the link between mindfulness and psychological well-being is summarized.

### *7.2.2 Research*

Research on the relation between mindfulness and psychological well-being may be divided into correlational studies and intervention studies.

In several correlational studies, self-reported mindfulness, as measured by questionnaires, has been found to correlate positively with various measures of psychological well-being, and negatively with psychological symptoms of distress, including negative correlations with symptoms of general distress, anxiety, and depression (Baer, Smith, & Allen, 2004; Baer, Smith, Hopkins, Krietemeyer, & Toney, 2006; Brown & Ryan, 2003; Feldman, Hayes, Kumar, Greeson, & Laurenceau, 2007). Of course, correlational studies do not provide any insights into the issue of causality. Experimental studies, including interventions, are the only kind of studies that may provide an answer to this issue.

Most experimental research has involved studies on the effectiveness of the MBSR protocol. This intervention usually involves 8 weekly sessions of 2.5 h and a silent retreat day, during which mindfulness psychoeducation is provided, and mindfulness is practiced during various exercises, such as mindful breathing, mindful moving (from hatha yoga), and vipassana (insight) meditation. In the early days of research, the studies were mainly uncontrolled trials, showing beneficial effects on the reduction of anxiety and pain symptoms (Kabat-Zinn, 1982; Kabat-Zinn, Lipworth, & Burney, 1985). More recently, well-performed randomized controlled trials (RCTs) in various patient and non-patient population, ranging from distressed students (Jain et al., 2007) to cancer patients (Speca, Carlson, Goodey, & Angen, 2000) have shown that MBSR is able to decrease symptoms of general distress, anxiety and depression, and enhance positive mood and quality of life (Jain et al., 2007; Lengacher et al., 2009; Nyklíček & Kuijpers, 2008; Speca et al., 2000).

Factually, one still does not know if the beneficial effects are due to an actual change in mindfulness. Perhaps nonspecific effects such as social support from the group may have resulted in the beneficial effects. In two recent RCTs, it was shown that change in self-reported mindfulness statistically at least partially mediates the beneficial effects of MBSR on perceived stress and quality of life (Bränström, Kvillemo, Brandberg, & Moskowitz, 2010; Nyklíček & Kuijpers, 2008). To provide a definite answer, an RCT should be performed using a control group in which all elements of MBSR but mindfulness are present or a design with multiple measurements of both mindfulness and well-being, providing an opportunity to unravel the temporal dynamics of changes in both variables. Despite the still unresolved issue of causality, the positive association between mindfulness and psychological well-being is well-established.

## 7.3 Emotion Regulation and Well-Being

ER is defined as the process of modulating one or more aspects of an emotional experience or response (Gross, 1998). It may take place either at a conscious or unconscious level.

ER is viewed as crucial for human psychological well-being (Consedine, this volume; Tamir & Mauss, this volume). In many forms of psychopathology, ranging from affective disorders to personality disorders, a deficit in ER has been identified (Gross & Muñoz, 1995). In addition, psychological interventions, including Cognitive Behavioral Therapy (CBT) and Dialectical Behavioral Therapy (DBT) often use tools to enhance ER and have shown to be effective in reducing psychological symptoms of various kinds (Hofmann & Asmundson, 2008; Linehan, 1993).

However, empirical research regarding which forms of ER are adaptive and which forms are maladaptive has not yielded unequivocal findings. Rather, more and more, the effects of ER are viewed as a complex process, heavily depending on the context in which ER takes place (Consadine, this volume). Nevertheless, for some forms of ER that have been extensively investigated, research findings do point in a certain direction, suggesting that some ER strategies are likely to promote or decrease psychological well-being across situations.

One such ER strategy is suppression of emotion. This strategy belongs to the group of *response-focused* ER strategies and involves the deliberate inhibition of emotional expression in the case one is emotionally aroused (Gross, 1998). Obviously, this strategy is very useful in all human societies in many circumstances in order not to disrupt social interactions. However, research has shown that this strategy is associated with decreased positive emotions (Gross & Levenson, 1997), interpersonal functioning (Butler et al., 2003), and well-being (Gross & John, 2003), and increased rumination regarding negative mood (Gross & John, 2003). Rumination or worry in themselves may be seen as emotion avoidant strategies as one function of rumination may be distraction from the emotional experience itself, paradoxically exacerbating the emotional experience (Roemer et al., 2009). Finally, evidence is also available for an association of emotion suppression with enhanced sympathetic nervous system reactivity to laboratory stressors, which under some conditions might lead to cardiovascular disease (Butler et al., 2003; Mauss & Gross, 2004). This has been especially shown to be the case regarding anger control, where however both anger suppression and anger expression (aggressive behavior, including a hostile attitude) have been linked with a larger cardiovascular risk (Mauss & Gross, 2004).

Another frequently researched ER strategy is cognitive reappraisal, an *antecedent-focused* strategy, which reflects the deliberate reinterpretation of emotive stimuli in order to modify the emotional impact (Gross, 1998). In contrast to emotional suppression, cognitive reappraisal has been found to be generally related to positive effects on psychological well-being, such as increased interpersonal functioning and positive mood (Gross & John, 2003) and decreased negative affect, without any accompanying sympathetic nervous system activation (Butler et al., 2003; Ochsner et al., 2004). Physiologically, cognitive reappraisal has been associated with lower blood pressure levels (Nyklíček & Vingerhoets, 2009) and with activation of prefrontal and anterior cingulate brain structures, which are known to be involved in adaptive ER (Ochsner et al., 2004).

In sum, although empirical research into this topic is still developing, findings suggest a link between several forms of ER and psychological and physical well-being. If both mindfulness and ER have shown to be beneficial for psychological well-being, and even therapies exist combining both (Linehan, 1993), one may wonder what the nature is of the relationship between the two and how they interrelate in their association with well-being.

In the next section, first, the relationship between the two is explored, both from a theoretical perspective as well as from available evidence.

## 7.4 Mindfulness and Emotion Regulation

### *7.4.1 Theory*

#### 7.4.1.1 Emotions Are Just Emotions

From a mindfulness perspective, emotions and thoughts feeding emotions are strongly interrelated mental phenomena that do not really need to be dealt with, *because they are just that: temporary mental events*, not having a clear correspondence to external reality (Blackledge & Hayes, 2001; Ekman et al., 2005). Sometimes it is even argued that too much emphasis on ER may be harmful, because the importance of emotions is overemphasized making (a) their impact larger than necessary and (b) as a consequence making people undertake often unsuccessful attempts to regulate them. "Attempts to regulate emotions actually can be a major cause of psychopathology" (Blackledge & Hayes, 2001, p. 243). In this view, emotions per se are not the problem, but the thoughts and actions following them resulting in attempts that can be summarized as *experiential avoidance.* Because negative emotions are viewed as undesirable, attempts are made to get rid of them in one way or another, which not only often is without success, but even often increase negative emotions, because of the failure to regulate them. When emotions can be seen as just emotions, temporary mental events ("a bit of our history brought into the present by the current context," Blackledge & Hayes, 2001), and accepted fully as such, there is no need for regulation (except in the case the associated action tendency is translated into action that harms other people, such as in the case of uncontrollable anger). Instead, acceptance of the emotion experience leads to instant relaxation in the emotion, making room for living one's life: "To feel feelings as feelings, to think thoughts as thoughts, fully and without defense, and get on with the business of living" (Blackledge & Hayes, 2001).

#### 7.4.1.2 The Examples of Suppression and Reappraisal

Regarding the two mostly investigated ER strategies to date discussed above, suppression and reappraisal, what is the relationship between mindfulness and these strategies? Mindfulness is incompatible with habitual suppression of emotion, because it involves a fundamental acceptance of what is taking place, including emotions as they unfold (Chambers et al., 2009). However, we should clearly make a distinction between suppression of *experience* and suppression of *expression* to the outside world. While mindfulness is accepting any *experience*, one may choose the degree to which one expresses the emotion behaviorally, depending on the appropriateness in a given situation. Thus, mindfulness is incompatible with suppression of emotional experience, but is not per se incompatible with behavioral suppression, independent of the former. One may argue that because emotional experience and expression most often are strongly interdependent, in most instances mindfulness will be also negatively related to emotional suppression on the behavioral level. This tendency is however counteracted by the naturally soothing effect of accepting mindfulness on emotional experience, often diminishing the need to express an emotion, of which the intensity is decreasing while being mindfully accepting (Nhat Hanh, 1991). On a more fundamental level discussed above, because the volitional regulation of emotional experience is not necessary from a mindfulness perspective, these regulatory effects that do occur as a result can be viewed as natural by-products of mindfulness.

Regarding cognitive reappraisal a similar argument may be provided. From a mindfulness perspective, there is no need to reappraise the situation, it is enough to just be aware of the appraisal without paying much importance to it (Kabat-Zinn, 1990). However, in a natural way, mindfulness leads to a kind of cognitive reappraisal at the moment one becomes aware of one's appraisals, either negative or positive. At that moment, these appraisals may be seen as just thoughts, often not well corresponding with external reality. This will loosen the importance of the appraisal, which may be released completely. This process may more accurately be termed as *deappraisal* rather than reappraisal, as no new appraisal has to occur instead. However, one may become aware of the fact that difficult situations may lead not only to unpleasant feelings (which per se are not a problem as we have seen), but also to positive outcomes such as personal growth or deepening interpersonal relationships. As a consequence, *reappraisal* may also occur, but as this new appraisal also may be viewed as just another thought, even such positive reappraisals may be released, leaving room for acceptance of the present reality just as it is.

A note of importance: This acceptance does not imply a surrender of the person to the situation. Acceptance includes the entirety of the reality, including acceptance of (potentially strong) personal feelings about a given situation, which may point to a natural need for action in order to enhance harmony in the person-environment interaction. Examples of such action may vary from simple walking away from a noisy environment to seeking help when being in an abusive relationship. Nevertheless, practicing accepting mindfulness does eventually lead to becoming comfortable in a wide range of situations, as many instances of person-environment mismatch stems from negatively colored mental phenomena, e.g. thoughts reflecting a rejecting attitude (Chambers et al., 2009; Kabat-Zinn, 1990).

In sum, although mindfulness is not aimed at explicit ER, including emotion suppression and cognitive reappraisal, theoretically it counteracts emotion suppression and enhances cognitive reappraisal and especially deappraisal in a natural way.

#### 7.4.1.3 Specific Mechanisms

According to Shapiro et al. (2006), there are several mechanisms by which mindfulness may be beneficial for one's well-being. Let's examine to what extent these mechanisms involve intentional or nonintentional ER processes. A central mechanism in their thinking is labeled "reperceiving," viewed as a meta-mechanism that comprises the other, subordinate, mechanisms. Reperceiving is conceptualized as a shift in perspective in which one is "able to disidentify from the contents of consciousness" (i.e. one's thoughts) and view his or her moment-by-moment experience with greater clarity and objectivity" (p. 377). In my view this actually reflects mindfulness itself, because mindfulness involves the clear, nonjudgmental perception of what is taking place in the moment, which implies disidentification, otherwise one cannot perceive clearly and nonjudgmentally (Krishnamurti, 1987). This view is supported by a recent study in which data on the relation between mindfulness and well-being testing Shapiro et al.'s model could be explained better when the reperceiving variable was combined with the mindfulness variable into a single variable, the correlation between the two being .74-.81 (Carmody, Baer, Lykins, & Olendzki, 2009). The disidentification process is the same as the one termed "cognitive defusion" in relational frame theory (Hayes, Luoma, Bond, Masuda, & Lillis, 2006) and "detached mindfulness" in metacognitive therapy (Wells, 2000). Thus, reperceiving and mindfulness are virtually identical concepts, implying the process of disidentification or cognitive defusion. Although this process is not intentionally aimed at regulating emotions, it does by the very process of seeing thoughts and emotions as just internal phenomena that can be observed, not identified with. Cognitive defusion is a central process in Acceptance and Commitment Therapy, leading to a decrease in negative affect, because negative affect is exacerbated by cognitive fusion of the self with ones thoughts (Blackledge & Hayes, 2001; Hayes et al., 2006).

What about the subordinate mechanisms? *Self-regulation* is a result of the reperceiving process, because as a consequence of disidentification with internal mental phenomena, one will be less ruled by the automatic patterns of thoughts and emotions that usually determine our behavior. As a result, one's degrees of freedom are substantially increased and behavior options expanded. An individual will therefore more likely choose behaviors that are congruent with well-being of the organism instead of behave according to the automatic, often maladaptive patterns. One may call this mechanism also behavioral freedom. *Values clarification* involves reconsidering the values that we have identified with and that have driven our behavior in the past. As values have been automatically formed through the influence of one's family, environment, and culture (Krishnamurti, 1987), disidentification helps to reconsider them, resulting again in greater degrees of freedom, this time regarding one's personal values. Those values that are in concordance with the being one is may start to be lived according to. Although not part of the conceptual area of emotional regulation, this will obviously influence one's affective state positively. *Cognitive, emotional, and behavioral flexibility* is a derivative from reperceiving or mindfulness that actually shows a large overlap with the first (self-regulation) as it involves the enhancement of one's options regarding cognitive, emotional, and other behavior as a direct result of disidentification from one's thoughts, emotions, and other internal events. ER, either volitional regulation of expression or non-volitional regulation of experience, may be viewed as part of this mechanism. The last mechanism discussed is *exposure*. It is clear that because of the willingness to attend to all phenomena unfolding in the present moment, be it external stimuli or internal ones, one exposes oneself to these phenomena, acknowledging them just as they manifest themselves, without defense. In this way, one learns that even strong emotions are not really as threatening as they seem to be, that they are only temporary phenomena in the mind and that one can tolerate them well. Exposure is effective in combating the consequences of experiential avoidance, driven by anxiety mainly, by some viewed as the most important factor leading to psychopathology (Blackledge & Hayes, 2001). Indeed, exposure is a well-known technique used especially in phobic anxiety patients, in whom symptoms diminish largely as a direct consequence of exposure (Barlow & Craske, 2000). Exposure directly leads to the decrease of negative emotions, especially anxiety-related.

In conclusion, potentially relevant mechanisms from this model may be summarized as flexible self-regulation, values clarification, and exposure.

#### 7.4.1.4 The RICH Central Direct Effects of Mindfulness

According to Chambers et al. (2009), mindfulness implies the following crucial processes related to ER that are not mentioned as such in the model by Shapiro et al. (2006): relaxation and metacognitive insight. Other relevant processes have been mentioned by Hayes and colleagues, claiming that mindfulness indirectly facilitates ER by decreasing both maladaptive overengagement (e.g., worry, rumination) and underengagement (e.g., experiential avoidance) with emotions (Hayes, Follette, & Linehan, 2004). These processes can be expected to be interrelated and associated with cognitive re/deappraisal, as discussed above. Thus, indirectly emotions are expected to be regulated by these processes as well. However, there may

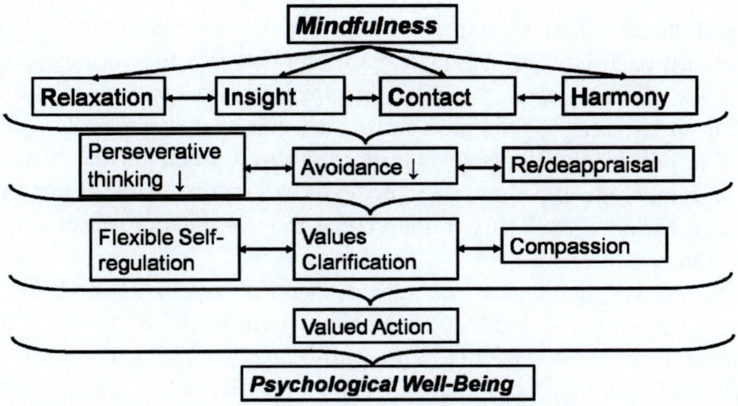


**Fig. 7.1** The RICH model of mindfulness and psychological well-being

be other important factors overlooked in the current models, reflecting central direct effects of mindfulness, which may form important intermediate paths between mindfulness and well-being. Therefore, a new model is proposed, incorporating four central direct effects of mindfulness, incorporating and expanding previous models, while simultaneously omitting redundant factors (see Fig. 7.1).

The first is Relaxation (R), a direct effect of the accepting and nonreactive attitude of mindfulness, although not always present in the first stages of mindfulness practice. Relaxation reflects relaxation of the whole body-mind system as a result of the release of (potentially disturbing) thoughts and other mental phenomena and acceptance of reality as it is (including the temporary potentially disturbing thoughts, emotions, etc.).

The second effect is Insight (I), also often not explicitly mentioned, except in the model by Chambers et al. (2009), although prominent in the original Buddhist thought (Nhat Hanh, 1988). According to Buddhist writings it is insight into the nature of phenomena (certainly including mental phenomena) which results in freedom from suffering. Insight involves insight into the various automatic mental processes, such as thoughts – including judgments – feelings, etc., and into the fact that the self is not identical to these processes (see cognitive defusion discussed above). This implies some distance between these mental processes and the awareness of them, which results in freedom of choice regarding the question to what extent it is favorable to get involved with these mental processes or just observe them passively and let them go.

The third direct effect is Contact with reality (C). Open, accepting mindfulness leads to being fully in touch with what is happening in the present moment, both internally in one's body-mind system and in the external environment. Where Insight refers to a somewhat distant perspective, as discussed above, contact implies fundamental intimacy with what is perceived. This contact leads to connectedness and compassion as discussed below. As such, this factor is strongly related to Shapiro et al.'s (2006) exposure, but explicitly including aspects of reality that are associated with neutral and positive affective states as well.

The final direct effect is Harmony (H), which involves a sense of positive resonance with what is in the moment: harmony between the various subsystems of one's body–mind system as well as between the system as a whole and the surrounding environment. This also is a direct effect of the open and accepting attitude of mindfulness. Where relaxation refers to a positive state of one's own system, harmony encompasses also the external reality. This factor, although usually not mentioned explicitly in theoretical models, is a known effect reported by meditation practitioners.

These four effects, which are interrelated, together comprise the RICH model of mindfulness' central direct effects, which are conceived as intermediate paths leading to other effects associated with well-being, which have been previously described, such as (self)compassion, behavioral flexibility, etc. (Baer, 2009; Kabat-Zinn, 1990; Shapiro et al., 2006). The model is conceived as a hierarchical model in which the higher order factors are most directly connected to mindfulness itself (most close: the direct RICH effects), while the lower order factors are more distant (most distant here: valued action). The lower order factors are under the influence of most higher-order factors of all higher levels, although one has to note that many associations are bidirectional as well. For instance, relaxation decreases rumination (a form of perseverative thinking, see below), but less rumination also enhances relaxation. Finally, psychological well-being, which in its broadest sense may be operationalized as general satisfaction with life, including low negative affect and high positive affect, is a result of all factors together.

#### 7.4.1.5 The Lower Level and Other Factors

One level below the direct RICH effects, four cognitive phenomena are present, most of which have been previously described as important factors enhancing psychological well-being and decreasing the risk of psychopathology in general.

The first is perseverative thinking, defined as repetitive maladaptive thought, including rumination and worry. Perseverative thinking is viewed as an important mechanism involved in the etiology of various psychiatric disorders such as depression (perseverative thinking usually called rumination here) and anxiety disorders (here usually called worry) (Borkovec, Ray, & Stöber, 1998; Brosschot, Pieper, & Thayer, 2005).

Experiential avoidance is also viewed as a central mechanism involved in psychopathology, as discussed above, via experiences of failure of unsuccessful attempts to avoid unpleasant aspects of life and decreased involvement in activities that are considered as having important values in life (Blackledge & Hayes, 2001; Hayes, 2004).

Cognitive appraisal has also been discussed above as an important factor in ER and well-being with cognitive reappraisal often having beneficial effects on well-being. As discussed above, mindfulness can involve both reappraisal, as one sees phenomena from a different perspective, and deappraisal: the letting go of unnecessary evaluations altogether.

One further level down, as a result of the preceding factors, notably the letting go of unnecessary and maladaptive thoughts, appraisals, and avoidance behaviors, flexible self-regulation emerges. Self-regulation here includes all forms of behavior: cognitive, emotional and overt behavior, which become less governed by automatic response patterns as developed across one's life. Another consequence is room for clarification of values that are truly important in one's life (Blackledge & Hayes, 2001; Hayes, 2004; Shapiro et al., 2006). This may lead to action enhancing living life congruent with these values. Finally, at this level, compassion, including self-compassion, emerges, as a result of all preceding factors, most notably insight into one's own and others' psychological processes, releasing judgments, and the accepting contact with what is present in the moment via a sense of connectedness with both oneself and other living beings.

Together the above factors, most directly stemming from the combination of factors described one level above, i.e. behavioral flexibility, clarification of values and (self)compassion, appropriate action follows that is congruent with one's personal values. All these factors together enhance ones psychological well-being.

One may question whether some factors should be included in the model and others excluded. One important example is acceptance. Should we consider it separately? One may argue that as a result of the multilevel nature of attention and awareness, one should. At one level, one may be judgmental about certain phenomena, either internal or external. When one is mindful, at a higher (meta) level one is acceptingly aware of this process, which will then be reducing the amount and severity of judgmental thoughts at the lower level, enhancing acceptance. However, albeit possibly present at several levels, because acceptance is part of the definition of mindfulness itself, it is not considered separately. The same holds for the process of decentering or cognitive defusion, meaning seeing internal mental phenomena such as thoughts, etc. as just mental phenomena, not as aspects of the self or objective truths (Baer, 2009). This also is an inseparable aspect of mindful perception, not a consequence of mindfulness. This view is supported by the fact that both aspects are present in the Five Factor Mindfulness Questionnaire (Baer et al., 2006) in the "accepting" and "non-reactivity" subscales, respectively.

Although experiential avoidance may be viewed similarly (as the opposite of mindfulness, which reflects fundamental experiential approach), experiential avoidance involves both fundamental mindlessness as well as an important consequence of mindfulness at the behavioral level. The practice of mindfulness decreases daily behaviors aimed at avoiding potentially unpleasant experiences, such as unpleasant emotions or anxiety-provoking social situations. This decreased experiential avoidance enhances behavioral flexibility, which is an important consequence of mindfulness practice, related to well-being. Therefore, this aspect is included as a separate factor in the model, albeit a part of it is included in the concept of mindfulness itself.

What about ER? Although ER is not mentioned explicitly in the model, it is present as part or result of several factors, mainly flexible self-regulation. Volitional ER especially pertains to regulation of expression of emotion that may be more effectively regulated. Emotional experience, as argued above, does not need to be regulated from a mindfulness perspective, although it usually indirectly is regulated as a result of a combination of the higher order factors, important drivers being relaxation, harmony, de/reappraisal, and less perseverative thinking and less avoidance.

Thus, the RICH model of mindfulness provides a new theoretical framework that may guide research into the working mechanisms of mindfulness regarding psychological well-being. ER is included in the model, although not as one separate explicit factor. Is empirical evidence available supporting an association between mindfulness and ER factors?

### 7.4.2 Research on Mindfulness and Emotion Regulation

In a recent theoretical article reviewing some evidence, it was suggested that mindfulness mediates effects on well-being, probably by decreasing rumination and experiential avoidance, and improving self-regulation (Baer, 2009). A number of illustrative studies are discussed below.

In some studies, relations have been reported between self-reported measures of mindfulness and general ER (Baer et al., 2006; Roemer et al., 2009). However, the instrument used to measure ER in these studies can be questioned in the context of examining the association between these two constructs. It is not a pure measure of ER as defined above, but includes aspects of emotional awareness, clarity, and acceptance (Roemer et al., 2009). Conceptually, these aspects are not aspects of *regulation* per se, but are either prerequisites for adequate ER (i.e., awareness and clarity) or even overlap with the definition of mindfulness (i.e., awareness and acceptance). This inflates correlations between mindfulness and ER making interpretations difficult. However, in a group of 342 students, mindfulness was found to be inversely related to passive and impulsive emotion-regulation strategies (Wupperman, Neumann, & Axelrod, 2008), suggesting more adequate self-regulation being associated with mindfulness. A related finding was obtained in a specific study in 33 married couples (Wachs & Cordova, 2007), showing that acting mindfully correlated with a greater control of anger expression.

Regarding the specific factors discussed in this chapter, self-reported mindfulness was found to correlate negatively with rumination, worry, thought suppression, alexithymia – poor insight into one's emotions – and experiential avoidance in various student samples (Baer et al., 2006; Brown & Ryan, 2003; Feldman et al., 2007). For instance, in one correlational study in 233 students, mindfulness was negatively associated with a measure of experiential avoidance, showing about 25% shared variance (Moore, Brody, & Dierberger, 2009).

Regarding acute effects of mindfulness practice, change in certain brain potential patterns (frontal fast theta EEG power), which is claimed to be associated with mindfulness, correlated with decreased scores on harm avoidance, which is related to experiential avoidance, during Zen meditation in novice meditators (Takahashi et al., 2005). In another experimental study, acute effects of a brief mindful breathing instruction were found to decrease negative affect intensity when viewing aversive slides, and also increase the willingness to view the slides, indicating decreased experiential avoidance (Arch & Craske, 2006).

DBT uses extensively both mindfulness and enhancement of ER skills as important aspects of the intervention. It is often used in patients with complex psychological problems, such as borderline personality, where DBT has been shown to enhance both mindfulness and ER skills, the interrelation of which, however, was not examined (Stepp, Epler, Jahng, & Trull, 2008).

In conclusion, although not many studies have been performed to date, the available evidence suggests an association between mindfulness and several ER factors. However, more research is needed on this topic, especially experimental studies and RCTs including measures of ER, which have been hardly performed to date.

## 7.5 Does Emotion Regulation Mediate the Relationship Between Mindfulness and Well-Being?

Only a few studies have been performed on the relationship between mindfulness, potentially mediating mechanisms related to ER and psychological well-being. In addition, most studies to date have not included formal mediation analyses to examine this issue. For instance, in the above mentioned study in 233 students, decreased avoidance and increased mindfulness predicted well-being after writing, but no mediation analyses were performed (Moore et al., 2009). This is also true for the other correlational studies discussed above (Baer et al., 2006; Brown & Ryan, 2003; Feldman et al., 2007). Another example is a study in chronic pain patients, in which mindfulness was positively correlated with pain acceptance, and values-based action, as well as negatively with pain and psychological symptoms (McCracken & Keogh, 2009). However, again, no mediation analyses were performed, not permitting any conclusions regarding possible paths between these factors.

One of the few exceptions is the study on the relationship between mindfulness and borderline features in a sample of 342 students (Wupperman et al., 2008). In this study, when ER strategies were controlled statistically, mindfulness still was associated with fewer symptoms of borderline features. This suggests a direct inverse link between mindfulness and these specific symptoms. In contrast, in the above mentioned small study of 33 couples (Wachs & Cordova, 2007), control of anger did statistically mediate the association between acting mindfully and marital quality, suggesting that control of anger may be a mechanism in this specific association.

Of course, more compelling evidence for the role of mediating variables has to come from experimental or intervention studies. An intervention combining mindfulness techniques and ER skill enhancement showed positive effects on psychological well-being and physician's ratings of joint tenderness in rheumatoid arthritis patients that had previous depressive episodes (Zautra et al., 2008). However, the relation between mindfulness and ER was not assessed. Similarly, several studies on the effectiveness of DBT have shown positive effects on mood and lower borderline symptoms (Harley, Sprich, Safren, Jacobo, & Fava, 2008; Stepp et al., 2008), but the components of mindfulness and ER were not analyzed separately, let alone interrelated. One exception is a very recent small randomized trial in patients with major depression receiving a DBT-based intervention or waitlist (Feldman, Harley, Kerrigan, Jacobo, & Fava, 2009), which found enhanced emotion processing to be associated with a larger decrease in depressive symptoms in the DBT group. However, this enhanced emotion processing did not mediate the intervention effect.

In an uncontrolled small trial, pre-to post-MBSR assessments showed both decreased mindfulness, decreased rumination and decreased depressive symptoms (Deyo, Wilson, Ong, & Koopman, 2009). Although changes in mindfulness correlated modestly with changes in rumination, no mediation analyses were performed. The same applies to another small uncontrolled study, in which mindfulness-based cognitive therapy was found to reduce insomnia, worry, and rumination in a group of patients with anxiety disorder (Yook et al., 2008).

In a small randomized intervention trial comparing MBSR with two control groups, increases in mindfulness were found to mediate decreases in rumination and distress (Shapiro, Oman, Thoresen, Plante, & Flinders, 2008). Potential mediation by rumination was not examined in that study, but it was in another investigation conducted by that research group (Jain et al., 2007). Here, mindfulness meditation was compared to a relaxation control group in a randomized trial conducted in 83 distressed students. Decrease in rumination was found to partially mediate the positive effects on stress reduction in this study.

In a controlled study on the effects of a mindfulness (vipassana) meditation course on alcohol use in 173 prisoners, avoidance of thoughts decreased, which partially mediated the effects of the meditation course on alcohol use and alcohol related problems in daily life (Bowen, Witkiewitz, Dillworth, & Marlatt, 2007).

In summary, the studies reviewed here suggest both direct effects of mindfulness and indirect effects of mindfulness via various mechanisms related to ER on various indices of psychological well-being. This is consistent with the presented RICH model of mindfulness effects. However, one must note that the number of well-conducted studies, especially the number of well-controlled trials and experiments applying mediation analyses is very small. More research is obviously needed to be able to draw firm conclusions.

## 7.6 Concluding Remarks

In this chapter, the associations between mindfulness, ER, and psychological well-being were examined. As both mindfulness and ER are related to well-being, it is worthwhile examining their interrelationship as well as the possibility that mindfulness exerts its effects on well-being via mechanisms of ER.

Theoretical perspectives on the issue were discussed and compared, showing a large diversity in viewpoints ranging from mindfulness being viewed as an ER strategy to ER being regarded as rather irrelevant from mindfulness perspective. It has become clear that although a link between mindfulness and ER does exist, this relation is not a straightforward one. Although for some mindfulness theorists ER per se is neither a goal in itself nor a mean towards a goal, emotions do get regulated when practicing mindfulness, albeit perhaps not in a volitional way. A new theoretical model of mindfulness effects on well-being via several pathway levels is proposed, in which ER is included at various levels of the model, finally influencing a person's well-being.

Empirical research pertaining to the various links between mindfulness, ER mechanisms, and well-being is reviewed. It has become clear that research in this field is young and that paucity exists of methodologically well-conducted studies. Especially studies examining the potentially mediating role of ER in the link between mindfulness and well-being are scarce. Future research should therefore focus on such studies including formal mediation analyses in controlled intervention trials. In addition, attempts should be made to examine to what extent ER related to mindfulness is explicit and volitional or an indirect and nonvolitional consequence of mindfulness.

Nevertheless, the available evidence does suggest that links exist between mindfulness and various ER strategies, notably lower use of suppression, avoidance, and rumination, which are included in the presented RICH model of mindfulness effects. Future studies should examine whether these, or other emotion regulatory processes, are indeed mechanisms in the mindfulness-well-being link.

## References

Arch, J. J., & Craske, M. G. (2006) Mechanisms of mindfulness: emotion regulation following a focused breathing induction. *Behaviour Research and Therapy*, *44*, 1849–1858.

Baer, R. A. (2009) Self-focused attention and mechanisms of change in mindfulness-based treatment. *Cognitive Behaviour Therapy, 38*, 15–20.

Baer, R. A., Smith, G. T., & Allen, K. B. (2004) Assessment of mindfulness by self-report: The Kentucky inventory of mindfulness skills. *Assessment, 11*, 191–206.

Baer, R. A., Smith, G. T., Hopkins, J., Krietemeyer, J., & Toney, L. (2006) Using self-report assessment methods to explore facets of mindfulness. *Assessment, 13*, 27–45.

Barlow, D. H., & Craske, M. G. (2000) *Mastery of your anxiety and panic* (3rd ed.). New York: Psychological Corporation.

Bishop, S. R., Lau, M. A., Shapiro, S., Carlson, L., Anderson, N. D., Carmody, J., Segal, Z. V., Abbey, S., Speca, M., Velting, D., & Devins, G. (2004) Mindfulness: A proposed operational definition. *Clinical Psychology: Science and Practice, 11*, 230–241.

Blackledge, J. T., & Hayes, S. C. (2001) Emotion regulation in acceptance and commitment therapy. *Journal of Clinical Psychology, 57*, 243–255.

Borkovec, T. D., Ray, W. J., & Stöber, J. (1998) Worry: A cognitive phenomenon intimately linked to affective, physiological, and interpersonal behavioral processes. *Cognitive Therapy and Research, 22*, 561–576.

Bowen, S., Witkiewitz, K., Dillworth, T. M., & Marlatt, G. A. (2007) The role of thought suppression in the relationship between mindfulness meditation and alcohol use. *Addictive Behaviors, 32*, 2324–2328.

Bränström, R., Kvillemo, P., Brandberg, Y., & Moskowitz, J. T. (2010) Mindfulness as a mediator of psychological well-being in a stress reduction intervention for cancer patients: a randomized study. *Annals of Behavioral Medicine*, 39, 151–161.

Brosschot, J. F., Pieper, S., & Thayer, J. F. (2005) Expanding stress theory: prolonged activation and perseverative cognition. *Psychoneuroendocrinology, 30*, 1043–1049.
Brown, K. W., & Ryan, R. M. (2003) The benefits of being present: Mindfulness and its role in psychological well-being. *Journal of Personality and Social Psychology, 84*, 822–848.
Butler, E. A., Egloff, B., Wilhelm, F. H., Smith, N. C., Erickson, E. A., & Gross, J. J. (2003) The social consequences of expressive suppression. *Emotion, 3*, 48–67.
Carmody, J., Baer, R. A., Lykins, L. E. B., & Olendzki, N. (2009) An empirical study of the mechanisms of mindfulness in a mindfulness-based stress reduction program. *Journal of Clinical Psychology, 65*, 613–626.
Chambers, R., Gullone, E., & Allen, N. B. (2009) Mindful emotion regulation: An integrative review. *Clinical Psychology Review, 29*, 560–572.
Deyo, M., Wilson, K. A., Ong, J., & Koopman, C. (2009) Mindfulness and rumination: does mindfulness training lead to reductions in the ruminative thinking associated with depression? *Explore (NY), 5*, 265–271.
Ekman, P., Davidson, R. J., Ricard, M., & Wallace, B. A. (2005) Buddhist and psychological perspectives on emotions and well-being. *Current Directions in Psychological Science, 14*, 59–63.
Feldman, G., Harley, R., Kerrigan, M., Jacobo, M., & Fava, M. (2009) Change in emotional processing during a dialectical behavior therapy-based skills group for major depressive disorder. *Behaviour Research and Therapy*, 47, 316–321.
Feldman, G., Hayes, A., Kumar, S., Greeson, J., & Laurenceau, J.-P. (2007) Mindfulness and emotion regulation: The development and initial validation of the Cognitive and Affective Mindfulness Scale-Revised (CAMS-R). *Journal of Psychopathology and Behavioral Assessment, 29*, 177–190.
Gross, J. J. (1998) Antecedent- and response-focused emotion regulation: Divergent consequences for experience, expression, and physiology. *Journal of Personality and Social Psychology, 74*, 224–237.
Gross, J. J., & John, O. P. (2003) Individual differences in two emotion regulation processes: Implications for affect, relationships, and well-being. *Journal of Personality and Social Psychology, 85*, 348–362.
Gross, J. J., & Levenson, R. W. (1997) Hiding feelings: the acute effects of inhibiting negative and positive emotion.*Journal of Abnormal Psychology 106*, 95–103.
Gross, J. J., & Muñoz, R. F. (1995) Emotion regulation and mental health. *Clinical Psychology: Science and Practice, 2*, 151–164.
Harley, R., Sprich, S., Safren, S., Jacobo, M., & Fava, M. (2008) Adaptation of dialectical behavior therapy skills training group for treatment-resistant depression. *Journal of Nervous and Mental Disease, 196*, 136–143.
Hayes, S. C. (2004) Acceptance and commitment therapy, relational frame theory, and the third wave of behavioral and cognitive therapies. *Behavior Therapy, 35*, 639–665.
Hayes, S. C., Follette, V. M., & Linehan, M. M. (Eds.). (2004) *Mindfulness and acceptance: Expanding the cognitive-behavioral tradition*. New York, NY: Guilford.
Hayes, S. C., Luoma, J. B., Bond, F. W., Masuda, A., & Lillis, J. (2006) Acceptance and commitment therapy: model, processes and outcomes. *Behaviour Research and Therapy, 44*, 1–25.
Hofmann, S. G., & Asmundson, G. J. G. (2008) Acceptance and mindfulness-based therapy: New wave or old hat? *Clinical Psychology Review, 28*, 1–16.
Jain, S., Shapiro, S. L., Swanick, S., Roesch, S. C., Mills, P. J., Bell, I., & Schwartz, G. E. (2007) A randomized controlled trial of mindfulness meditation versus relaxation training: Effects on distress, positive states of mind, rumination, and distraction. *Annals of Behavioral Medicine, 33*, 11–21.
Kabat-Zinn, J. (1982) An outpatient program in behavioral medicine for chronic pain patients based on the practice of mindfulness meditation: theoretical considerations and preliminary results. *General Hospital Psychiatry, 4*, 33–47.
Kabat-Zinn, J. (1990) *Full catastrophe living: Using the wisdom of your body and mind to face stress, pain, and illness*. New York: Delacourt.

Kabat-Zinn, J. (1994)*Wherever you go, there you are: Mindfulness meditation in everyday life*. New York: Hyperion.

Kabat-Zinn, J., Lipworth, L., & Burney, R. (1985) The clinical use of mindfulness meditation for the self-regulation of chronic pain. *Journal of Behavioral Medicine, 8*, 163–190.

Krishnamurti, J. (1987) *The awakening of intelligence*. San Francisco: Harper.

Lengacher, C. A., Johnson-Mallard, V., Post-White, J., Moscoso, M. S., Jacobsen, P. B., Klein, T. W., Widen, R. H., Fitzgerald, S. G., Shelton, M. M., Barta, M., Goodman, M., Cox, C. E., & Kip, K. E. (2009) Randomized controlled trial of mindfulness-based stress reduction (MBSR) for survivors of breast cancer. *Psycho-Oncology, 18*, 1261–1272.

Linehan, M. M. (1993) *Cognitive-behavioral treatment of borderline personality disorder*. New York: Guilford.

Mauss, I. B., & Gross, J. J. (2004) Emotion suppression and cardiovascular disease: Is hiding feelings bad for your heart? In I. Nyklíček, L. Temoshok &, A. J. Vingerhoets (Eds.), *Emotional expression and health: Advances in theory, assessment and clinical applications* (pp. 61–81). Hove: Brunner-Routledge.

McCracken, L. M., & Keogh, E. (2009) Acceptance, mindfulness, and values-based action may counteract fear and avoidance of emotions in chronic pain: An analysis of anxiety sensitivity. *Journal of Pain, 10*, 408–415.

Moore, S. D., Brody, L. R., & Dierberger, A. E. (2009) Mindfulness and experiential avoidance as predictors and outcomes of the narrative emotional disclosure task. *Journal of Clinical Psychology, 65*, 971–988.

Nhat Hanh, T. (1976) *Miracle of mindfulness: A manual for meditation*. Boston: Beacon.

Nhat Hanh, T. (1988) *The heart of understanding: Commentaries on the Prajnaparamita Heart Sutra*. Berkeley, CA: Parallax.

Nhat Hanh, T. (1991) *Peace is every step: The path of mindfulness in everyday life*. New York: Bantam.

Nyklíček, I., & Kuijpers, K. F. (2008) Effects of mindfulness-based stress reduction intervention on psychological well-being and quality of life: Is increased mindfulness indeed the mechanism? *Annals of Behavioral Medicine, 35*, 331–340.

Nyklíček, I., & Vingerhoets, A. (2009) "Adaptive" psychosocial factors in relation to home blood pressure: A study in the general population of southern Netherlands. *International Journal of Behavioral Medicine, 16*, 212–218.

Ochsner, K. N., Ray, R. D., Cooper, J. C., Robertson, E. R., Chopra, S., Gabrieli, J. D., & Gross, J. J. (2004) For better or for worse: neural systems supporting the cognitive down- and up-regulation of negative emotion. *Neuroimage, 23*, 483–499.

Roemer, L., Lee, J. K., Salters-Pedneault, K., Erisman, S. M., Orsillo, S. M., & Mennin, D. S. (2009) Mindfulness and emotion regulation difficulties in generalized anxiety disorder: preliminary evidence for independent and overlapping contributions. *Behavior Therapy, 40*, 142–154.

Ryan, R. M., & Brown, K. W. (2003) Why we don't need self-Esteem: On fundamental needs, contingent love, and mindfulness: Comment. *Psychological Inquiry, 14*, 71–76.

Ryan, R. M., & Deci, E. L. (2000) Self-determination theory and the facilitation of intrinsic motivation, social development, and well-being. *American Psychologist, 55*, 68–78.

Shapiro, S. L., Carlson, L. E., Astin, J. A., & Freedman, B. (2006) Mechanisms of mindfulness. *Journal of Clinical Psychology, 62*, 373–386.

Shapiro, S. L., Oman, D., Thoresen, C. E., Plante, T. G., & Flinders, T. (2008) Cultivating mindfulness: effects on well-being. *Journal of Clinical Psychology, 64*, 840–862.

Speca, M., Carlson, L. E., Goodey, E., & Angen, M. (2000) A randomized, wait-list controlled clinical trial: The effect of a mindfulness meditation-based stress reduction program on mood and symptoms of stress in cancer outpatients. *Psychosomatic Medicine, 62*, 613–622.

Stepp, S. D., Epler, A. J., Jahng, S., & Trull, T. J. (2008) The effect of dialectical behavior therapy skills use on borderline personality disorder features. *Journal of Personality Disorders, 22*, 549–563.

Takahashi, T., Murata, T., Hamada, T., Omori, M., Kosaka, H., Kikuchi, M., Yoshida, H., & Wada, Y. (2005) Changes in EEG and autonomic nervous activity during meditation and their association with personality traits. *International Journal of Psychophysiology, 55*, 199–207.

Thera, N. (1972) *The power of mindfulness*. San Francisco, CA: Unity Press.
Wachs, K., & Cordova, J. V. (2007) Mindful relating: Exploring mindfulness and emotion repertoires in intimate relationships. *Journal of Marital & Family Therapy, 33*, 464–481.
Wallace, B. A., & Shapiro, S. L. (2006) Mental balance and well-being: Building bridges between buddhism and western psychology. *American Psychologist, 61*, 690–701.
Wells, A. (2000) *Emotional disorders and metacognition: Innovative cognitive therapy*. Chichester: Wiley.
Wupperman, P., Neumann, C. S., & Axelrod, S. R. (2008) Do deficits in mindfulness underlie borderline personality features and core difficulties. *Journal of Personality Disorders, 22*, 466–482.
Yook, K., Lee, S. H., Ryu, M., Kim, K. H., Choi, T. K., Suh, S. Y., Kim, Y. W., Kim, B., Kim, M. Y., & Kim, M. J. (2008) Usefulness of mindfulness-based cognitive therapy for treating insomnia in patients with anxiety disorders: a pilot study. *Journal of Nervous and Mental Disease, 196*, 501–503.
Zautra, A. J., Davis, M. C., Reich, J. W., Nicassario, P., Tennen, H., Finan, P., Kratz, A., Parrish, B., & Irwin, M. R. (2008) Comparison of cognitive behavioral and mindfulness meditation interventions on adaptation to rheumatoid arthritis for patients with and without history of recurrent depression. *Journal of Consulting and Clinical Psychology, 76*, 408–421.

# Part II
# Social Perspective

# Chapter 8
# Intergroup Emotions: More than the Sum of the Parts

**Russell Spears, Colin Leach, Martijn van Zomeren, Alexa Ispas, Joseph Sweetman, and Nicole Tausch**

## 8.1 Introduction and Overview

In this chapter, we present a range of evidence on intergroup emotions from our own lab' with the aim of showing that the intersection of research of groups and emotions enriches both research domains. The study of intergroup emotions is a relatively new "niche" area that can be thought of both as part of the realm of emotion research and also a subarea within the field of intergroup relations. Rather than seeing this development simply as an area of specialization or specification, we try to make the case that bringing these two fields together leads to insights that are more than the sum of the parts. Given our background, the main focus here will be on how emotion extends our understanding of intergroup relations in various ways. However, the very extension of emotion into the intergroup realm can in itself be seen as part of the synergic value that also potentially feeds back into emotion theory. In keeping with the focus in this volume on the role of emotion in regulating behavior, the intergroup focus shows the importance of shared emotions as validating experience, and regulating, and explaining behavior at the group level.

After outlining the background and basis for intergroup emotion, we present research addressing the following two specific questions relating to two key domains of intergroup relations: (1) What does the emotion-based approach add to our understanding of prejudice and discrimination, and the extreme forms this can take? (2) What do group emotions add to our understanding of social change and collective action by disadvantaged groups? Our choice of topics is not entirely arbitrary or opportunistic. The focus on prejudice and discrimination and conflict between groups, and the question of how low status or disadvantaged

R. Spears (✉)
School of Psychology, Cardiff University, Tower Building, 70 Park Place, Cardiff, CF10 3AT, UK
e-mail: SpearsR@Cardiff.ac.uk

I. Nyklíček et al. (eds.), *Emotion Regulation and Well-Being*,
DOI 10.1007/978-1-4419-6953-8_8, © Springer Science+Business Media, LLC 2011

groups contest their position, have been two central topics with the field of intergroup relations. They have also been perhaps *the* two central focal themes of social identity theory (SIT; Tajfel & Turner, 1979), which forms the starting foundation for much work reported here, as well as for the influential intergroup emotion theory (Smith, 1993). However, these themes are also central to many other approaches to intergroup relations including relative deprivation theory, realistic conflict theory, social dominance theory and various interdependence approaches.

Because of the centrality of social identity theory to our own research, and as a basis for intergroup emotion theory, we provide a brief overview of this theory here. This is important because although SIT does not furnish an approach explicitly couched in terms of emotions in its original form, it does arguably provide the foundations of the appraisals that do *afford* an emotion based analysis, and the behavior that follows them (see e.g., Leach, Snider & Iyer, 2002; Smith, 1993; Van Zomeren, Spears, Fischer & Leach, 2004). The concept of social identity was introduced in part to makes sense of discrimination, or more precisely differentiation, in the minimal group studies (Tajfel 1978). The social identity explanation is couched in terms of the positive differentiation that reward allocations provide, creating a positive sense of group distinctiveness, and thus a meaningful sense of group identity per se (Spears, Jetten, Scheepers & Cihangir, 2009). This part of social identity theory clearly relates to our first theme. Social identity theory also aims to understand the conditions under which disadvantaged groups try to change their circumstances, relating to our second theme. The classical analysis of the circumstances of when low status or disadvantaged groups will challenge the status quo depends on perceptions of the stability of their status disadvantage and its perceived legitimacy. When the situation is seen as unstable and illegitimate, people are more likely to perceive the situation as changeable, to perceive cognitive alternatives to the status quo, and to challenge the out-group. Tajfel described such social comparisons as insecure and the perception of cognitive alternatives was the key psychological motive to engage in strategies of social change.

Framed in these terms, social identity theory can be seen as an incipient theory of emotion, having two of the key elements of the classical tripartite formulation: appraisals and action tendencies. In line with appraisal theories, the perceptions of (in)stability and legitimacy are psychologically mediated interpretations of the social reality. The coping potential implied by counterfactuals to the status quo capitalizing on instability can be seen as a secondary appraisal that sit very well with the stress and coping model (see Lazarus & Folkman, 1984; Van Zomeren et al., 2004). That these appraisals are translated in to action tendencies is a further clear parallel to emotion theory (Frijda, 1986). The "only" thing missing is an *explicit* specification of the admittedly nontrivial, intervening emotion states (e.g., hope, anger). Much of the theory and research presented below is about filling in the emotional gaps, so to speak, which help to explain and specify the ensuing behavior.

## 8.2 An Emotion-Based Approach: From Individual Prejudice to Intergroup Prejudices

Research on intergroup emotions is often traced back to the seminal chapter by Smith (1993), in which he set out a framework for understanding aspects of intergroup relations, and in particular prejudice and discrimination, in terms of emotion theory. Smith's approach also recognized the importance of taking a group-level (albeit psychological) approach to understanding these phenomena. In this respect, he acknowledges the importance of the social identity approach (social identity and self-categorization theory) and the value of considering identity of both self and other, at the intergroup level. The new element here was to introduce the specification that emotion theory could provide to an analysis of these intergroup relations.

It would not be fair to say that emotions was completely lacking in previous approaches to prejudice and discrimination; some of the earliest explanations, such as Adorno et al.'s work on the authoritarian personality (1950), had explored the powerful emotions that could underlie prejudice and discrimination. However, work in this tradition was quite individualistic, conceptualizing prejudice as arising from a process of personality development from a psychoanalytic perspective. As the cognitive revolution replaced the New Look in psychology generally and social psychology in particular, the motivational and emotional bases of prejudice took a back seat (Hamilton, 1981). Ironically, Tajfel's early work on the cognitive aspects of prejudice (1969) was cited as a key influence by the protagonists of the cognitive approach, in which prejudice was seen as arising from stereotypic biases (e.g., social categorization, illusory correlation; see Hamilton, 1981), and where the role of motivation and emotion as driving forces in prejudice were somewhat thrown out with the bathwater (Pettigrew, 1981).

The cognitive approach also neglected the intergroup level of analysis reasserted in social identity theory and Tajfel left no doubt as to the importance of more motivational and emotional processes factors in this framework. In his definition of social identity, he refers to the social identity as "that part of the self-concept referring to group membership … together with its emotional significance" (1978). However, as we have already noted, it is also fair to say that this emotional significance was never fully realized by social identity theory. Thus, like other approaches to prejudice and discrimination that recognized the importance of motivational aspects of prejudice (e.g., attitude-based approaches), prejudice or in-group bias was conceptualized as a rather uni-dimensional affective reaction, which was positive to the in-group and more negative towards out-groups, with discrimination, the behavioral manifestation of this in-group bias, simply following on from this.

Once again, the value of the intergroup focus of the social identity approach (above attitudinal approaches) was to recognize the intergroup dimension to prejudice and discrimination; not just in defining the target of prejudice, but in defining the (group) nature of the perceiver and their relation to the target: prejudice is not just an individual attitude, it reflects a collective orientation that takes into account the dynamics of the social structure and the perceiver's relation to it. However, the limitations of this approach become apparent when we move from the simplicity of minimal groups in the lab,' to the complexity of real world intergroup relations. Although the broader statement of social identity theory was attuned to group differences and identity threats defined by inequalities in status, because the response to such threats to group identity remains couched in terms of a positive evaluative differentiation from the out-group, there is a danger, what we underestimate variety, both in the nature of the group response to such threats and indeed variety in the very nature of such threats. A related limitation of the social identity theory noted by Brewer (1999) is her claim that it is better equipped to explain in-group favoritism (or "in-group love") rather than out-group derogation (or "out-group hate"), and so does not adequately explain the more extreme and malicious forms that prejudice and discrimination can take.

With the development of intergroup emotion theory, the stage was set for explanations of prejudice that fully recognized the group level and emotional bases of prejudice and discrimination. Taking an emotion-based approach opens the door to a broad repertoire of intergroup relationships that could be analyzed in terms of a range of appraisal dimensions. It is important to acknowledge the early seminal work of Dijker (1987) who used emotion theory to analyze the different forms of prejudice to different ethnic minorities in Dutch society. Applying appraisal theory, (Lazarus & Folkman, 1984; Lazarus, 1991) Smith (1993) argued that different appraisals of intergroup relations could lead to a variety of different emotional prejudices and indeed different discriminatory action tendencies (Frijda, 1986) characteristic of these emotions (e.g., confrontation, avoidance).

Thus, Mackie, Devos and Smith (2000) showed that appraisals of relative in-group strength led to anger, which mediated offensive action tendencies towards the out-group. By contrast, in later work they showed that appraisals of in-group weakness predicted fear, which mediated avoidant action tendencies (see Mackie, Silver & Smith, 2004; Maitner, Mackie & Smith, 2006). In both cases it makes sense to talk of "emotional prejudice" given the negative affective orientation towards the out-group, but the emotional experience and resulting behavior is quite different in each case. Thus emotion regulates group behavior in meaningful and appropriate ways that reflect the in-group's situation and coping resources. That this emotional reaction to the out-group is a group level reaction based on social identity has been made perhaps most evident in a program of research in which the authors manipulated the anger directed at a target by varying the salience of the in-group identity (Gordijn, Wigboldus & Yzerbyt, 2001). Students at the University of Amsterdam reacted with anger towards a computer hacker (a Maths student) who caused a disruptive computer crash at the rival Free University when their shared identity as students had been made salient (Psychology vs. Maths students); compared to when their university identity was made salient, rendering the very same victims of the crash out-group rather than in-group.

The key new insight of intergroup emotion theory was to recognize the potential power of the emotion based analysis in helping us to extend and understand that range of experience and behavioral reactions that might characterize prejudice and discrimination in its different forms. Thus, the signature of prejudice and discrimination associated with racism, sexism, homophobia, and so forth may be quite different, and indeed we can distinguish different forms of racism and even sexism, depending on the nature of the target, the nature of the in-group, and the perceiver's appraisal of the intergroup relationship.

This approach allows us not only to reappraise the variety of forms of prejudice, but also indeed to question its traditional conceptualization as a negative affective orientation towards an out-group. It had been clear for some time that some forms of prejudice did not fit neatly into the simple mould in which the out-group is negatively evaluated or downgraded compared to the in-group. Some forms of prejudice clearly positively valued the out-group at least on certain key dimensions. Take the classic case of anti-Semitism for example. This out-group is often rated highly on the dimension of competence (which contributes in important ways to identity threats). For some forms of sexism the positive evaluation associated with prejudice can be even more apparent. The case of benevolent sexism (Glick & Fiske, 2001), for example, reflects a positive evaluation of women by men, but particularly on the dimension of warmth (and less so on competence) – the mirror opposite of the profile for anti-Semitism just described. In this case reacting positively to women can go hand in hand with paternalism, which reinforces their power disadvantage – "the iron fist in the velvet glove" to use Jackman's (1994) evocative phrase. According to this view prejudices relates not only to the evaluation of the target group, but the *type* of evaluation and the intergroup status and power relations that the prejudice might serve, and reinforce.

Such examples are more compatible with the multidimensional approach represented by intergroup emotion theory and prompted the development of various multidimensional models that have attempted to examine the appraisal dimensions that better account for this diversity of prejudice. We will consider three such briefly here. The stereotype content model of Fiske et al. (2002) proposed a taxonomy in terms of competence and warmth that captures well the different examples of anti-Semitism (high competence, low warmth), and benevolent sexism (high warmth, low competence). These refer to envious and paternalistic forms of prejudice respectively. Completing the quadrant are target groups that are evaluated low on both (e.g., homeless people) resulting in contemptuous prejudice, whereas groups high in both warmth and competence are likely to be those we admire and of course generally include the in-group itself.

A second influential model that perhaps takes an even more explicitly emotion-focused approach to understanding the different forms of prejudice raises in intergroup relations is group image theory (Alexander, Brewer & Hermann, 1999). This model combines three appraisal dimensions (group goals, status, and power relations) to analyze the diverse images of an out-group that can emerge, and explain the different kinds of prejudice associate with each group image. Thus "allies" are characterized by compatible goals and equal status and power, but with incompatible goals (e.g., competition for valued resources) quickly become "enemies," resulting in emotions such as anger and action tendencies such as attack or containment. Incompatible goals combined with status inferiority and power superiority evoke the "barbarian" image, fear, and protective or avoidant behavior. Out-groups that are superior in terms of power and status evoke an "imperialist" image associated with envy or resentment, and resistance or rebellion.

Another important taxonomic model broadly grounded in the social identity approach is that of Leach et al. (2002) who focus on high status or advantaged groups in their relation to disadvantaged groups and add to the two-key appraisal dimensions of legitimacy and stability furnished by social identity theory. They introduce appraisals of the control of the high status groups over the outcomes of the low status other, and whether the emotional reaction is self-focused or other-focused in nature. Applying this to the case of the high status group's perspective, thus results in a taxonomy of (2 × 2 × 2 × 2=) 16 different cells or combinations, many of which can be characterized by emotional states. Those associated prejudice and discrimination are concentrated in, but not confined to cases where the superior in-group's status is seen as legitimate.

Thus, they predict that legitimate high status, which is however unstable, other-focused, but not under the high status in-group's control can lead to indignation, whereas high control for a similar combination is more likely to be associated with feelings of disdain. As noted above, emotion-based prejudice is not always justified by legitimacy. Unstable status advantage that is illegitimate, where there is little control over the others' outcomes, and a self-focused perspective, is associated with fear and worry that one's disadvantage could disappear (comparable to the insecure social comparisons predicted by social identity theory for the perspective of the disadvantaged group, as demonstrated by Mackie et al., 2004 above). However, a similar combination with a *stable* status advantage and greater control over the other's outcomes may lead to gloating. Of course, not all of the outcomes are likely to be prejudiced or discriminatory in nature (e.g., pity, sympathy and moral outrage are all cases of other-focused emotions predicted to arise from specific combinations of this matrix), but this reminds us that prejudice and discrimination are not inevitable outcomes of intergroup relations.

This overview of intergroup emotion theories is far from exhaustive. For example, in another influential model Cottrell and Neuberg (2005) have developed a socio-functional approach that also specifies the different kinds of threat appraisals that can underlie different forms of prejudice. However, the general value of the emotion-based approach should be clear; specifying the appraisal dimensions that can be used to understand the specific emotional reactions of one group to another provides many insights into the diversity of prejudice and discrimination, but also other forms of group relation (including harmony). Although there is already much research in the literature that speaks to such framework, these theories also function as generative programs, identifying gaps to be filled. Our aim in the next section is not to provide a definitive test of these theoretical frameworks, but to use the principles from intergroup emotion theories to illustrate the "add-on" value of this approach to prejudice and discrimination that lack a group-level and emotion-based analysis.

## 8.3 Putting the Passion in Prejudice: What Does Group Emotion Add to the Mix?

In this section we present some evidence that further illustrates and extends the emotion-based view of prejudice and discrimination outlined in the theoretical overview. As the previous section makes clear, in many ways, the general case for the value of a group-emotion based approach to prejudice has already been made. Here, we address the specific argument that emotion-based approaches can help us to understand the more extreme and derogatory forms that prejudice and discrimination can take, and that cannot easily be explained by more cognitive, attitudinal and individualistic approaches, and also group-based approaches that lack emotion specification. With this in mind we focus on two general examples to make our case. First, we develop the analysis of prejudices based on anger and fear described earlier (Mackie et al., 2000, 2004; Gordijn et al., 2001; Smith, 1993), but argue that the *combination* of these two emotions can form a particularly potent mixture in terms of prejudice and discrimination towards certain out-groups, especially when we also take into account perceptions of these emotions in the groups concerned (or "meta-emotions" in the case of the out-group target). Second, we examine in some detail a more specifically malicious emotion, schadenfreude, that we argue can constitute a quite distinct form of prejudice when experienced at the group level, and which clearly moves us in to the realm of out-group derogation.

### *8.3.1 Anger Fear and Loathing*

In the previous section, we briefly presented evidence that anger and fear, and the appraisals underlying them could form different bases of prejudice with distinct sequelae in terms of action tendencies (e.g., Mackie et al., 2000, 2004). Perhaps, because these forms of emotional prejudice are seen as distinct, no previous research to our knowledge has considered whether and how these emotions might combine and even interact. A major reason for this hinges on the analysis that a key appraisal for anger is in-group strength or power and out-group weakness, whereas for fear the key appraisal is its opposite: in-group weakness and out-group strength. In so far as these emotions are seen as mutually exclusive, we think this reasoning may be limiting our analysis.

First, relative group strength can be seen in continuous and relative terms, making it possible for a mixture of emotions to co-occur (indeed the notion of "mixed emotions" has at least lay validity in everyday discourse). Second, as we shall argue, there are conditions under which weakness can become strength (and evoke fear) where there is a perception that the other has "nothing to lose." A third argument relates specifically to anger. In this case we argue that strength is perhaps not even the most important appraisal associated with anger, and it may not always even be necessary for it to be experienced (although it may limit its expression and action tendencies in various ways). We argue that appraisals of injustice, or being wronged in some way is the more important and primary appraisal for anger, and not necessarily whether one has the strength to do something about this (a secondary or coping appraisal; Lazarus & Folkman, 1984). This issue is not just important in this section, but resurfaces when we consider the emotional basis for collective action on the part of the disadvantaged and disempowered in our second section.

In a series of unpublished studies, Ispas (2007) examined the different signatures of prejudice associated with group-based fear and anger. However, this research differs in an important respect from previous work on intergroup emotions in so far as it focuses on the attribution of emotions to in-groups and out-groups together with perceived control over these emotions, rather than self-reports of these intergroup emotions experienced as group members. This work had shown a close relation between one's own and attributed group emotions in intergroup contexts (Ispas, 2007): emotions attributed to groups, and also prototypical group members, tend to be even stronger, and less under control (especially for the out-group) than self-reported group-based emotions. These findings provide further evidence of the group level of analysis of emotional prejudice and point to the importance of the perceptions (stereotypes) of emotions at the group level in shaping and validating the experience of these emotions as group members. Our focus here is thus on the attribution of fear and anger to in-group and out-groups, which are important social appraisals in their own right (Manstead & Fischer, 2001), reflecting and feeding into the emotional experience of intergroup relations.

This research was conducted primarily in Romania, with some comparative British data, and made use of the various social and ethnic groups represented in that country. To provide the relevant background, the main relevant groups in this society are the Romanian majority group and three minority groups; Moldovans, Hungarians, and Roma people. Moldovans form a relativity low status group compared to the majority Romanians, but are culturally similar and not perceived as threatening. Hungarians are a relatively high status group with a different language and, beyond some mild status rivalry, also not threatening. In contrast, the Roma people (sometimes pejoratively referred to as gypsies) are very negatively perceived by Romanians and other groups, and also evoke high levels of threat; the stereotypes are that they are perceived as neither having nor wanting proper jobs, dependent on state handouts, as being a source of petty crime, being hostile, and so forth. Although this group also attracts quite high levels of prejudice and discrimination in many other European countries, prejudice and discrimination seems to be particularly tolerated and even blatant among Romanians in Romania. This seems to be related to the fact that the Roma people form a much larger minority in Romania than in any other country (they are a negligible minority in Britain), confirmed by group strength appraisals. In short, for Romanians, the Roma people fulfill some of the conditions for Alexander and Brewer's "barbarian" group image (low status but some numerical power).

In a first study conducted on Romanian people (the in-group) Ispas (2007) examined attributions of fear and anger by Romanians to the in-group and to Moldovans. Results revealed greater attributions of fear to the out-group, reflecting their relative weakness, but low levels of anger and no differences between the groups on this emotion was consistent with their relatively harmonious non-threatening intergroup relation. A second study with Romanian and Hungarian participants also resulted in low levels of attributed fear and anger by both groups to each other although both groups reported that Romanians were more likely to oppose than avoid Hungarians, consistent with their relative power and the mild status threat.

However, the interesting contrast comes from a third study in which Romanians rated their perceptions of the Roma out-group, with a British sample rating the same group in Britain. Both samples attribute high levels anger to the in-group and the Roma out-group reflecting the hostile intergroup relations. However, more fear was attributed to the Roma out-group in the British sample, whereas the Romanian sample also rated their in-group as having somewhat more fear towards Roma people than the British sample. These relatively high ratings for fear in the in-group and low fear for the out-group for the Romanians reflect the relative size and power of this minority compared to the British case, and convey the level of threat posed by this out-group in the Romanian sample. Consistent with this, the Roma out-group were seen as more likely to actively oppose than avoid Romanians (reflecting their lack of fear) and the Romanian in-group were equally likely to oppose and avoid the Roma out-group, action tendencies associated with anger and fear respectively. This combination of in-group and anger and fear, together with low out-group fear, helps to explain the high levels hostile prejudice toward the Roma people in Romania (compared to a British comparison in-group) and the open discrimination to which they are exposed in that society. Whereas previous research has tended to focus on either anger *or* fear, this study shows that in combination, these emotions can also intensify prejudice and discrimination and help to explain the particular pattern of behavioral responses.

However, for a group to prove a threat and evoke fear does not mean it has to have structural power or strength. The appraisal of out-group threat/strength could relate to ideology and symbolic threat, and a willingness to engage in acts of extremism associated with this. Groups such as Al Qaeda form a potent example of this kind of perceived threat and concerns about Islamic extremism might lead to greater generalized (emotional) prejudice toward Muslims, than a comparable out-group. This was the objective of a further study that investigated emotions among (non-Muslim) British people towards Muslims (Ispas, 2007). As predicted, results confirmed both greater fear- and anger-based emotional reactions towards a Muslim religious minority (British people of Pakistani origin) than towards a comparable non-Muslim religious minority (British people of Indian origin, Hindus), as well as greater avoidance of the Muslim minority. This is a clear example of where an emotion-based account has a clear explanatory advantage over traditional accounts of racism that assume prejudice towards non-white people or ethnic minorities in general to be the same. The emotional prejudice towards Muslims in particular can be understood in terms of the perceived threat that some people perceive radical Islam to pose at this point in history and over-generalize this to the Muslims as a whole.

Another example of the combinative power of anger and fear, or more precisely how fear or anxiety can amplify anger-based prejudice, is provided in recent research by Van Zomeren et al. (2007). This research examined emotional prejudice towards the homeless. Recall, this is a group that falls in the most negative "contemptuous prejudice" quadrant of Fiske et al.'s (2002) stereotype content model, characterized by low warmth and low competence. However, in terms of more specific emotional reactions, it is another out-group that may, under certain conditions, evoke the potent combination of fear and anger that can underlie more extreme forms of prejudice and discrimination. In this study, we measured or manipulated factors relevant to both of these emotions. Specifically in Study 1, participants were asked to imagine a scenario in which they were confronted with some homeless people who either committed a rather mild social transgression (singing and asking for money) or, in a separate condition a much stronger and threatening transgression (demanding money in an intimidating fashion) calculated to evoke anger and also some fear (in this case weakness becomes strength to the extent that homeless people are perceived to have little to lose by confronting those who are well off). We also measured intergroup anxiety beforehand as a continuous indicator of fear. Reported anger towards the homeless people in the scenario was the main dependent variable.

As predicted, an interaction pattern emerged such that anger was generally high for the strong norm transgression across high and low levels of anxiety, but the anger sloped away more steeply as intergroup anxiety reduced for the milder transgression. This interaction pattern was replicated in a second study with a similar norm manipulation, in which participants actually expected to interact with a homeless person. Moreover, offensive action tendencies showed an identical interactive pattern. In this case, higher levels of fear (intergroup anxiety) combined with appraisals of high threat in the situation intensified the anger and confrontational approach behavior towards the homeless that resulted.

To summarize, although there is much value in looking at emotion "main effects" as explanations of prejudice, emotional combinations like fear and anger can help to explain the particular intensity of prejudice and discrimination towards groups that evoke these emotions. However, some emotions are quite pernicious in their own right and we now turn to one such emotion: schadenfreude.

### 8.3.2 *Malicious Emotions: Intergroup Schadenfreude as Prejudice*

In the previous section we considered the emotions of anger and fear as emotional dimensions of prejudice. Although we have argued this has much value from the perspective of group emotions theory, there is still a sense in which these emotions, although part of a pattern of prejudice, are not prejudiced in themselves. Prejudice after all means to "prejudge," and anger and fear are primary or basic emotions that we share with other animals, and so there is perhaps not the element of intention or malice aforethought that we associate with prejudice (Spears & Leach, 2004). Emotions specifically designed to harm the out-group would help us to explain the more pernicious forms of prejudice and out-group hate (Brewer, 1999). Perhaps the archetypal malicious emotion is schadenfreude: the pleasure one feels at the misfortune or downfall of another. In this section, we describe a program of research that examines evidence for schadenfreude at the intergroup level as a form of emotional prejudice (Leach, Spears, Branscombe & Doosje, 2003, Leach & Spears, 2008; Spears & Leach, 2004, 2008).

Our research on schadenfreude has been influenced by the writing of Friedrich Nietzsche who saw schadenfreude as a form of imaginary revenge against a rival

(Nietzsche, 1887/1967) on the part of those who are not in a position to exact revenge directly. He referred to the "vengefulness of the impotent" (1967, p. 37) to refer to the fact that those who feel a sense of inferiority, and therefore are powerless in competing with the target group, can derive satisfaction at seeing the rival fall. In this respect schadenfreude is an emotion experienced from the sidelines as a passive bystander, distinguishing it from the more active emotion of gloating, which results from defeating or bettering the rival directly. To paraphrase Nietzsche, schadenfreude is about seeing others suffer, not making them suffer. The Nietzschean analysis is relevant as much to the intergroup level of social comparison and rivalry, although most previous research on this emotion has focused on the interpersonal level (e.g., Feather, 1994; Smith, Turner, Garonzik, Leach, Urch & Weston, 1996; Van Dijk, Ouwerkerk, Goslinga, Nieweg & Galluci, 2006). However, we think our Nietzschean view of schadenfreude makes it particularly relevant to the understanding of prejudice at the group level. In particular, this phenomenon might provide compelling evidence for the displacement models of prejudice that were popular in the psychodynamic era, such as scapegoating (e.g., Fromm, 1941; see Glick, 2008). Whereas the earlier approaches were individualistic and personality based, the group emotion approach, grounded in the social identity principles, allows us to revisit these ideas with a fresh theoretical impetus.

As with other group-based emotions, a first theoretical step is to show that schadenfreude can be experienced at the group level. This is important because not only was much earlier work on schadenfreude demonstrated at the interpersonal level, but some research in which group and category boundaries have been examined suggests that people may be more inclined to show schadenfreude towards (members of) the in-group or own category than towards the out-group. For example, recent research by Van Dijk et al. (2006), adapting a paradigm developed by Smith et al. (1996), showed that people tended to show more schadenfreude to a high-performing other who failed, when this was someone of their own gender rather than the opposite gender. This finding was interpreted in terms of the greater comparative relevance of others from one's own gender group (Tesser, 1988).

However, in these studies we think that the gender dimension as an intergroup context was not particularly salient and so (in some unpublished studies) we examined some conditions under which intergroup schadenfreude might be more likely. In the first study in this program we used the paradigm of Smith et al. and Van Dijk et al., in which women participants were told about a high-flying, but overconfident student who fails in an exam (a schadenfreude opportunity). We varied the gender of this target, and also manipulated the salience of gender. In the low salience conditions, prior to the schadenfreude opportunity, the participants read a Wikipedia article about global warming, whereas in the high gender salience condition they read an article about feminism. In the low gender salience condition we found slightly more schadenfreude to the female target, consistent with Van Dijk et al.'s findings, but for high gender salience this effect reversed with reliably more schadenfreude towards the male target.

Because we only engaged women participants in this study, the design was "incomplete," so in a further study we recruited both women and men as participants and chose a context in which we thought gender would be more chronically salient, namely a business domain (Newberry, 2006). Participants read a scenario in which a biased male team leader chose the target to head up a work-group according to his preference rather than on merit. This preferred person subsequently underperformed and was demoted, providing the schadenfreude opportunity. In this case we found clear evidence for inter-gender schadenfreude for both men and women: schadenfreude was higher towards the target of the *opposite* gender although this effect was somewhat stronger for women. In another study (Fuller, 2005) we looked at inter-gender schadenfreude in the realm of driving, another domain in which we thought gender might be quite salient, because of stereotypical male prejudice to women drivers in particular. In this case both men and women read about a (non-fatal) car accident suffered by a target male or female driver. Once again we found clear evidence of an inter-gender schadenfreude effect although in this case the effect was somewhat stronger for our male participants.

To summarize, these studies with gender, especially those using complete designs, provide compelling evidence that intergroup schadenfreude can occur and under the right conditions (e.g. high gender salience) can be stronger than intra-group schadenfreude effects. It could be that some of the asymmetries we found (greater intergroup schadenfreude for women in the business domain, but stronger for men in the driving domain) reflect the higher salience of perceived threat for these gender groups in these respective domains (the sense of disadvantage or sexism by women in the business domain, and encroachment by women of the "male" domain of driving). This remains speculative of course, but relevant to this issue, it is now time to return to our argument that intergroup schadenfreude may be particularly likely when the subject is suffering a threat to identity, and particularly where there is some sense of inferiority compared to the rival, which makes direct competition more dangerous and thus less opportune.

Our first attempt to examine this (and indeed our first attempt to demonstrate intergroup schadenfreude) used the domain of international soccer rivalry of the Dutch towards Germany as a context in which to examine evidence for the role of inferiority-based threat (Leach, Spears, Branscombe & Doosje, 2003). In our first study conducted in the aftermath of the 1998 soccer world cup, we manipulated inferiority threat in two different ways (in a 2 × 2 design). First, we manipulated chronic inferiority threat by asking our Dutch respondents a series of questions about the success of various nations in previous world cup tournaments, including the in-group (the Netherlands), and also Brazil and England (but not the target rival, Germany). The Dutch have never won the world cup and so this manipulation formed a painful reminder of this fact, while being forced to acknowledge the most successful team historically, Brazil (their nemesis in many tournaments), and even the fact that England has won the tournament once. In the acute inferiority threat condition, we simply asked respondents to rate how they felt about the game where Brazil had knocked them out of the tournament earlier that summer. These manipulations were then followed by the schadenfreude opportunity, rating their emotional reactions to the elimination of Germany by Croatia. As predicted, both manipulations of inferiority threat led to increases in subsequent ratings of schadenfreude, the pleasure at Germany's loss (and the effect of acute inferiority threat on schadenfreude was replicated in a second study).

In subsequent research (Leach & Spears, 2008) we went about gathering further direct evidence that it is the experience of the pain of in-group inferiority, which primarily predicts and explains intergroup schadenfreude towards third-party rivals. It is important to note that this forms a self-focused explanation (using the loss of the other to compensate for the pain of one's one inferiority), because most other established explanations of schadenfreude tend to take an other-focused perspective, variously explaining schadenfreude in terms of envy or coveting of the successful other (e.g., Smith et al., 1996), the anger and resentment at undeserved success of the target who get their come-uppance (e.g., Feather, 1991; Feather & Sherman, 2002), or dislike-based anger directed at the target (Hareli & Weiner, 2002). Reminiscent of some of the classical psychodynamic theories of prejudice, we were interested in showing that schadenfreude says as much or more about the *experiencer* than about the target.

In some preliminary (and as yet unpublished) studies we remained in the same sporting domain of Dutch soccer of the earlier studies. The first study took advantage of the fact that the Dutch had failed to qualify for the 2002 World Cup, a very painful and shaming experience for such a proud soccer nation. We measured this shame (albeit with a single item) after reading about the painful loss to Ireland in the qualifying competition that put them out of this tournament and then subsequently measured pleasure towards a German loss to England in another qualifying game – the schadenfreude opportunity. As predicted, the pain of the inferiority was a reliable predictor of schadenfreude and this was much stronger than and unmoderated by other predictors of schadenfreude, such as the dislike of the out-group (cf. Hareli & Weiner, 2002).

Despite this loss Germany progressed to the tournament stage of the World Cup and despite their poor form going in, they made it to the final, which they then lost. This provided us with another schadenfreude opportunity for our Dutch participants, examined in a further follow-up study. We measured the pain of in-group inferiority among the Dutch with a better multiple-item scale and also assessed a fuller range of the competing (other-focused) explanations for schadenfreude. Once again the pain of chronic inferiority was the strongest predictor of schadenfreude towards the out-group loss including out-group dislike (cf. Hareli & Weiner, 2002) and the perceived illegitimacy of the rival's success (cf. Feather & Sherman, 2002), which was only marginally significant.

In subsequent studies (Leach & Spears, 2008) we gathered additional evidence for our theoretical model with its central predictive role for the pain of in-group inferiority, addressing some of the limitations of the earlier studies in the process. First we developed an inter-university quiz competition paradigm that allowed us to get greater experimental control over some of the key variables (see also Spears & Leach, 2004, 2007, 2008). In particular, our goal was to experimentally tease apart in-group failure from out-group success, which are typically confounded, and more specifically to set up in-group inferiority before any knowledge of the rival's success becomes apparent. This paradigm also allowed us to examine the illegitimacy of in-group inferiority (as opposed to the pain about this) as well as the illegitimacy of out-group success, together with a range of the other (other-focused) explanations for schadenfreude (envy, anger at the rival's success, but also the pain of inferiority *implied by the rival's success*: a feeling Nietzsche referred to as *ressentiment*).

In this paradigm, we explained that the Dutch inter-university quiz tournament involved two separate pools, A and B, comprising separate round-robin leagues within each pool, and with the top two teams meeting in the grand final (similar to two league format for the "World Series" of baseball). This allowed us to set up the inferiority of the in-group (University of Amsterdam: UvA), who displayed a poor performance playing in Pool A, independently from the success of the cross-town rival (the Free University: VU) who won Pool B, before proceeding to the grand final (where they lost: the schadenfreude opportunity).

In the first study we varied the order in which participants heard about in-group failure and the rival out-group's success. In one condition, these were both presented before the schadenfreude opportunity (and could therefore causally affect this) and in a second condition, the information about in-group inferiority was only presented after the schadenfreude opportunity and so could not affect it. As predicted, in the condition where the pain of in-group inferiority could affect subsequent schadenfreude in this performance domain, it was a strong predictor of this emotion, whereas none of the other-focused explanations produced notable effects. Moreover, in the condition where the pain of inferiority was assessed *after* schadenfreude and where the other-focused explanations were thus advantaged, their effects were not stronger.

In a follow-up study that further refined the paradigm, we manipulated the (il) legitimacy of both in-group failure, and also the illegitimacy of out-group success relevant to this explanation as a basis for schadenfreude (Feather & Sherman, 2002). Specifically we provided feedback that the questions used during the inter-university quiz were provided by Professors at the home university (an illegitimate advantage) or not (a legitimate procedure). Once again the pain of domain inferiority was a strong predictor of schadenfreude. Also, consistent with the *ressentiment* pathway, the pain of inferiority had an indirect effect on schadenfreude via anger at the out-group's success. However, the illegitimacy of in-group pain was not a reliable predictor, and the various other-focused explanations did not produce notable effects either.

To summarize, this line of research shows that actual inferiority threats provided by past poor performance (Leach et al., 2003) and the perceived pain of inferiority felt as a result of such appraisals (Leach & Spears, 2008) are key factors that explain the occurrence and intensity of schadenfreude felt at the failure of a third party, who was not even responsible for establishing this inferiority. In this sense we provide some evidence for a self-focused account of emotional prejudice that is reminiscent of classic psychoanalytic accounts of prejudice based on displacement and scapegoating (e.g., Fromm, 1941; see Glick, 2008). Although the psychodynamic and personality accounts underlying these earlier theories have fallen from favor, we show that taking an group-level emotion-based approach can be fruitful in understanding how prejudice can arise, even towards groups where there is no obvious direct case for the prejudice other than rivalry. This perhaps says much more about the prejudiced perceiver than it says about the target. This is not to say that intergroup schadenfreude will never arise in cases where there is a more direct relation with rivals who are directly responsible for inflicting defeat on the out-group. In such cases we have also found evidence that direct losses to the out-group rival can increase subsequent schadenfreude towards misfortunes suffered by the rival, and that this is mediated by the dejection at the past loss, the more specific form of pain at in-group inferiority in such situations (Leach & Spears, 2009; Spears & Leach, 2004, 2007, 2008).

More recently, we have moved back from the control of the laboratory to see how our approach to intergroup schadenfreude can be applied to real life groups where there may be status and/or power differences that feed an inferiority complex that might make direct challenges to the out-group difficult, but schadenfreude a more viable form of "imaginary revenge." One context in which we have been studying this is the relation between the Welsh and their more powerful English neighbors within the UK. In a number of studies, the evidence we have gathered so far is that the Welsh do indeed show evidence of greater schadenfreude towards English misfortune (in the sporting domains of soccer and rugby for example) than the English do towards the Welsh. For example, in one study, the Welsh were much more likely to derive satisfaction from an English sporting loss (both in soccer and rugby) than towards an equivalent loss by either Scottish or Irish national teams, whereas the English reported low levels of schadenfreude to losses by Welsh, Scottish and Irish teams. Further research points to the important role of emotions associated with rivalry and disempowerment (inferiority, "impotence"), and a perceived lack of respect as key factors in the high levels of Welsh schadenfreude towards the English.

It is perhaps noticeable that we have mentioned little in the way of action tendencies or behavior in this section on schadenfreude. This is largely because the behavioral signature of this emotion, consistent with this passive bystander perspective, is to do very little beyond (often secretly) enjoying the misfortune of the rival. Indeed our research comparing schadenfreude and gloating – the more active pleasure derived from defeating a rival – confirms schadenfreude to be a much more passive and less intense emotion with few clear behavioral tendencies (Leach, Spears, Manstead, Thompson & Thatcher, 2009). However, it is interesting to consider the relationship between schadenfreude and more general forms of prejudice and discrimination, and their associated action tendencies (e.g. in terms of approach and avoidance). This was one objective of research by Heim (2007), who examined English feelings of schadenfreude towards the loss of their big rival Germany (again) to Italy in the 2006 world cup, after first being reminded of the English loss to Portugal (an acute inferiority threat). There are two interesting possibilities here concerning the relationship between schadenfreude and more general measures of prejudice. On the one hand, as an emotional form a prejudice in itself, schadenfreude could be expected to be associated with high levels of prejudice and related behavior. However, it could also be that having the opportunity to express schadenfreude serves the self-focused goal of exacting the imaginary revenge that assuages one's group inferiority, thereby reducing the need to feel or express more general forms of prejudice (i.e., negative attitudes towards the out-group). To test this idea, this study manipulated the order in which schadenfreude and prejudice were measured after the acute inferiority threat. We also introduced a norm manipulation in which in the experimental condition participants received feedback that other English people had shown pleasure at the German loss, to see if this would increase schadenfreude and prejudice (although this condition could of course only affect prejudice where it was measured after schadenfreude).

This study actually provides support for both of these ideas. First, the degree of schadenfreude and prejudice were related: those reporting higher levels of schadenfreude also reported more negative attitudes towards Germany, and also higher levels of both approach and avoidance action tendencies. Schadenfreude was also more strongly predictive of negative intergroup attitudes towards Germany in the condition with normative feedback of high schadenfreude, legitimating this emotion, than in control condition. Approach and avoidance action tendencies also showed a stronger relation with schadenfreude when validated by the norm than not. More interesting perhaps was the finding that, in the condition where schadenfreude preceded the prejudice measures, it actually significantly *reduced* the prejudiced attitudes towards Germany, although approach and avoidance action tendencies were unaffected. A second study in which we again manipulated the norm validating in-group schadenfreude once again showed a clear relation between schadenfreude and prejudice measures in general.

In summary, this study shows that schadenfreude hangs together with other more general and blatant forms of prejudice and prejudice-related action tendencies (Mackie et al., 2000), and this relation can be strengthened when normatively validated. However, interestingly, there is also some evidence that having the opportunity to express schadenfreude can reduce more general prejudiced attitudes. Although we have been promoting here the idea that schadenfreude is a malign emotion and form of prejudice, it may also have a more benign side, if it acts as an outlet preventing more overt forms of prejudices under certain conditions. Once again this fits with the classical displacement ideas of prejudice – once this is satisfied, it may not be necessary (Crandall & Eshleman, 2003; Glick, 2008).

### *8.3.3 Summary*

In this section we have presented evidence from our lab' supporting the group emotion approach to prejudice and discrimination and argued that this framework adds much to our understanding and specification of prejudice, and the conflict between groups more generally. In the first subsection we extended earlier work that has distinguished between anger and fear-based emotional prejudice (e.g., Mackie et al., 2000, 2004) to argue that the combination of these emotions may be particularly potent and help to explain (and justify) some of the more extreme and blatant forms of prejudice, such as that directed at Roma people in Romania, Muslims, and the homeless. In the second subsection we focused on a single emotion that is more malicious in its own right, namely (intergroup) schadenfreude. Here we argue, in contrast to most other explanations of schadenfreude that are largely concerned with the interpersonal domain, and that emphasize aspects of the target (other-focused explanations), schadenfreude at the intergroup level, especially when more intensely experienced, can often reflect and indeed address more self-focused concerns such as perceived inferiority. There is clear link here to displacement models of prejudice, albeit framed in a more social and emotionally grounded framework. In this respect, the emotion based group level analysis breaks new ground while reinvigorating some old themes.

## 8.4 Intergroup Emotion and Social Change: Putting the Passion into Protest

We now address the second key theme that emerges from the field of intergroup relations, and social identity theory, namely the question of when and how disadvantaged groups challenge their position through collective action. Once again our main theoretical and empirical argument is that introducing group emotion provides added analytic and explanatory value to the social identity framework. However, before we develop this argument it is important to acknowledge a theoretical debt to another influential intergroup approach that does accord a role to group level emotions, and also predates intergroup emotion theory and social identity theory, namely relative deprivation theory. Although the early research in this tradition did not always explicitly measure emotion, the concept of resentment at group disadvantage was implied in early accounts of fraternal deprivation (Runciman, 1966) and has become increasingly central to the assessment of this concept (e.g., Crosby, 1976; Mummendey et al., 1999; Smith & Kessler, 2004). Such work has therefore also been an important influence on our attempts to specify the role of emotion in mediating reactions of group disadvantage, along with the analyses provided by social identity theory. Recall that the basic SIT analysis of disadvantaged groups is that under conditions of illegitimacy and instability they will envisage cognitive alternatives to the status quo, and engage in direct social competition aimed at social change, such as collective action. It is apposite that these two elements of illegitimacy and instability correspond to two separate paths in our model, incorporating group-based emotions, designed to explain such motivations to engage in collective action (Van Zomeren, Spears, Fischer & Leach, 2004).

The dual path model also builds on the distinction made by Lazarus in his appraisal theory between emotion-focused coping and problem-focused coping (e.g., Lazarus, 1991). Translating these ideas to the plight of the disadvantaged and the conditions under which they might engage in collective action, Van Zomeren et al. (2004) proposed that problem-focused coping will arise when positive appraisals of the group's ability to challenge the higher status group or powerful authority are made. In terms of social identity theory this might occur under conditions of instability, although the more agent-centered or self-focused appraisal of the power to transform one's situation is group strength, power, or "collective efficacy." Our research confirms that perceptions of group efficacy, buttressed by appraisals of "social action support," the perception that others are also willing to stand up and be counted, is one key process route predicting collective action (Van Zomeren et al., 2004).

However, because our main focus in this chapter is on group-based emotions, we will focus here primarily on the second, emotion-focused coping route to collective action. A key appraisal predicting emotional reactions of the disadvantaged is clearly the perceived injustice of the situation (or indeed the unjust behavior of the out-group itself). This reasoning is again very reminiscent of social identity theory where the illegitimacy of status relations are a key component in generating the cognitive alternatives to the status quo that motivate striving towards social change. However, as in the case of emotional prejudice, there is no explicit group emotion-based account in SIT of how the perception of injustice might be translated into action. The dual path model, building on relative deprivation themes, intergroup emotion theory, and especially the emotion-focused coping principles of the stress and coping model, argues that group anger will be a key emotion that mediates the appraisals of injustice or illegitimacy on collective action.

It is interesting to note here a difference with the reasoning of Mackie and colleagues (2000, 2004) who argued that group strength is a key appraisal underlying anger (in contrast to fear for example; see the earlier section on prejudice). As already described, group strength, qua group efficacy, forms part of a separate path to group action in our model, that does not necessarily involve group-based emotion (if you have group efficacy there is no need to invoke anger or indeed emotion, so our reasoning goes). Although we are *not* claiming that group strength *never* feeds into anger, we do think that the injustice appraisal is more fundamental or primary in evoking anger, hence our separation of these two routes in the dual path model. Of course this is partly an empirical question and one, which we test empirically in a number of studies, reported below. However, before getting to these details, it is useful to note that the dual path model elaborates and extends the social identity based account of collective action based on appraisals of illegitimacy and instability; whereas status instability has close conceptual links to appraisal of group efficacy, the addition of emotions to the illegitimacy appraisal clearly adds a missing mediating link that puts the passion into protest.

In the first study testing these ideas Van Zomeren et al. (2004), a student sample at the University of Amsterdam were presented with the prospect of cuts and a proposal to raise student fees by € 600 to add to the existing fees of around € 1,500, something clearly expected to anger the students. However, we predicted this anger to be exacerbated by a manipulation of procedural injustice in which students would not be consulted over this proposal (i.e. no voice; high procedural injustice) versus were to be consulted (voice, a more legitimate procedure). We expected the unjust procedure to spark anger leading to stronger intentions to engage in collective action. In a second manipulation, designed to establish the group-based nature of the emotion (cf. Gordijn et al., 2001), we presented these proposals as applying at their own university and thus affecting their own group, or being implemented at a rival university (the Free, VU) and therefore being less group-relevant.

Results clearly supported the dual path model for the conditions in which the in-group (UvA students) was disadvantaged. Group efficacy predicted collective action, and group efficacy was predicted by perceptions of social action support in line with the model. Importantly, the manipulation of injustice had little effect on this efficacy route to action. By contrast it did provoke group-based anger, although interestingly the path model showed this effect to be mediated by perceptions of opinion support (the belief that other students shared participants' own views opposing the proposal). Anger also then predicted collective action tendencies. The overall path model representing these two paths (and without any predicted path between anger and efficacy) exhibited very good overall fit. By contrast, the comparable model for the out-group disadvantaged condition revealed few of these paths to be significant and exhibited poor model fit, consistent with the argument that the in-group (and in-group emotions) are not invoked in this case.

An interesting feature of this study is that, in addition to showing the clear and contrasting routes to collective action based on efficacy and emotion, there was also a clear differentiation between the role of social action support and opinion support feeding into these two different routes respectively. We had anticipated the role of action support (which relates to appraisals of efficacy after all: putting your money where your mouth is, to quote the title of our paper). Perhaps less obvious was the role played by perception of opinion support in relation to appraisals of illegitimacy and its effect on anger. However, in retrospect, this makes a lot of sense: knowing that others share your opinion, and appraisals of injustice, make it likely they will share your anger, and this may indeed socially validate this emotional response (it is group-based anger after all). This is an example of a "social appraisal" (Manstead & Fischer, 2001) appropriate to the group level of analysis regulating group behavior via a group emotion. However, opinion support and the anger experienced do not necessarily say anything about the group's efficacy, or ability to follow up on this (although the idea that collective anger is socially validating and therefore empowering is an interesting possibility that requires research attention).

In two follow-up studies we aimed to replicate the basic effects and structural model of our first experiment, while systematically manipulating opinion support (Study 2) and social action support (Study 3) and maintaining the same procedural injustice manipulation designed to evoke the group based anger in both studies. To cut a long story short, these studies replicated the overall dual path model in both cases, and distinguished anger-based and efficacy-based routes to collective action tendencies. Moreover, as predicted, social opinion support fed into the anger route in both studies whereas social action support fed into the efficacy route (although opinion support also had an effect on group efficacy in Study 3).

One possible criticism of these studies is that they focus on intentions to engage in collective action (i.e. action tendencies rather than actual behavior). While this is true it is well known that intentions do reliably predict behavior and this is confirmed by a meta-analysis of the collective action literature (Van Zomeren, Postmes & Spears, 2008). Further work using the dual path model confirms that collective behavior is predicted by action tendencies (Sweetman, Spears & Livingstone, 2009a).

Subsequent research developed within the dual path framework has extended the model in various ways. For example, a series of studies by Sweetman, Spears, and Livingstone (2009b), has applied the model to what we call "solidarity based collective action," that is action on behalf of the disadvantaged group from those in the advantaged group, or a third party of intermediate or ambivalent status (see also Thomas & McGarty, 2009). These studies employed both minimal group identities and existing university-based group identities to test these ideas. The goal here was to show that members of privileged groups could themselves also be motivated to engage in support for disadvantaged groups, at least when they perceive their plight as illegitimate, thereby provoking similar emotions such as anger, albeit vicariously on their behalf. For example, one study examined how Cardiff University students felt and reacted towards feedback in an official report that graduates from their university were likely to enjoy many career benefits shared with other top UK universities (Oxford and Cambridge), or were categorized as part of groups of universities whose graduates would suffer disadvantage, or were not represented in the survey at all (a third party or intermediate position).

Importantly, although the *means* differed, the overall (dual path) structural model did not differ for advantaged and third party groups in the studies. Moreover, if the privileged group was characterized as being responsible for the disadvantaged position of the lower status group, the appraisal of injustice and consequent anger and action tendencies were strengthened. There is an interesting comparison to be made here with the study of Van Zomeren et al. (2004; Study 1b) reported above, in which the dual path model did *not* hold for a rival out-group (cf. Gordijn et al., 2001). However, in that case, the out-group manipulation made it clear that the issue was of little direct relevance to the participants themselves, and the target group was a rival of equal status and so did not evoke the injustice appraisal of illegitimate inequality as here. A study by Thomas and McGarty (2009), which found moral outrage at environmental damage to be a significant predictor of collective action intentions is also slightly different to the solidarity-based collective action found here: whereas moral outrage is an other-focused emotion (Leach, Snider & Iyer, 2002), the anger found in the case of the advantaged group is likely to be self-focused, especially where the in-group is seen as responsible for the out-group's disadvantage. It is heartening that bystander groups and even the advantaged groups themselves can feel and act on behalf of the disadvantaged group, and this points to the fact that many liberation struggles for group equality have also involved the support of members of the privileged and powerful groups themselves.

Extending the process model to the advantaged and third party groups also alerted us to the possibility that group emotions other than anger (and moral outrage) might play a role in motivated group based action, or just as relevant, in impeding it. In contrast, emotions such as admiration and awe (see Haidt, 2003) may serve to justify and legitimate the position of the advantaged group, thereby reducing the tendency to act on its behalf. Indeed, this possibility need not only apply to the advantaged and third party groups, but could be a factor in helping to explain why disadvantaged groups themselves do not always act collectively in their own interests (an important part of the puzzle, as much as explaining action). A series of studies have now produced support for other-praising emotions such as admiration and awe in attenuating collective action tendencies, and once again this forms part of a process model that differs little depending on where people are members of advantaged, disadvantaged, or an intermediate group (Sweetman et al., 2009a, b).

Nor is anger the only emotion that can positively motivate forms of collective action on behalf of the group. Recent research by Tausch et al. (2008) shows that where the appraisals of a group disadvantage go beyond mere injustice and suggest that the out-group has acted immorally, and thus in ways that confer some moral superiority to the aggrieved group, this can stimulate emotions such as contempt that justify forms of group action that are more extreme and aggressive. We put this idea to the test in the context of students in Germany who were (in some cases quite literally) up in arms about the proposal to allow regional states to charge for student fees, overturning federal law, and making the chance to study at university more difficult for many. This led to a wave of protests and we gathered data on a representative student sample in Hessen in 2007. As well as measuring support for normative or constitutional acceptable forms of protest (e.g. signing petitions, going on marches), we also distinguished this from more anti-normative forms of action such as resistance (unconstitutional but non-violent action such as boycotts, blocking buildings, etc.) and violence (e.g., arson, attacks on police).

In line with the dual path model, anger (and efficacy) led to greater support for protest and resistance, but not to support for the more extreme forms of violent action. However, perceptions injustice were also strongly associated with a sense of moral superiority, which fed feelings of contempt for the authorities that reliably predicted support for violence (but not the more constitutional forms of action). Interestingly, whereas group efficacy was positively related to protest and resistance, it *negatively* predicted violence, suggesting that people engaging this strategy are likely to see their situations as more desperate and requiring more desperate measures (Spears, Scheepers & van Zomeren, 2009).

To summarize, although originally conceptualized to focus on anger as the motivator of collective behavior, the subsequent research makes clear that the dual path model can be extended to include a wider repertoire of group-based emotions that help to explain the motivation to engage in action, but also to withdraw or even oppose it and the different kinds behaviors that may be motivated by them. This model works well for the groups most directly affected, but can also be applied to cases of vicarious emotional support on their behalf by third parties and even members of the advantaged or powerful out-group themselves. This provides a richer model for analyzing the specificity of behaviors involved in collective action and social change that extends earlier intergroup approaches that lack this emotional specification such as social identity theory, or which have a more limited emotional focus, such as relative deprivation theory.

## 8.5 Concluding Remarks

In this chapter we have tried to make a case that the realm of intergroup emotions is more than the sum of the parts. An analysis of group-based emotions clearly extends and enriches our understanding of intergroup relations. Although less explicitly focused on the benefits to emotion theory, we think there is also a strong case that taking an intergroup perspective emphasizes the social nature of emotions in validating experience and regulating behavior at the group level, in ways that are perhaps not acknowledged by more intra-psychic and even interpersonal approaches to emotion. For example the concept of social appraisal (Manstead & Fischer, 2001), the idea that the emotional reactions of others inform our own emotional experience, has hitherto largely been studied in interpersonal contexts. Returning to our main intergroup focus, group emotions help to explain the intensity and extremity of some forms prejudice and discrimination, and also the diverse forms these can take. However, emotions are not restricted to malicious and malign aspects of intergroup life, but consistent with the social change agenda of social identity theory, they are also at the heart of attempts to liberate the group from its disadvantage.

## References

Adorno, T.W., Frenkel-Brunswick, E., Levinson, D.J., & Sanford, R.N. (1950) *The authoritarian personality*. New York: Harper and Row.

Alexander, M.G., Brewer, M.B., & Hermann, R.K. (1999) Images and affect: A functional analysis of out-group stereotypes. *Journal of Personality and Social Psychology*, 77, 78–93.

Brewer, M.B. (1999) The psychology of prejudice: In-group love or out-group hate? *Journal of Social Issues*, 55, 429–444.

Cottrell, C.A., Neuberg, S.L. (2005) Different emotional reactions to different groups: A sociofunctional threat-based approach to "prejudice." *Journal of Personality and Social Psychology*, 88, 770–789.

Crandall, C.S. & Eshleman, A. (2003) A justification-suppression model of the expression and experience of prejudice. *Psychological Bulletin*, 129, 414–446.

Crosby, F.J. (1976) A model of egotistical relative deprivation. *Psychological Review*, 83, 85–113.

Dijker, A. (1987) Emotional reactions to ethnic minorities. *European Journal of Social Psychology*, 17, 305–325.

Doosje, B., Branscombe, N.R., Spears, R., & Manstead, A.S.R. (1998) Guilty by association: When one's group has a negative history. *Journal of Personality and Social Psychology*, 75, 872–886.

Feather, N.T. (1994) Attitudes toward high achievers and reactions to their fall: Theory and research concerning tall poppies. *Advances in Experimental Social Psychology*, 26, 1–73.

Feather, N.T. & Sherman, R. (2002) Envy, resentment, *schadenfreude*, and sympathy: Reactions to deserved and undeserved achievement and subsequent failure. *Personality and Social Psychology Bulletin*, 28, 953–961.

Fiske, S.T., Cuddy, A.J.C., Glick, P., & Xu, J. (2002) A model of (often mixed) stereotype content: Competence and warmth respectively follow from perceived status and competition. *Journal of Personality and Social Psychology*, 82, 878–902.
Frijda, N.H. (1986) *The emotions*. Cambridge: University Press.
Fromm, E. (1941) *Escape from freedom*. New York, NY: Holt, Rinehart & Winston.
Fuller, D. (2005) Gender and intergroup schadenfreude in the driving domain. Unpublished project report, Cardiff: Cardiff University.
Glick, P. (2008) When neighbors blame neighbors: Scapegoating and the breakdown of ethnic relations. In V.M. Esses & R.A. Vernon (Eds.). *Why neighbors kill: Explaining the breakdown of ethnic relations* (pp. 123–146). Oxford: Blackwell.
Glick, P. & Fiske, S.T. (2001) Ambivalent sexism. In M.P. Zanna (Ed.). *Advances in experimental social psychology* (vol. 33, pp. 115–188). Thousand Oaks, CA: Academic Press.
Gordijn, E.H., Wigboldus, D., & Yzerbyt, V.Y. (2001) Emotional consequences of categorizing victims of negative out-group behavior as in-group or out-group. *Group Processes and Intergroup Relations*, 4, 317–326.
Haidt, J. (2003) The moral emotions. In R.J. Davidson, K.R. Scherer & H.H. Goldsmith (Eds.). *Handbook of affective sciences* (pp. 852–870). Oxford: Oxford University Press.
Hamilton, D.L. (1981) Stereotyping and intergroup behavior: some thoughts on the cognitive approach. In D.L. Hamilton (Ed.). *Cognitive processes in stereotyping and intergroup behavior.* Hillsdale, NJ: Erlbaum.
Hareli, S. & Weiner, B. (2002) Dislike and envy as antecedents of pleasure at another's misfortune. *Motivation and Emotion*, 26, 257–277.
Heim, H. (2007) *Intergroup schadenfreude, attitudes and discrimination; the effect of norm, opportunity and audience*. Unpublished project report. Cardiff: Cardiff University.
Ispas, A. (2007) *Prejudice and intergroup conflict: the strategic attribution of anger and fear in the context of intergroup relations*. Unpublished MPhil dissertation. Cardiff: Cardiff University.
Jackman, M.R. (1994) *The velvet glove: Paternalism and conflict in gender, class, and race relations*. Berkeley, CA: University of California Press.
Lazarus, R.S. (1991) *Emotion and adaptation*. New York, NY: Oxford University Press.
Lazarus, R. S. & Folkman, S. F. (1984). Stress, Appraisal, and Coping. New York: Springer.
Leach, C.W., Snider, S., & Iyer, A. (2002) "Poisoning the consciences of the fortunate": The experience of relative advantage and support for social equality. In I. Walker & H.J. Smith (Eds.). *Relative deprivation: specification, development, and integration* (pp. 136–163). New York, NY: Cambridge University.
Leach, C.W. & Spears, R. (2008) "A vengefulness of the impotent": The pain of in-group inferiority and schadenfreude toward successful out-groups. *Journal of Personality and Social Psychology*, 95, 1383–1396.
Leach, C.W. & Spears, R. (2009) Dejection at in-group defeat and schadenfreude toward second- and third-party out-groups. *Emotion*, 9, 659–665.
Leach, C.W., Spears, R., Branscombe, N.R., & Doosje, B. (2003) Malicious pleasure: Schadenfreude at the suffering of another group. *Journal of Personality and Social Psychology*, 84, 932–943.
Leach, C.W., Spears, R., Manstead, A.S.R., Thompson, R., & Thatcher, B. (2009) *Schadenfreude versus gloating at interpersonal and intergroup levels*. Manuscript in preparation. Cardiff: Cardiff University.
Mackie, D.M., Devos, T., & Smith, E.R. (2000) Intergroup emotions: Explaining offensive action tendencies in an intergroup context. *Journal of Personality and Social Psychology*, 79,602–616.
Mackie, D.M., Silver, L.A., & Smith, E.R. (2004) Intergroup emotions: Emotion as an intergroup phenomenon. In C.W. Leach, & L.Z. Tiedens (Eds.). *The social life of emotions* (pp. 227–245). Cambridge: Cambridge University Press.
Maitner, A.T., Mackie, D.M., & Smith, E.R. (2006) Evidence for the regulatory function of intergroup emotion: Emotional consequences of implemented or impeded intergroup action tendencies. *Journal of Experimental Social Psychology*, 42, 720–728.

Manstead, A.S.R., & Fischer, A.H. (2001) Social appraisal: The social world as object of and influence on appraisal processes. In K.R. Scherer & A. Schorr (Eds.). *Appraisal processes in emotion: Theory, methods, research* (pp. 221–232). London: Oxford University Press.

Mummendey, A., Kessler, T., Klink, A., & Mielke, R. (1999) Strategies to cope with negative social identity: Predictions by social identity theory and relative deprivation theory. *Journal of Personality and Social Psychology*, 76, 229–245.

Newberry, J. (2006) *The salience of sexism in reversing the gender bias in schadenfreude*. Unpublished project report. Cardiff: Cardiff University.

Nietzsche, F. (1887/1967, 1996) *On the genealogy of morals* (Translated by W. Kaufmann & R.J. Hollingdale, originally published 1887). New York: Random House.

Pettigrew, T.F. (1981) Extending the stereotype concept. In D.L. Hamilton (Ed.). *Cognitive processes in stereotyping and intergroup behavior* (pp. 303–331). Hillsdale, NJ: Erlbaum.

Runciman, W.G. (1966) *Relative deprivation and social justice: A study of attitudes to social inequality in twentieth-century England*. Berkeley: University of California Press.

Smith, E.R. (1993) Social identity and social emotions: Toward a new conceptualization of prejudice. In D.M. Mackie & D.L. Hamilton (Eds.). *Affect, cognition, and stereotyping* (pp. 297–315). San Diego, CA: Academic Press.

Smith, H.J. & Kessler, T. (2004) Group-based emotions and intergroup behavior: The case of relative deprivation (pp. 292–313). In L.Z. Tiedens & C.W. Leach (Eds.). *The social life of emotions*. New York: Cambridge University Press.

Smith, R.H., Turner, T.J., Garonzik, R., Leach, C.W., Urch, V., & Weston, C. (1996) Envy and *schadenfreude*. *Personality and Social Psychology Bulletin*, 22, 158–168.

Spears, R. & Leach, C.W. (2007) *Inter-group schadenfreude through the bogus pipeline: A portal to the pleasure and the pain*. Unpublished Manuscript. Cardiff: Cardiff University.

Spears, R. & Leach, C.W. (2004) Intergroup schadenfreude: conditions and consequences. In L.Z. Tiedens & C.W. Leach (Eds.). *The social life of emotions* (pp. 336–355). New York: Cambridge University Press.

Spears, R. & Leach, C.W. (2008) Why neighbors don't stop the killing: Group-based schadenfreude. In V.M. Esses & R.A. Vernon (Eds.). *Why neighbors kill: Explaining the breakdown of ethnic relations* (pp. 93–120). Oxford: Blackwell.

Spears, R., Jetten, J., Scheepers, D., & Cihangir, S. (2009) Creative distinctiveness: Explaining in-group bias in minimal groups. In: S. Otten, T. Kessler & K. Sassenberg (Eds.). *Intergroup relations: the role of motivation and emotion* (pp.23–40). New York: Psychology Press.

Spears, R., Scheepers, D., & van Zomeren, M. (2009) *Nothing to lose*. Ms in preparation. Cardiff: Cardiff University.

Sweetman, J.P., Spears, R. & Livingstone, A.G. (2009a) *Salience of intragroup power relations leads to intergroup solidarity: The role of anger and other praising emotions in protest behavior*. Ms in preparation. Cardiff: Cardiff University.

Sweetman, J.P., Spears, R. & Livingstone, A.G. (2009b) *Independent Effects of Ideology, Responsibility and Group Status on Collective Action: Anger Leads to Challenge While Admiration Promotes Apathy Towards Inequality*. Ms in preparation. Cardiff: Cardiff University.

Tajfel, H. (1978) Interindividual behavior and intergroup behavior. In H. Tajfel (Ed.). *Differentiation between groups: Studies in the social psychology of intergroup relations* (pp. 27–60). London: Academic Press.

Tajfel, H. & Turner, J.C. (1979) An integrative theory of intergroup conflict. In W.G. Austin & S. Worchel (Eds.). *The social psychology of intergroup relations* (pp. 33–47). Monterey: Brooks/Cole.

Tausch, N., Becker, J., Spears, R., & Christ, O. (2008) *Emotion and efficacy pathways to normative and non-normative collective action: A study in the context of student protests in Germany*. Paper presented at Groups pre-conference, EASP, Croatia.

Tesser, A. (1988) Toward a self-evaluation maintenance model of social behavior. In L. Berkowitz (Ed.). *Advances in experimental social psychology*, 21, 181–227. San Diego, CA: Academic Press.

Thomas, E.F. & McGarty, C.A. (2009) The role of efficacy and moral outrage norms in creating the potential for international development activism through group-based interaction. *British Journal of Social Psychology*, 48, 115–134.

Van Dijk, W., Ouwerkerk, J.W., Goslinga, Nieweg, M., & Gallucci, M. (2006) When people fall from grace: Reconsidering the role of envy in schadenfreude. *Emotion*, 6, 156–160.

Van Zomeren, M., Fischer, A., & Spears, R. (2007) Testing the limits of tolerance: How intergroup anxiety amplifies negative and offensive responses to out-group-initiated contact. *Personality and Social Psychology Bulletin*, 33. 1686–1699.

Van Zomeren, M., Postmes, T., & Spears, R. (2008) Toward an integrative social identity model of collective action: A quantitative research synthesis of three socio-psychological perspectives. *Psychological Bulletin*, 34, 504–535.

Van Zomeren, M., Spears, R., Fischer, A., & Leach, C.W. (2004) Put your money where your mouth is! Explaining collective action tendencies through group-based anger and group efficacy. *Journal of Personality and Social Psychology*, 87, 649–664.

# Chapter 9
# The Social Sharing of Emotions in Interpersonal and in Collective Situations: Common Psychosocial Consequences

**Bernard Rimé, Dario Paez, Patrick Kanyangara, and Vincent Yzerbyt**

## 9.1 Introduction

Research on "the social sharing of emotion" documented the fact that following an emotional episode, the person who experienced it talks with others about this episode in 80–95% of the cases (for reviews, see Rimé, 2009; Rimé, Philippot, Boca, & Mesquita, 1992; Rimé, Finkenauer, Luminet, Zech, & Philippot, 1998). This propensity is not dependent on the subject's level of education. It was observed at comparable importance in countries as diverse as Asian, North American, and European ones (Mesquita, 1993; Rimé, Yogo, & Pennebaker, 1996; Singh-Manoux, 1998; Singh-Manoux & Finkenauer, 2001; Yogo & Onoe, 1998). Episodes which involved fear, or anger, or sadness were shared as often as episodes of happiness or of love. However, emotional episodes involving shame and guilt were shared at a somewhat lesser degree (Finkenauer & Rimé, 1998). Laboratory studies confirmed that exposure to an emotion-eliciting condition provokes sharing (Luminet, Bouts, Delie, Manstead, & Rimé, 2000). Progressive extinction is the normal fate of social sharing. More intense episodes are shared more repetitively and for a longer period (Rimé et al., 1998).

## 9.2 The Cathartic View of Emotional Expression

A widespread belief holds that *merely talking* about an emotional experience would dissolve the emotional impact of this experience and would thus grant emotional recovery. Various studies examined how far the mere fact of sharing a given emotional experience had such an effect. The impact of the emotional experience was assessed using indices, such as felt emotions when reaccessing the specific episode,

B. Rimé (✉)
Department of Psychology, University of Louvain, 10, Place Cardinal Mercier,
B 1348 Louvain-la-Neuve, Belgium
e-mail: Bernard.Rime@uclouvain.be

I. Nyklíček et al. (eds.), *Emotion Regulation and Well-Being*,
DOI 10.1007/978-1-4419-6953-8_9, © Springer Science+Business Media, LLC 2011

or frequency of intrusive thoughts, and mental rumination about this episode. Two types of research methods were involved: (1) monitoring the extent of sharing of specified emotional episodes, and (2) experimentally inducing social sharing specified emotional episodes.

In studies of the first type, the research design generally involved assessing (1) the initial intensity of emotions elicited by the episode, (2) the extent of sharing that developed after, and (3) the intensity of emotions elicited when the memory of the episode was activated later. It was tested whether a positive correlation occurred between the amount of social sharing after the emotional event and the degree of emotional recovery – or the difference between (1) and (3). Surprisingly, these studies failed to yield such a correlation and thus failed to support the prediction that sharing an emotion would reduce the emotional load (Rimé et al., 1998). In studies of the second type, experiments involving various types of sharing were conducted (Zech, 2000; Zech & Rimé, 2005). In some studies, psychology students interviewed relatives about a negative emotional event of their recent past. In other studies, participants extensively shared with an experimenter the most upsetting event of their life. In each of these studies, sharing conditions were created by instructing participants to emphasize either the factual aspects of the episode or the feelings. Control conditions involved talking about a nonemotional topic. Consistently across studies and whatever the condition, sharing emotional experiences failed to alleviate the load of the emotional memory. Yet, in a paradoxical manner, compared to the controls, participants who shared their emotions reported that the experience was ultimately beneficial, both from a cognitive standpoint (e.g., it helped in putting order in themselves) and from a social standpoint (e.g., they experienced comforting behaviors from the part of the recipient).

To sum up, both correlative and experimental studies failed to support the belief that sharing an emotion brings emotional relief. Recent clinical research conducted on the effects of psychological debriefing techniques provided data in the same direction. Psychological debriefing is a very popular group technique implemented among exposed individuals immediately after catastrophes with the purpose (PTSD) (see Dyregrov, 1997; Mitchell & Everly, 1995, for overviews). Participants describe in detail their experience. The technique clearly involves "putting emotions into words," and its purpose is to prevent posttraumatic stress disorder. It is thus perfectly suited to test how far talking about an emotional experience is conducive to emotional recovery. Meta-analytic reviews of controlled trials consistently concluded that debriefings have no efficacy in reducing trauma-related symptoms (Arendt & Elklit, 2001; Rose & Bisson, 1998; Van Emmerik, Kamphuis, Hulsbosch, & Emmelkamp, 2002). Adverse effects were even found in some studies. Nevertheless, victims or professionals who had been exposed to a traumatic situation generally reported that taking part in a psychological debriefing was useful and beneficial to them. Thus, in line with the findings of social sharing studies, debriefing participants failed to manifest a significant alleviation of the emotional impact that the eliciting event had, but they generally reported the feelings of relief or other benefits that they attributed to the debriefing situation.

## 9.3 What Sharing Emotions Brings and What Sharing Emotions Does Not Bring

There are thus consistent observations according to which the social sharing of an emotion fails to bring a sizeable emotional recovery for the shared emotional experience. We proposed that a sharing situation fails to bring this effect because the cognitive ingredients requested to achieve emotional recovery are generally absent from sharing interactions (Rimé, 2009). Early after an emotion – which is precisely when most sharing takes place – people do not engage yet in the cognitive processing of their recent emotional experience. They generally refuse to abandon their frustrated goals (Klinger, 1975; Martin & Tesser, 1989). They do not consider modifying their hierarchy of motives. They stick to their existing schemas. They do not want to change their representations. They stand by their initial appraisal of the emotional situation. They do not feel ready to reframe it nor to change their perspective. Yet, the completion of these various cognitive needs is critical to emotional recovery. Thus, except when they intentionally target the cognitive processing of the emotional experience (Nils & Rimé, 2009), social sharing situations are not bound to open upon emotional recovery. Writing methods, in which participants write about traumas of their distant past (e.g., Pennebaker, 1997) are probably much more likely to stimulate a cognitive processing of these experiences and thus to favor such a recovery.

What are the benefits people find in sharing emotion? The investigation of listeners' responses in social sharing situations suggested that an interesting interpersonal dynamic develops in such situations (Christophe & Rimé, 1997). First, when they rated the intensity of their primary emotions while listening, sharing listeners manifested a remarkable salience of the emotion of interest. This finding is consistent with observations showing that emotional materials fascinate human beings (Rimé, Delfosse, & Corsini, 2005). Second, a positive linear relation occurred between the emotional intensity of the episode heard and the intensity of the listeners' emotion. Thus, listening to an emotional story is emotion eliciting. Third, responses displayed by sharing listeners varied dramatically as a function of the intensity of the shared episode. For low intensity episodes, listeners' responses mostly consisted of verbal manifestations. Conversely, the higher the intensity of the episode heard was, the more listeners displayed nonverbal behaviors (e.g., touching, hugging, kissing …). In sum, at increasing levels of emotional intensity, sharing interactions became decreasingly verbal and increasingly nonverbal.

The interpersonal dynamic which develops in the sharing of emotions can thus be sketched as follows. A person A who experienced an emotion feels the need to share this experience and shares it effectively with a person B. The latter manifests a strong interest for the narrative. This stimulates sharing and person A consequently expresses emotions more and more. The enhanced expression arouses emotions in person B. A reciprocal stimulation of emotion develops in this manner in the dyad which leads to enhanced empathy and to emotional communion. The empathetic feelings experienced by person B stimulate a willingness to help and support person A. If the emotional intensity of the episode shared is high, person B is likely to reduce his or her verbal communication and to switch to a nonverbal mode, with body contact or touching. In sum, emotional sharing has the potential to bring the sender and the receiver closer to one another. Both empirical and theoretical arguments support such a view. Studies of self-disclosure interactions led to views exactly in the same direction (e.g., Reis & Patrick, 1996). Laurenceau, Feldman-Barrett, and Pietromonaco (1998) concluded from their studies that self-disclosure of emotion emerged as a more important predictor of intimacy than did self-disclosure of facts and information. A meta-analytic review of 94 studies about self-disclosure and liking led Collins and Miller (1994) to consider that (a) people who engage in intimate disclosures tend to be liked more than people who disclose at lower levels and (b) people like others as a result of having disclosed to them. The developmental background of the human species supports this sharing-intimacy model. The infants' capacity to regulate one's emotion originated in the context of attachment – a resource that infants activate when under stress (Bowlby, 1969). Thus, in stressful situations, attachment figures provided the child with presence, appeasement, contact, comfort, support, and meaning. It may then not come as a surprise that when later in life, individuals confront an emotional experience, their typical response is to turn to the social milieu in order to find among intimates ingredients, such as appeasement, contact, comfort, support, and meaning.

Thus, social sharing interactions favor manifestations of empathy, emotional fusion, feelings of unity, prosocial behavior, social recognition and validation, consolidation of social ties, and social integration. In this manner, such interactions meet the ingredients requested to buffer the temporary destabilization of the person – insecurity, anxiety, and helplessness – which any negative emotional experience generally entails. This sheds a light on the question of the marked subjective benefits people report after having shared an emotion. They reflect the improvement in subjective well-being which results from the alleviation of the insecurity, anxiety, and helplessness elicited by the negative emotional episode.

## 9.4 Collective Consequences of Dyadic Sharing

Psychosocial consequences of sharing an emotional experience extend far beyond the social integration of the initial interactants. As the social sharing of emotion arouses emotion in the target and as emotion elicits social sharing, targets of social sharing then incline to share what they heard with third persons. In other words, a process of *secondary social sharing* develops. This was first documented by Christophe and Rimé (1997), and then abundantly replicated and extended by Curci and Bellelli (2004). The latter authors' data led to conclude that some three-quarters of episodes personally confided to someone were then shared by the latter with new targets. Psychosocial consequences of sharing an emotion extend even further.

As targets of secondary sharing also experience emotion, they incline to tertiary sharing. Episodes heard in a secondary sharing were shared again with several new listeners for one third of participants and with one new listener for another third (Rimé & Christophe, 1997). Emotional episodes thus open upon a process of spreading of emotional information across social networks. When an intense emotional event affects a given individual, innumerable members of this person's community are informed of it within the next hours by virtue of this sharing propagation. That such a process actually develops in real life was nicely confirmed in a field study wherein 33 college students visited a hospital morgue (Harber & Cohen, 2005). Students' emotional reactions to this experience predicted how many people they told (primary sharing), how many people their friends told (secondary sharing), and how many people their friends' friends told (tertiary sharing). Within 10 days, nearly 900 people had heard about the morgue visit through the cascade of social sharing.

To sum up, through the spreading of emotional information, most people in a community will know what happened to one of them. This propagation of emotional information has many implications. It means that emotion elicits intragroup communication. It means that members of a community keep track of the emotional experiences affecting their peers. It means that every emotional episode of some importance happening in their community open upon a sharing process likely to strengthen members' social ties. It also means that in a group, the shared social knowledge about emotional events and emotional reactions is continuously updated as a function of new individual experiences.

## 9.5 Effects of Reviving Emotions in Collective Rituals

Human beings also share emotions in collective contexts. Collective emotional events, such as a victory, defeat, loss, or a disaster, indeed elicit collective rituals under the form of celebrations or commemorations. As was the case for interpersonal sharing situations, it is commonly considered that collective rituals involving emotional reexposure have the power to "liquidate" the emotional impact. Paralleling what we did earlier, we now examine the validity of this cathartic explanation of collective rituals.

A prototypical case emotional expression in a collective context is found in Truth and Reconciliation Commissions. Such commissions were developed in countries where major violations of human rights happened – e.g., Northern Ireland, South Africa, Israël-Palestine, Guatemala, Argentine, Chile, Bosnia, Serbia-Kosovo, Haiti, East Timor, Sierra Leone, Rwanda, and El Salvador. In Truth and Reconciliation Commissions, victims express publicly the facts from which they or their relatives suffered. Similarly, perpetrators are expected to express publicly the facts as they occurred. Experience with truth and reconciliation revealed that participation in such tribunals may end up in a retraumatization of victims (Bronéus, 2008; Byrne, 2004; Kaminer, Stein, Mbanga, & Zungu-Dirwayi, 2001). These conclusions are thus at odd with a cathartic view of social rituals and are perfectly consistent with the findings from social sharing studies. Yet, at the same time, positive effects have also been mentioned among the outcomes of Truth and Reconciliation Commissions. Survivors reported pride, relief, and a feeling of completion from public expression of their sufferings in a solemn setting. Thus, in the collective context too, sharing an emotional experience failed to reduce the emotional upset, but participants who did so manifested important cognitive and social benefits. A theory proposed a century ago by a founding father of sociology can make sense from these contrasted findings (Paez, Rimé, & Basabe, 2005).

Durkheim (1912) argued in favor of the socially functional nature of shared activities of recall of emotional events, especially when they regard events which affected the social group or community. Though primarily focused on religious cults, his analysis addressed as well any collective manifestations gathering members of a given society in a ceremony proper to recreate the moral community to which they belong. Collective events, such as commemorations, celebrations, feasts, and demonstrations, all fit such a definition. They generally involve the presence of the group symbols (flags, emblems …) and collective expressions (singing, yelling, telling words or sentences, shared movements, music, and dance) which aptly awaken the latent social dimension of every human being. Particularly central to Durkheim's view was that in such a context, individuals' consciousnesses echo one another. Any expression of emotions among participants vividly elicits analogous feelings in people around them so that a reciprocal stimulation of emotion follows. Such a circular process is particularly propitious to instal a collective state of emotional communion. In this state, participants' salience of their self is lowered and their collective identity is enhanced. They thus end up experiencing unity and similarity. This is how, according to Durkheim, social rituals have the capacity to boost participants' feelings of group belonging and of social integration. By the same token, shared beliefs and collective representations are set at the foreground, thus consolidating participants' faith in their cultural beliefs and confidence in collective action. As a consequence, participants will be able to return to their individual life endowed with feelings of self-confidence, strength, and enhanced trust in life.

Durkheim's model of the psychosocial consequences of expressing emotions in a collective context parallels our model of the effects of emotional expression in dyadic situations. In both models, social integration of participants is achieved via a process of emotional reactivation, emotional contagion, and emotional communion. Despite the fact that it is now about a century old, no study to date tested Durkheim's reasoning. And yet, it involves a number of quite testable predictions. The model first leads to expect that taking part in a ritual would end up in reactivating emotional upset among all participants. A second set of consequences resulting from participation in collective rituals regards social variables. After participation in a ritual, participants' perceived societal cohesion and feelings of group belonging should be enhanced, reinforcing the perception of positive personal, interpersonal, and collective reactions (i.e., posttraumatic growth), and increasing the perception of hope and solidarity (i.e., higher positive climate). Third, those individuals who participated in a ritual should manifest enhanced subjective social support, positive affectivity, openness to experience, self-esteem, self-confidence, and trust, as well as prosocial behaviors. Hereafter, we will expose studies we conducted with the purpose to assess the aspects of these predictions.

## 9.6 Collective Rituals and Assimilation of Collective Violence

Paez, Basabe, Ubillos, and Gonzalez-Castro (2007) examined the effects of participating in political demonstrations and protests held in reaction to the 11 March 2004 train bombings in Madrid, Spain. On that day, bomb attacks on several commuter trains had a death toll of nearly 200 people. These events triggered scenes of protest and socio-political turmoil in the country. Some 25% of the Spanish population participated in repeated massive protest demonstrations. College students (63% of sample) and their relatives (37%) ($N = 661$) from five Spanish regions and eight universities completed questionnaires 1, 3, and 8 weeks, respectively, after the bombing. One week after the events, respondents first rated their extent of participation in demonstrations of the previous days. They then completed scales assessing negative emotional arousal and emotional climate. Three weeks after the events, they rated scales assessing subjective social support, loneliness, posttraumatic growth and positive affects. Finally, 8 weeks after the events, they rated again all the previous psychological scales. Twenty-two percent of the respondents reported not participating in demonstrations, 11% reported attending sometimes, 14.8% a lot of times, and 52.5% replied that they attended all demonstrations. Participants were dichotomized into nondemonstrators (score 1 "not at all participating in demonstrations") and demonstrators (scores 2, 3, and 4). Mean comparisons were carried out in order to test if differences in outcomes discriminated these two groups.

The findings supported the positive interpersonal and social effects of taking part in demonstrations. Participation in demonstrations was associated with (1) enhanced perception of social integration (perceived social support and positive affect) 3 weeks later, (2) enhanced beliefs regarding positive life changes in response to trauma, and (3) enhanced perception of a positive emotional climate (perceived hope, solidarity, and trust) 2 months later. Results also evidenced direct effects of communal coping on posttraumatic growth and social support. Taking part in demonstrations was associated with a higher social support and a lower loneliness in later weeks, thus suggesting that it reinforced people's social resources. In addition, participating in demonstrations enhanced the belief that there can be both personal and social benefits from dealing with the trauma (posttraumatic growth), thus suggesting that it broadened cognitive resources. A structural equation analysis confirmed that the latter effect was the primary mediator of the perception of a positive emotional climate. These results fit well within a social functionalist framework of understanding participation in ceremonies and rituals. In the aftermath of a collective trauma, demonstrations reinforced feelings of collective solidarity as was proposed by Durkheim.

We reasoned that sharing emotions after a collective trauma would fulfill exactly the same function as participation in ceremonies and rituals. Social sharing would be functional because it contributes to the enhancement of interpersonal integration and social cohesion and to the strengthening of positive shared beliefs about society. These processes would compensate the increase in negative affect elicited by the traumatic event and maintained by the reactivation involved in social sharing. In order to test these propositions, Rimé, Paez, Martínez, and Basabe (2006) investigated effects of the social sharing of emotions on psychosocial responses of Spanish respondents to the terrorist attacks of 11 March 2004. The predictions were twofold. One the one hand, we hypothesized that repeated verbal emotional expression about Madrid's events sustained the intensity of the events-related emotional arousal and mental rumination. On the other hand, we expected more extended verbal emotional expression about these events to be associated with (1) enhanced social integration (i.e., lower perceived loneliness and higher perceived social support), (2) higher positive affect, (3) higher positive view of life changes or benefits from the trauma, particularly posttraumatic growth of the collective type, (4) higher similarity with others, higher social cohesion, and more positive perception of emotional climate, and (5) better knowledge of the collective traumatic event.

Data were collected from a large sample of respondents first 1 week after Madrid's events, then 3 weeks after the events, and finally 8 weeks after the events. These events had a very high emotional impact on participants. As we expected (Rimé et al., 1998), their initial emotional responses measured 1 week after these events involved overabundant mental rumination and social sharing of emotions. An analysis of correlations between the measures of social sharing and emotional impact of 11th March events made immediately apparent that sharing emotions was associated with a higher initial emotional impact and was also predictive of a higher emotional impact at later measurement times, as predicted by our first side hypothesis. Moreover, concurrent correlations indicated that people who were still sharing emotions 2 months after the events were also higher on variables reflecting the emotional impact these events still had. These observations are in line with previous studies showing that sharing emotions has reactivating effects with regard to the shared emotional experience (Rimé et al., 1998) and that it fails to yield positive effects for emotional recovery. All in all, thus the findings totally contradicted the cathartic or discharge view of emotional expression. They were fully consistent with views that *merely* sharing an emotion yields emotional arousal and emotional reactivation (Rimé et al., 1998; Zech & Rimé, 2005) and that sharing an emotion cannot lead to emotional resolution unless it involves a *systematic cognitive processing* of the shared emotional experience (Rimé, 2009).

Paradoxically, however, as was predicted by the second side of Durkheim's model, socially sharing emotions in the first week after March 11 events was also found associated with a good number of markers of social integration and well-being assessed in later weeks. Thus, the initial sharing of emotions was related with (1) enhanced perception of social support, reduced the feelings of loneliness and enhanced positive affect at 3 and 8 weeks, (2) enhanced perception of positive changes in reaction to trauma (i.e., posttraumatic growth), and (3) enhanced perception of contentment, hope, solidarity, and confidence in the emotional climate. Multivariate analysis by means of structural equation modeling showed that social sharing effects at time 1 on posttraumatic growth were indirect and mediated by social sharing at time 2 and by emotional arousal or intensity at time 2. Positive effect of social sharing at time 2 on positive emotional climate were mediated by posttraumatic growth. Thus, direct and indirect effects of social sharing on positive outcomes were observed. These results support theoretical views according to which the social sharing of emotions fulfils important functions to the enhancement of social cohesion and to the reconstruction of positive beliefs about the group (Rimé et al., 1998; Rimé, 2009). They also fit findings from experimental studies showing that even though sharing emotions was not conducive to emotional recovery, participants in sharing sessions reported a good number of positive benefits from such sessions (Zech & Rimé, 2005).

The above results thus supported the predictions from Durkheim's model. On the one hand, initial social sharing of emotions was found predictive of enhanced emotional arousal and the perception of a negative emotional climate. On the other hand, the same indicator of initial sharing of emotion also predicted effects in the other direction, with enhanced social integration, positive affect, and posttraumatic growth.

## 9.7 Collective Rituals and Assimilation of a Genocide

We wondered whether collective rituals that instigated at a socio-political level could affect in a significant manner emotions and the emotional climate instaled in a population as a result of past conflicts, violations of human rights, or massacres.

Gasparre, Bosco, Bellelli, & Paez (in press) examined the correlates of participation in secular commemorations, funerary rituals, and transitional justice in Guatemala. This country survived four decades (1960–1996) of internal armed conflict and massive political repression. Overall, between 100,000 and 200,000 people (women, children, and the elderly in their majority) were violently killed during this conflict. Some 83% of these victims were Maya. More than half of those killed were assassinated in group massacres aimed at destroying communities. Specifically, during the 1970s and 1980s, the Guatemalan army developed a "scorched earth" policy and burned to the ground over 400 villages of the Highland indigenous population. Many of those who participated in these massacres had been forced into military service. Consequences of this state-sponsored violence included the displacement of hundreds of thousands of peasants and the militarization of the countryside. According to the Commission for Historical Clarification, one million people – approximately 25% of the population of the Guatemalan Highlands – were displaced between 1981 and 1983. Peace Accords were signed in 1996, but were hardly implemented in reforms. Participation in human rights social movement, including commemorations, rituals, demonstrations, and memorials was the collective response of Maya's communities to the impunity and obstacles to obtain reparation and changes.

Gasparre et al. (in press) explored the psychosocial effects that participation in different types of rituals had on individuals who had been directly affected in the Guatemala genocide. The sample consisted of 59 individuals (41 women, 18 men) ranging in age from 29 to 90 years ($Mean_{age}$ = 49.0; SD = 15.4), with 93% of them identifying themselves as *Maya*. Participants rated items assessing how often they did participate (1) in secular commemorations (e.g., celebrations set up in memory of the events), (2) in a Truth and Reconciliation Commission (Truth Commission or Rehmi project), and (3) in funerary and commemorative religious rituals. Following the framework proposed by Durkheim (1912), Gasparre et al. hypothesized that higher levels of participation in rituals should be associated to higher levels of social support, altruistic coping, posttraumatic growth, and engagement in human rights social movement. First of all, participation in rituals did not decrease personal negative emotions related to the collective violence experience. It was also related to higher level of rumination and to a higher social sharing about the past traumatic events. These various results all support Durkheim's contention that participation in rituals entails a reactivation of the commemorated emotions rather than their extinction. In clear support of the second side of Durkheim's model, however, for each of the three types of rites considered, higher participation was associated to higher social support, to a superior coping by means of social support, enhanced altruistic behavior, communal coping or engagement in political action and human rights social movement, and a lesser avoidance of thoughts and responses related to the traumatic event. Moreover, participation in rituals was associated to posttraumatic growth, thus confirming that rituals reinforce positive beliefs about the self, others, and the society. This study confirms the absence of positive effects of social rituals on reminiscence and emotions related to the traumatic event as well as the positive effects the rituals entail for social variables. Moreover, they manifested that the level of participation in rituals was related to social sharing and coping by social support, confirming that interpersonal communication is embedded in collective forms of coping with a traumatic emotion. These results are important because they rest on participants who have lived through a profound social tragedy. However, the study is limited by the fact that it was retrospective based upon volunteers. The studies to be examined hereafter were adopted longitudinal designs. They were based on large samples of both victims and authors of collective violence.

In Rwanda, it is estimated that some 1,000,000 Tutsis were killed in a genocide occurred between April and July 1994. Some 130,000 persons were then accused of participation in the genocide. To deal with this past, a traditional community-based conflict resolution system called *Gacaca* was adapted as a Rwandan version of Truth and Reconciliation Commissions. We examined whether the Gacaca tribunals exerted an impact on emotions, emotional climate, and social variables. Based upon Durkheim's (1912) theory, it was predicted that participation in the Gacaca would involve a reactivation of negative emotions in both groups and would also impact negatively on perceived emotional climate. However, positive consequences were expected for social integration. We thus predicted that participation would impact upon intergroup perception under the form of the reduction of (1) the prejudicial reactions of survivors and prisoners toward each other and (2) the perceived homogeneity of outgroup members. In a first study, 50 survivors of the 1994 genocide in Rwanda and 50 prisoners accused of being responsible for genocidal acts completed four scales 45 days before and 45 days after their participation in the Gacaca trial (Kanyangara, Rimé, Philippot, & Yzerbyt, 2007). The scales assessed (1) negative emotions presently felt with regard to the genocide, (2) perceived emotional climate, (3) negative stereotypes of the outgroup, and (4) perceived similarity among outgroup members.

As regarded individual emotions, it was found that negative emotions (sadness, fear, disgust, anxiety, and shame) were significantly enhanced after participation in the Gacaca, especially among survivors. Regarding emotional climate, given the reactivation of the negative memories of extreme intergroups conflicts entailed by the Gacaca, we predicted that negative emotion would prevail. This was indeed the case. Emotional climate worsened after the Gacaca, and the decline was more marked among the survivors than among the prisoners. Thus, all the variables indexing negative emotion reflected the emotional reactivation effects predicted by Durkheim's model. As for social variables, before Gacaca, survivors were more stereotyped against prisoners than the other way round. However, in line with the predicted effects of enhanced social integration, the negative stereotype toward the other group markedly decreased after the Gacaca, both among survivors and among prisoners. This effect was particularly pronounced for the stereotypes held by survivors toward the prisoners. As regarded outgroup homogeneity, research on stereotyping and intergroup relations has demonstrated that one signature of intergroup prejudice is to consider the members of the outgroup as being similar to each other (Yzerbyt, Judd, & Corneille, 2004). Building on Durkheim's insights, our hypothesis was that outgroup similarity should decrease after the Gacaca. This is indeed what our results revealed, both in the survivors' and the prisoners' samples. Results for both indices of social cohesion were thus totally in line with Durkheim's hypothesis. The emotionally intense social ritual of Gacaca increased social cohesion at least in two ways: by lessening the negative stereotypes attributed to the outgroup and by reducing the perceived similarity attached to outgroup members.

To sum up, the results of this first study suggested that Durkheim's theory of social rituals can integrate positive and negative consequences of truth and reconciliation situations in a reconciling theoretical framework. However, a major weakness of our first study was the absence of control groups of participants not yet exposed to Gacaca. This limitation did not allow to ascertain that the effects observed in the before and after comparisons were attributable to participation in the Gacaca. Therefore, we conducted a new study, including such controls, both for victims and prisoners as well as much larger number of participants (Rimé, Kanyangara, & Yzerbyt, Paez, 2010). The data were collected between February and April 2006 in four of the five Rwandan Provinces. Victims and perpetrators belonged either to the experimental or to the control conditions. In contrast to experimental participants, control participants came from a neighborhood where no Gacaca trial had yet taken place and where no such trial was being planned within the next year. Also, control participants had not taken part in any other Gacaca trial outside of their neighborhood. Both experimental and control participants responded twice, once before and once after the Gacaca trial that took place for the experimental participants. The two sets of ratings were collected within a period of 10 weeks. In total, 755 persons took part in the study. The experimental group comprised 384 participants of whom 200 were victims and 184 were perpetrators. The control group involved 371 participants of whom 195 were victims and 176 were perpetrators.

The collected results again fully supported Durkheim's view that participation in a ritual entails reactivation of negative emotions. Whereas victims in the control condition did not evidence changes, victims who participated in the Gacaca subsequently manifested an increase virtually in all the assessed negative emotions. Specifically, marked significant increases were observed for anger, disgust, fear, anxiety, and sadness. At the same time, however, participation in the Gacaca led to an important decrease in self-reported shame among victims. This suggests that social rituals contribute to restore the victims' dignity. As for perpetrators, the pattern of results for negative emotions closely resembled the one observed on victims. Consistent with the prediction, perpetrators who participated in Gacaca manifested an increase of the negative emotions of fear, sadness, and anxiety. Also, participation in the Gacaca ended up in augmenting shame among perpetrators. Their profile was thus opposite to the profile of the victims in one important respect. In sum, participation in a transitional justice ritual, such as the Gacaca, clearly has a marked emotional cost, both for victims and perpetrators. Such findings corroborate the frequent clinical observations according to which participation in a truth and reconciliation procedure involves a risk of retraumatization (Daley, 1997; Hamber, 2001, 2006; Hayner, 2001). They fully support Durkheim's (1912) view that the emotional reactivation resulting from participants' reciprocal stimulation are at the core of social rituals.

Psychosocial effects were indexed by means of four dependent variables: (1) ingroup identification, (2) positive stereotypes about the outgroup, (3) negative stereotypes about the outgroup, and (4) perceived outgroup homogeneity. In line with the model derived from Durkheim (1912), we expected that each of these variables would reveal that participation in the Gacaca improved social cohesion. The data supported this prediction in three out of the four tests. First, whereas ingroup identification decreased among both victims and perpetrators after the trial, their respective control groups showed a trend in the opposite direction. The only participants who reported being moderately attached to their groups were the victims in the control group. This suggests that rituals involving collective emotional expressions and the recognition of collective past misdeeds contributed to weaken Hutu and Tutsi's "ethnic" identification and to construct an integrative superordinate identity. Second, an important ingredient of intergroup reconciliation is a change in stereotypes. The pattern obtained for positive stereotypes was remarkable. Indeed, both victims and perpetrators in the experimental groups started off being less positive but ended up being more positive than those in the control groups. This suggests that, at least as far as stereotypic representations of the other group are concerned, the

Gacaca process had a beneficial impact on the parties involved. Negative stereotypes decreased considerably after the Gacaca, but this effect was not found in the experimental groups alone. The general decrease in negative stereotypes may partly result from the fact that the norms toward reconciliation gained in popularity in the country as time passed by. Third, we found a considerable decrement in the perceived homogeneity of the outgroup after participation in the Gacaca, both among victims and prisoners in the experimental groups. In contrast, we observed no such change for victims and perpetrators in the control groups. Thus, in line with Durkheim's insights, these results provide yet another piece of evidence in support of the social integrative impact of participation in these social rituals. A perception of the outgroup as being homogeneous denies individual and personal characteristics to outgroup members and reduces them to a mere instantiation of their category, thus sustaining prejudice and hostile social relations.

In sum, the various results recorded for our psychosocial variables strongly support the view that participation in the Gacaca ritual enhances the social cohesion of groups which, in the past, were opposed to each other in the most dramatic way.

## 9.8 The Validity of Durkheim's Model of Social Rituals

We can now formulate conclusions about the theoretical model upon which the described studies relied. Durkheim's (1912) model of the effects of participation in a collective ritual predicts two consequences. On the one hand, rituals are expected to trigger strong reactivation of the emotions associated with the commemorated event. On the other hand, rituals are predicted to contribute to the reconstruction of participants' collective identity by boosting group cohesion and participants' feelings of social integration.

With respect to emotional reactivation, our findings globally supported the prediction of the model. Participation in rituals was unrelated to negative emotions in the case of Guatemala and was associated to rumination – in fact, the association was positive but nonsignificant because of the low degrees of freedom. Participation in demonstrations in Spain increased negative emotions and rumination. Both victims and perpetrators who participated in the Gacaca manifested a considerable increase in their negative emotions in the period which followed participation and, compared to before the Gacaca, victims' perception of a negative emotional climate was higher after their participation. These findings are in perfect agreement with both the clinical observations (Daley, 1997; Hamber, 2001; Hayner, 2001) and the rare pieces of empirical evidence concerning the consequences of truth and reconciliation situations (Brounéus, 2008; Byrne, 2004; Kaminer et al., 2001). The unanimous view thus runs against a "cathartic" or discharge perspective of the expression of emotion in social context. This conclusion is consistent with the findings emerging from the research on the emotional expression between individuals (Kennedy-Moore & Watson, 1999; Rimé, 2009). At the same time, the reactivation of negative emotions resulting from rituals like

Gacaca involved a series of constructive consequences. The findings supported the positive psychosocial effects anticipated by Durkheim (1912). Participation in rituals in Guatemala was associated to (in Guatemala) or predicted (in Spain) positive effects at interpersonal and group level, including higher social support, adaptive coping, and posttraumatic growth. It also had positive effects on the perception of collective hope and solidarity in Spain. Moreover, even in the case of adversarial rituals, such as popular trials in the Gacaca, positive intergroup effects were confirmed. In spite of enhancing a negative emotional climate among victims, participation in the Gacaca improved participants' national identification by decreasing their identification with the ethnic group, increasing their positive view of the other group, favoring a more individualized perception of members of the outgroup – and by reinforcing a positive emotional climate among perpetrators. We interpret these effects as reflecting the improvement of social cohesion which was predicted by Durkheim. To conclude, a clear understanding of a procedure such as the Gacaca requires taking into account not only the various emotions experienced before and after participation, but also the emotional climate as well as a series of psychosocial variables.

## 9.9 General Conclusion

It could be argued for long whether the social sharing of emotion represents a person to person version of collective rituals or whether collective rituals constitute a collective version of the interpersonal sharing of emotion. Our preliminary data testing hypotheses according to which social sharing of emotion and collective rituals encompass essentially the same psychosocial ingredients seemed promising. Both processes result from a similar compulsion to share emotional experiences with one's peers. Neither social sharing nor collective rituals have the capacity to terminate the related emotional experience and to bring emotional recovery. Both processes necessarily induce the reactivation of the emotional episode upon which they focus and in the case of negative emotions at least, this will inevitably elicit a temporary rise of negative emotions. When shared with others, however, the temporary reactivation of emotions is instrumental in eliciting emotional contagion and emotional fusion among those who are involved, whether they are intimate social sharing partners or members of a large crowd. Theory and facts converged in showing that the empathic process thus elicited is instrumental in bringing interactants closer together. The resulting social integration has a good number of emotional, social, and cognitive consequences, for the group as well as for involved individuals. These consequences seem well appropriate to buffer the destabilizing effects that emotional events, whether private or collective, have for those who experience them. It can be concluded that after emotional expression in a social context, *agony is relieved but not put to rest* (Daley, 1997). In this framework, social processes are thus evidencing their most fundamental function: rendering individual life possible.

## References

Arendt, M., & Elklit, A. (2001) Effectiveness of psychological debriefing. *Acta Psychiatrica Scandinavia, 104*, 423–437.

Bowlby, J. (1969) *Attachment and loss. Vol. 1: Attachment*. London: Hogarth Press.

Brounéus, K. (2008) Truth-telling as talking cure? Insecurity and retraumatization in the Rwandan Gacaca courts. *Security Dialogue, 39*, 55–76.

Byrne, C. C. (2004) Benefit or burden: Victims' reflections on TRC participation. *Peace and Conflict: Journal of Peace Psychology, 10*, 237–256.

Christophe, V., & Rimé, B. (1997) Exposure to the social sharing of emotion: Emotional impact, listener responses and the secondary social sharing. *European Journal of Social Psychology, 27*, 37–54.

Collins, N. L., & Miller, L. C. (1994) Self-disclosure and liking: A meta-analytic review. *Psychological Bulletin, 116*, 457–475.

Curci, A., & Bellelli, G. (2004) Cognitive and social consequences of exposure to emotional narratives: Two studies on secondary social sharing of emotions. *Cognition and Emotion, 18*, 881–900.

Daley, S. (1997, July 17) In apartheid inquiry, agony is relieved but not put to rest. *New York Times*, p. A1.

Durkheim, E. (1912) *Les formes élémentaires de la vie religieuse [The elementary forms of religious life]*. Paris: Alcan.

Dyregrov, A. (1997) The process in psychological debriefings. *Journal of Traumatic Stress, 10*, 589–605.

Finkenauer, C., & Rimé, B. (1998) Socially shared emotional experiences vs. emotional experiences kept secret: Differential characteristics and consequences. *Journal of Social and Clinical Psychology, 17*, 295–318.

Gasparre, A., Bosco, S., Bellelli, G., & Paez, D. (in press) Cognitive and social consequences of participations in social rites: Collective coping, social support and posttraumatic growth in Guatemala Genocide's victims. *Revista de Psicologia Social.*

Hamber, B. (2001) Does the truth heal: A psychological perspective on the political strategies for dealing with the legacy of political violence. In N. Biggar (Ed.), *Burying the past: Making peace and doing justice after civil conflict* (pp. 131–148). Washington: Georgetown University Press.

Hamber, B. (2006) *'Nunca mass' and the politics of person: Can truth telling prevent the recurrence of violence?* Notre Dame, IN: University of Notre Dame Press.

Harber, K. D., & Cohen, D. J. (2005) The emotional broadcaster theory of social sharing. *Journal of Language and Social Psychology, 24*, 382–400.

Hayner, P. B. (2001) *Unspeakable truths: Confronting state terror and atrocity*. New York: Routledge.

Kaminer, D., Stein, D. J., Mbanga, I., & Zungu-Dirwayi, N. (2001) The Truth and Reconciliation Commission in South Africa: Relation to psychiatric status and forgiveness among survivors of human rights abuses. *British Journal of Psychiatry, 178*, 373–377.

Kanyangara, P., Rimé, B., Philippot, P., & Yzerbyt, V. (2007) Collective rituals, intergroup perception and emotional climate: Participation in "Gacaca" tribunals and assimilation of the Rwandan Genocide. *Journal of Social Issues, 63*, 387–403.

Kennedy-Moore, E., & Watson, J. C. (1999) *Expressing emotion: Myths, realities, and therapeutic strategies*. New York: Guilford Press.

Klinger, E. (1975) Consequences of commitment to and disengagement from incentives. *Psychological Review, 82*, 1–25.

Laurenceau, J. P., Feldman-Barrett, L., & Pietromonaco, P. R. (1998) Intimacy as an interpersonal process: The importance of self-disclosure, partner disclosure, and perceived partner responsiveness in interpersonal exchanges. *Journal of Personality and Social Psychology, 74*, 1238–1251.

Luminet, O., Bouts, P., Delie, F., Manstead, A. S. R., & Rimé, B. (2000) Social sharing of emotion following exposure to a negatively valenced situation. *Cognition and Emotion, 14*, 661–688.

Martin, L. L., & Tesser A., (1989) Toward a motivational and structural theory of ruminative thought. In J. S. Uleman & J. A. Bargh (Eds.), *Unintended thought* (pp. 306–326). New York: Guilford.
Mesquita, B. (1993) *Cultural variations in emotion: A comparative study of Dutch, Surinamese and Turkish people in the Netherlands.* Unpublished doctoral dissertation, University of Amsterdam, The Netherlands.
Mitchell, J. T., & Everly, G. S. (1995) Critical incident stress debriefing (CISD) and the prevention of work-related traumatic stress among high risk occupational groups. In G. S. Everly & J. M. Lating (Eds.), *Psychotraumatology. Key papers and core concepts in post-traumatic stress* (pp. 267–280). New York: Plenum Press.
Nils, F., & Rimé, B. (2009) *Social sharing of emotion, listeners' responses and emotion regulation.* Manuscript submitted for publication.
Paez, D, Basabe, N, Ubillos, S., & Gonzalez-Castro, J. L. (2007) Social sharing, participation in demonstrations, emotional climate, and coping with collective violence after the March 11th Madrid bombings. *Journal of Social Issues, 63*, 323–338.
Paez, D., Rimé, B., & Basabe, N. (2005) Un modelo socio-cultural de los rituales: efectos y procesos psico-sociales de la participacion en manifestaciones después del atentado del 11.de Marzo. *Revista de Psicología Social, 17*, 369–375.
Pennebaker, J. W. (1997) Writing about emotional experiences as a therapeutic process. *Psychological Science, 8*, 162–166.
Reis, H. T., & Patrick, B. C. (1996) Attachment and intimacy: Component processes. In E. T. Higgins & A. W. Kruglanski (Eds.), *Social psychology: Handbook of basic principles* (pp. 523–563). New York: Guilford Press.
Rimé, B. (2009) Emotion elicits the social sharing of emotion: Theory and empirical review. *Emotion Review, 1*, 60–85.
Rimé, B., & Christophe, V. (1997) How individual emotional episodes feed collective memory. In J. W. Pennebaker, D. Paez, & B. Rimé (Eds.), *Collective memory of political events: Social and psychological perspectives* (pp. 131–146). Hillsdale, NJ: Erlbaum.
Rimé, B., Delfosse, C., & Corsini, S. (2005) Emotional fascination. Responses elicited by viewing pictures of September 11 attack. *Cognition and Emotion, 19*, 923–932.
Rimé, B., Finkenauer, C., Luminet, O., Zech, E., & Philippot, P. (1998) Social sharing of emotion: New evidence and new questions. In W. Stroebe & M. Hewstone (Eds.), *European review of social psychology* (Vol. 9, pp. 145–189). Chichester, UK: Wiley.
Rimé, B., Paez, D., Martinez, F., & Basabe, N. (2006) *Social sharing of emotion, posttraumatic growth and emotional climate: Follow-up of 644 Spanish citizen's response to the collective trauma of March 11th terrorist attacks in Madrid.* Manuscript submitted for publication.
Rimé, B., Philippot, P., Boca, S., & Mesquita, B. (1992) Long lasting cognitive and social consequences of emotion: Social sharing and rumination. In W. Stroebe & M. Hewstone (Eds.), *European review of social psychology* (Vol. 3, pp. 225–258). Chichester, UK: Wiley.
Rimé, B., Yogo, M., & Pennebaker, J. W. (1996) Social sharing of emotion across cultures. Unpublished raw data.
Rimé, B., Kanyangara, P., Yzerbyt, V., & Paez, D. (2010) *Emotional, social, and intergroup consequences of participation in a Truth and Reconciliation process after a genocide: Asssessing effects of Gacaca tribunals in Rwanda.* Manuscript submitted for publication.
Rose, S., & Bisson, J. (1998) Brief early psychological interventions following trauma: A systematic review of the literature. *Journal of Traumatic Stress, 11*, 697–710.
Singh-Manoux, A., & Finkenauer, C. (2001) Cultural variations in social sharing of emotions: An intercultural perspective on a universal phenomenon. *Journal of Cross-Cultural Psychology, 32*, 647–661.
Singh-Manoux, A. (1998) *Les variations culturelles dans le partage social des émotions* [Cultural variations in social sharing of emotions]. Unpublished doctoral dissertation, Université de Paris X-Nanterre, France.
Van Emmerik, A. A., Kamphuis, J. H., Hulsbosch, A. M., & Emmelkamp, P. M. (2002) Single session debriefing after psychological trauma: A meta-analysis. *The Lancet, 360*, 766–771.

Yogo, M., & Onoe, K. (1998) *The social sharing of emotion among Japanese students.* Poster session presented at ISRE '98, The Biannual conference of the International Society for Research on Emotion, held in Wuerzburg, Germany, August 4–8, 1998.

Yzerbyt, V. Y., Judd, C. M., & Corneille, O. (2004) *The psychology of group perception: Perceived variability, entitativity, and essentialism.* London: Psychology Press.

Zech, E., & Rimé, B. (2005) Is it talking about an emotional experience helpful? Effects on emotional recovery and perceived benefits. *Clinical Psychology and Psychotherapy, 12,* 270–287.

Zech, E. (2000) *The effects of the communication of emotional experiences.* Unpublished doctoral dissertation. Louvain-la-Neuve, Belgium: University of Louvain.

# Chapter 10
# The Experience and Regulation of Regret Across the Adult Life Span

**Daniel Västfjäll, Ellen Peters, and Pär Bjälkebring**

## 10.1 Introduction

Regret is a decision-related emotion that arises when a chosen outcome is, or is believed to be, worse than a non-chosen alternative (Connolly & Zeelenberg, 2002). The experience and anticipation of regret has been linked to important real-life decisions such as health behaviors (medical screening, condom use) and financial decisions (Zeelenberg, 1999). The behavioral consequences of regret include both risk aversion and risk taking, decision avoidance, and non-optimal decision making (Anderson, 2003; Gilovich & Medvec, 1995; Zeelenberg & Pieters, 2007). Moreover, enduring negative emotions like regret may have a negative impact on psychological and physical health (Fredrickson, 2001). Thus, understanding how and why we experience regret and how regret influences choices and behaviors are important research questions. However, previous research on regret has, to a large extent, relied on younger participants and to date little is known about how and if the experience and anticipation of regret changes over the adult life-span. In this chapter we review the available evidence for how the experience and regulation of regret vary with age. The aim of this chapter is to merge existing findings and develop a set of novel hypotheses of how aging, emotional experience, and regulation may interact in everyday life. This is an important task since older adults today are asked to make an increasing number of decisions and the older population is rapidly growing. Identifying factors that may differentially influence the decisions of younger and older adults is an important task that will help in understanding how older adults make decisions (Peters, Hess, Västfjäll, & Auman, 2007).

D. Västfjäll (✉)
Decision Research, 1201 Oak St, Suite 200, 97401 Eugene, Oregon, USA
e-mail: daniel.vastfjall@psy.gu.se

I. Nyklíček et al. (eds.), *Emotion Regulation and Well-Being*,
DOI 10.1007/978-1-4419-6953-8_10, © Springer Science+Business Media, LLC 2011

### 10.1.1 Regret, Age, and Emotion Regulation

A recent definition suggest that the emotion regret is "…an aversive, cognitive emotion that people are motivated to regulate in order to maximize outcomes in the short term and learn maximizing them in the long run" (Zeelenberg & Pieters, 2007). Regret, like other emotions, has several different functions (Peters, 2006; Peters, Västfjäll, Gärling, & Slovic, 2006). Emotions can be helpful, providing crucial information about the state of our interactions with the world (Clore, 1994) or speeding our responses in life-threatening situations (Frijda, 1986). However, we frequently experience strong emotions that need to be managed if we are to optimally function. Much research has investigated the determinants of experienced and anticipated regret among younger adults (for an overview see Zeelenberg, 1999). In contrast, very little research has thus far addressed the prevention and management of regret (here called regret regulation; see Zeelenberg & Pieters, 2007) in decision making and, especially, age differences in such regulation. There are good reasons to expect that older and younger adults may differ in their experience, anticipation, and regulation of regret since, among other things, the opportunities to overcome regrets decline with age. This is illustrated by recent research of Wrosch and Heckhausen (2002; see also, Wrosch, Bauer, & Scheier, 2005; Wrosch, Bauer, Miller, & Lupien, 2007). These authors asked participants to report activities that they regretted not having pursued during their lives and to indicate the amount of personal control that they had on the situation at the time. Both the experience and regulation of regret differed between the age groups. Younger adults used internal-control attributions associated with active attempts to change the regrettable behavior, attenuating the regret and lowering rumination. For older adults, these attributions were instead associated with more intense regrets and as a consequence, they actively attributed control to an external agent in a self-protective manner and thereby attenuated their regrets. These findings suggest that regret experience and regulation may be systematically linked to aging.

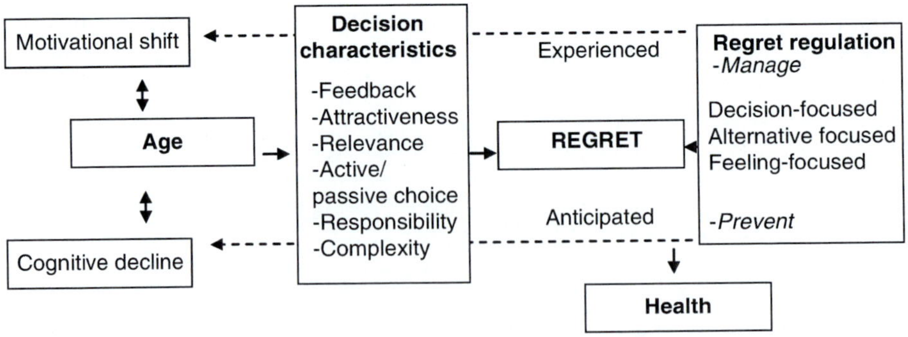


**Fig. 10.1** Framework for studies on age differences in the experience, anticipation, and regulation of regret

Not only does chronological age decrease time to undo the consequences of a decision, but with increasing age changes take place in both emotional and cognitive processes that are potentially relevant to the experience, anticipation, and regulation of regret. We review two areas of research, age-related cognitive decline and age-related motivational shifts, which are potentially relevant to the relationship between aging and the experience, anticipation, and regulation of regret (Fig. 10.1).

### *10.1.2 Cognitive Decline*

A powerful determinant of emotional reactions to a decision outcome is whether the outcome was compared with alternative outcomes or other states of the world (Boninger, Gleicher, & Stratham, 1994; Gleicher et al., 1990; Kahneman & Miller, 1986). This counterfactual thinking thus refers to the mental simulation of comparing the present state with other possible, but unobtained states (Roese, 1997). Counter factual thoughts are common in everyday experience and may exert a substantial influence (McMullen, 1997). Research on outcome evaluation has shown that participants feel more strongly about an alternative if counterfactual alternatives are salient (Gleicher et al., 1990). A further distinction is made between counterfactuals that improve reality (thinking about how things could have been better), and counterfactuals that worsen reality (thinking about how things could have been worse) (Landman, 1993; Sanna, 1998). Regret is a negative emotion experienced when the present state of affairs is compared to a better counterfactual reality (what could have been better: Roese, 1997; Van Dijk & Zeelenberg, 2005). Regret, like other counterfactual emotions, thus relies on mentally simulating various alternative outcomes. Such cognitive activities also require deliberative capacity, and in this sense, regret can be seen as a higher-order cognitive emotion (Russell, 2003). Several lines of research suggest age-related declines in the controlled processes of the deliberative system such as decreased speed of processing (e.g., Salthouse, 1996), and deficits in explicit memory and learning (Cohen, 1996). These changes are evident at a neural system level where the prefrontal cortex (related to working memory and executive functions such as the control and regulation of cognition) deteriorates with normal aging (MacPherson, Phillips, & Della Sala, 2002). Since regret is a cognitive emotion relying on comparison (Zeelenberg & Pieters, 2007) that involves orbitofrontal and prefrontal activation of the cortex (Camille et al., 2004; Coricelli et al., 2005), this line of research suggests that the experience of regret should decline with age and co-vary with age-related declines in deliberative capabilities. This is also consistent with research by Hess, who has hypothesized that aging is associated with increasing selectivity in task engagement because of actual or perceived declines in cognitive resources (Hess, 2000, 2006). Anticipation of regret has not, so far, been extensively studied across the adult life span, but given that anticipation is defined as "primarily cognitive expectations about future emotions, without actually experience them in the present" (Loewenstein, Weber, Hsee, & Welch, 2001) it may be expected that cognitive decline should lead to decreased anticipation of regret. Similarly, emotion regulation is cognitively and physically demanding (Gross, 2008) and so a purely cognitive perspective on emotion regulation suggests that emotion regulation should be less often employed and be less successful among older adults. However, recent research has shown that emotion regulation in fact increases with age and that older adults often are very skilled in regulating emotion (Charles & Carstensen, 2007; Magai, 2008; Gross, 2008). Thus, decreased anticipated and experienced regret are expected for cognitive reasons.

### *10.1.3 Motivational Shift and Increased Emotion Regulation*

Some recent research has shown that changes in time perspective result in emotional goals that are becoming increasingly important as the end of life nears, which in turn results in greater monitoring of emotional information (Carstensen, 2006). Because older adults are closer to the end of life, age should be associated with an increased importance of emotional goals, increased attention to emotional content, and an increased focus on positive information that can be used to optimize emotional experience (Peters et al., 2007). Supporting this, Mather et al. (2004) found that older adults (compared to younger adults) had disproportionately greater activation in the amygdala in response to positive vs. negative information, suggesting an age-related shift in processing styles (i.e., a positivity bias; see also Mather & Carstensen, 2003). Other research has suggested an age-related increase in maintaining positive affect – older adults tend to be in more positive and less negative mood states compared to younger adults (Mroczek, 2001). Thus, research focusing on age-related motivational shifts also predicts that older adults will experience relatively less regret than younger adults.

However, interestingly, one of the functions of regret is to help learning so as to prevent repeating decisions that lead to regret (Zeelenberg & Pieters, 2007; functional aspect of regret). Emotional memory is thus likely to play a major role. Research on age-related motivational shifts suggests that emotional memory among older adults is relatively intact, but that positive emotional memories are given disproportionate weight compared to negative memories. Thus, the same event occurring some time earlier may be remembered differently by older and younger adults. Specifically, it is more likely that older adults will have "come to terms with" the regret-inducing event (i.e., retained the positive aspects of an event or reinterpreted it more positively; also called choice-supportive memory; Kryla-Lighthall & Mather, 2009; Mather & Johnson, 2000). Kennedy, Mather, and Carstensen (2004), in fact, found that older adults showed a tendency to remember events from the same time period in the past more positively than did younger adults. As a result, predictions from a motivational perspective are mixed. We used these opposing predictions to make novel predictions in the pilot study below.

## 10.2 Studies on the Experience of Regret Across Adult Life

In a pilot study we examined how the experience of regret may change with age (Västfjäll, Peters, & Johanson, 2009). Both cognitive and motivational theories suggest that regret should diminish with age, whereas much of the available empirical data points toward the opposite (Roese & Summerville, 2005; Timmers, Westerhof, & Dittmann-Kohli, 2005). However, prior research has generally investigated only life regrets – major important events that can have long lasting consequences (Roese & Summerville, 2005; long-term regrets; Gilovich & Medvec, 1995). We submit that a critical factor determining the intensity of regret is the irreversibility of the decision. With increasing age, the time available to undo the consequences of a major event (life regrets such as realizing that you would have wanted children) will lead to an amplification of regret. We thus expect an interaction with age where "life" regrets seem more reversible in young age than in older age. An action leading to regret early in life may lead to amplification in older age simply because the possibility of reversing the consequence of the decision has been lost. Finally, older adults have simply had more time to think about and perhaps ruminate on the negative outcome. This combination (more time for rumination and more limited opportunity to undo the consequences) can amplify the experience of regret. However, also due to older adults' selectivity in their emotional responses (maintaining positive affect and prioritizing meaningful goals; Fung & Carstensen, 2004, 2006), their diminished cognitive resources and greater experience with decisions and their outcomes over a life time (hence knowing which decisions matter the most), we predict that for minor everyday events (short-term regrets), aging may be related to less intense regret. Thus, younger adults may (relative to older adults) have greater short-term regrets, but by dint of less life experience, they may also overestimate the regret everyday decisions actually will cause. This is consistent with some recent research demonstrating that older adults (relative to younger adults) are more correct in their affective forecasts for everyday decisions (i.e., ratings of affect for winning or losing gambles; Nielsen, Knutson, & Carstensen, 2008).

We thus believe that the critical difference between everyday and life regrets is the perception of the reversibility of decision outcomes. Older adults may recognize that major life events are those worth prioritizing, but at the same time the possibility to undo the event will become more and more limited with age. Younger adults may not have or recognize this need to prioritize resource allocation to a selected number of decisions and at the same time likely have more possibilities to undo possible negative outcomes. Our conception of life and everyday regrets is similar to that of Wrosch and Heckhausen (2002) who note that undoing the consequences of regrettable behaviors is not always possible, given that some life paths cannot be changed when people advance in age (e.g., having a different career, establishing a family).

A sample of 825 Swedish adults (18–85 years) rated the frequency of everyday regrets, as well as the intensity and duration of a recalled regret-inducing event (everyday regret) and what they regret the most (life regret). In addition to chronological age, we included a measure of self-perceived available future time to undo the event (future time perspective; FTP). Overall, we expected that the frequency of experienced regret, as well as the intensity of regret, for everyday events would decrease with chronological age. However, the intensity of life regrets was expected to increase with chronological age. In both cases, having an open-ended FTP was expected to lead to less intense regret.

To test these hypotheses, regression analyses were performed to predict experienced regrets with sex, educational background and income as control variables and age as predictor. The regression of the frequency of experienced everyday regrets during the past 3 months was significant, $F(6{,}773) = 13.13$, $p < 0.001$, $R^2_{adj} = 0.09$. As expected, the frequency of reported regret decreased with increasing age ($b = -0.30$, $p < 0.01$). In addition, age was significantly associated with a decrease in intensity ($b = -0.42$, $p < 0.01$) and duration ($b = -0.28$, $p < 0.01$) of everyday regrets, $F(6{,}733) = 15{,}37$, $p < 0.001$, $R^2_{adj} = 0.17$ (intensity) and $F(6{,}733) = 3{,}96$, $p < 0.01$, $R^2_{adj} = 0.04$ (duration). Instead for life regrets, age increased the intensity of regret ($b = 0.20$, $p < 0.01$; $F(6{,}725) = 8.12$, $p < 0.01$, $R^2_{adj} = 0.11$). The effect of age on duration of life regrets was not significant. Overall, these findings support the hypothesis that older adults experience regret more strongly for life regrets, but less strongly for everyday events. Further support for this comes from an analysis of the mental age measure. Since chronological and mental age (as measured by the FTP measure) showed a relatively moderate intercorrelation, the FTP measure was examined separately. Consistent with our expectations, the FTP measure showed results conceptually similar to the effect of age on life regrets – having an open-ended FTP covaried with lower intensity (beta weight $-0.39$, $p < 0.001$), and shorter duration ($-0.18$, $p < 0.01$) for life regrets. Thus, both old age and a limited FTP appear to produce a similar effect on the experience of life regrets. We interpreted this as initial evidence that the time remaining in life and the possibilities to undo the negative consequences of a decision are determining factors for the experience of regret in later life.

This study showed that age modulates the experience of regret, and that motivational shifts may partly account for this. However, measures of cognitive decline were not included so that the role of deliberative processing in determining regret cannot be properly assessed with this data. Moreover, this study only examined retrospective regrets and did not include anticipation of future regret. Most importantly, it did not directly examine the role of regret regulation, a topic that we turn to next.

### *10.2.1 Regret Regulation Across the Adult Life Span*

Among younger adults, the consequences of experienced regret and the possibility of future regrets are managed by a number of systematic strategies. Zeelenberg and Pieters (2007) summarized them into three categories; decision-focused, alternative-focused, and feeling focused prevention and management strategies (see Table 10.1).

Examples of strategies to prevent future regret involve avoiding feedback about non-chosen outcomes, deliberately anticipate regret, and delaying the decision.

Strategies to mitigate experienced regret include justification, reversal of the decision, and emotion regulation or suppression. Zeelenberg and Pieters noted that these strategies are used and implemented (among younger adults) based on "their accessibility and their instrumentality to the current overarching goal." We propose that the accessibility, instrumentality, as well as goals related to regret may differ between younger and older adults, in that these age groups differ in:

1. Emotion regulation goals (older adults avoid negative and prioritize positive information to a larger extent than younger adults; Magai, 2008)
2. Cognitive abilities needed to carry out emotion regulation
3. Choice priorities (older adults prefer qualitative over quantitative experiences; Fung & Carstensen, 2004).

It should also be noted that the regulation strategies described in Table 10.1 are mainly derived from laboratory studies, and it is still an empirical question what strategies are actually employed to regulate regret in everyday life.

In summary, based on previous empirical and theoretical work (including our pilot study as well as motivational and cognitive theories of aging) it appears plausible that older and younger adults differ in the experience, anticipation and regulation of regret.

**Table 10.1** Strategies for regulating regret among younger adults

| |
|---|
| Prevent future regret |
| *Decision-focused prevention strategies* |
| Increase decision quality |
| Increase decision justifiability |
| Transfer decision responsibility |
| Delay or avoid decision |
| *Alternative-focused prevention strategies* |
| Ensure decision reversibility |
| Avoid feedback about forgone alternatives |
| *Feeling-focused prevention strategies* |
| Anticipate regret |
| Manage current regret |
| *Decision-focused management strategies* |
| Undo decision |
| Justify decision |
| Deny responsibility for the decision |
| *Alternative-focused management strategies* |
| Reverse decision (switch to alternative) |
| Re-appraise quality of alternative |
| *Feeling-focused management strategies* |
| Psychological repair work |
| Suppress or deny regret |

From Zeelenberg and Pieters (2007)

## 10.3 Some Novel Hypotheses About Regret Regulation and Suggestions for Ways of Testing Them

How do younger and older adults differ in the regulation of regret? Little previous research has been performed on this topic and an initial step may be to develop a testable framework. In an ongoing research project we examine these questions and address them by looking at how various decision characteristics influence age-related differences in the experience, anticipation, and regulation of regret. In the following section we describe how we intend to test this framework empirically.

### *10.3.1 Experience and Regulation of Regret in Everyday Life*

While it is believed that regret is a frequently experienced emotion in everyday life, no studies have so far adequately sampled everyday regret experiences (studies of decision experiences among younger adults have been performed but these have not measured regret, for example, Hogarth, Portell, & Cuxart, 2007; Hogarth, Portell, Cuxart, & Kolev, 2008). Similarly, studies of emotional experiences with older adults exist, but they did not measure regret or examined decisions, for example, Carstensen, Pasupathi, Mayr, & Nessleroad, 2000). The experience sampling method (ESM) may be a particularly useful method to assess regret, other emotional experiences, and decisions simultaneously (e.g., Conner, Barrett, Bliss-Moreau, Lebo, & Kashub, 2003). This technique requires participants to carry a small, hand-held computer or palmtop with them at all waking hours, for a specified period (e.g., a week). During the week, the palmtop emits sound signals at predetermined or randomized intervals. Each time the participant hears this signal, he or she is supposed to immediately respond to various questions administered by the palmtop about his or her latest experience. One advantage of the ESM is that it permits one to study personal events as they unfold in their natural and spontaneous context. Another advantage is that it renders possible repeated measurements over time, so that one may obtain a better sense of whether a specific phenomenon occurs in particular recurrent patterns – for instance at specific times of the day. When frequency estimates of specific emotions (and the determinants/consequences of the emotion) are needed, the ESM may yield more reliable data than the aggregated, retrospective, and cognitively biased data obtained in survey studies (Ready, Weinberger, & Jones, 2007).

The ESM is consistent with Brunswik's (1956) notion of *representative design*, which involves randomly sampling stimuli from the environment, so that environmental properties are preserved. The method seems promising for decision researchers who are concerned about the limited external validity of data from laboratory-based studies. Clearly, then, a representative sampling of decision situations is important to ensure generalizability of findings from studies of the importance of regret for everyday behavior. Hogarth et al. (2007) successfully studied everyday risk and

**Table 10.2** Example questions in the ESM

| |
|---|
| 1. Have you made or thought about making a decision (since beeped last time)? (yes/no) |
| 2. What was the decision about? (health, money, consumption, social relationships, etc.) (multiple choice) |
| 3. If yes, was it a decision you are thinking about but have not made yet? (branch to 4) Or a decision that you already made? (branch to 5). How long ago/when will the decision be made? Have you reported about it before? Common to both are measures of the characteristics of the decision; agency (who will make the decision), responsibility, omission/commission, importance, attractiveness (these are important both for prevention and managements strategies). Examples items "if somebody else could affect your decision or if somebody else could be blamed or praised for it?" What information do you think is worth attending to, what not to consider? (multiple choice/rating scales) |
| 4. Pre-decision phase (prevention of regret) |
| Information search questions: to what extent "have you compared the alternative to others?," "Have you actively been searching for more information" "tried to ignore information about other alternatives" (multiple choice) |
| Thoughts: "how often have you thought about this decision" "how often have you considered that the decision could have a bad outcome?" "thought about delaying the decision?" (multiple choice/rating scales) |
| Anticipated feelings: likert ratings of anticipation of specific emotions such as regret, anger, disappointment,, sadness, happiness, elation 16 emotion-related terms that sample the entire affective space will be selected (Västfjäll, Friman, Gärling, & Kleiner, 2002). In this way, both specific emotions and dimensional representations of valence/arousal can be used in predicting choice |
| 5. Post-decision phase (management of regret) (note here we can further differentiate pre- and post-outcome) |
| Similar to 4, but thoughts also include decision justifiability |

benefit perception for activities occurring naturally in people's lives. Interestingly, Hogarth et al. found that many of the risks that people reported were not consistent with what had been obtained in previous survey research. For example, participants in the ESM study rarely mentioned risk of terrorism while this was frequently mentioned in survey responses (Hogarth et al., 2007).

Using this method, participants can report their experience at the time of the beep (since the last time they responded) about decisions they made or will make. A branching procedure following the logic outlined in Table 10.2 could be used. Table 10.2 gives sample questions (modeled after Zeelenberg & Pieters,' 2007) regret-regulation themes (see Table 10.1). The basic concept described here is to cover both pre-decision and post-decision phases as well as capture what the decision is about.

This method is possible to use with older adults. Riis et al. (2005) have demonstrated successful use of this procedure with middle aged to older adults with significant health problems. Moor, Connelly, and Rogers (2004) conducted a usability study with younger (25–30 years) and older adult adults (75–85 years). They concluded that older adults can complete tasks such as pressing buttons and identifying and pressing detailed icons just as well as younger individuals although they do need additional practice time. The older adult also preferred larger icons although they could read smaller sizes of even detailed picture icons at 10 mm.

Using this method it may be expected to find differences in:

1. What the participants feel regret about: Older adults are expected to experience stronger regret for irreversible life regrets, whereas younger adults may experience more regret about everyday choices, consistent with our pilot study. Similarly, both age groups will experience more regret for decisions that are important to them (although the content of important decisions will, however, be different on both an individual and a group level).
2. The frequency of regret: older adults (due to motivational forces aimed at promoting positive affect) will experience regret less often.
3. Regret prevention strategies – to prevent regret, older adults (relative to younger adults) are expected to search for less information, make fewer comparisons, focus more on positive information, avoid negative information, anticipate regret more, and be more prone to avoid or delay decision.
4. Regret management strategies – to manage regret, older adults will view their choices as more positive (choice-supportive memory; Mather & Johnson, 2000).

## 10.4 Laboratory Studies of the Experience, Anticipation, and Regulation of Regret

In experimental laboratory studies, determinants of regret and regret regulation can be more carefully delineated, manipulated, and tested. For instance, self-report measures of decision processes may not always yield reliable data due to limited introspective ability (Västfjäll, in press).We propose that to understand the mechanisms of regret regulation in different age groups, experimental manipulations of the basic determinants of regret are needed. At the core of regret theory lays the notion that the chosen (or to-be-chosen) alternative is compared with other alternatives (Van Dijk & Zeelenberg, 2005). As evident in Table 10.2, many regret regulation strategies also involve making or not making these counterfactual comparisons (e.g., seeking or avoiding feedback about foregone options). It is possible to experimentally investigate the role of counterfactual comparisons and its interaction with regret and aging. For example, in a series of studies, Mellers et al. demonstrated that the emotional utility of an outcome critically depended on unobtained outcomes (Mellers, Schwartz, Ho, & Ritov, 1997; Mellers & McGraw, 2001). So, getting a salary raise is a positive emotional experience, but knowing that you could have gotten even higher salary will deflate that emotion (Kahneman, 1992). Larsen, McGraw, Mellers, and Cacioppo (2004) investigated such mixed emotions to outcomes. They had participants playing binary gambles. Half the gambles involved a 50–50 chance of winning either of two amounts; the remaining gambles involved a 50–50 chance of losing either of two amounts. Disappointing wins were wins of $5 when the alternative was a $6, $9, or $12 win. Losing gambles were constructed by reversing the signs of the outcomes. This resulted in relieving losses of $5 when the alternative was a $6, $9, or $12 loss, and a single outright loss of $5 instead of $3. Larsen et al.

found that participants indeed experienced mixed emotions about outcomes, once the unobtained outcome was known. This procedure may be used to investigate age differences in regret. It may be expected that older adults will experience less regret; however, recent research has shown that older adults experience more complex blends of emotions (Ersner-Hershfield, Mikels, Sullivan, & Carstensen, 2008) so that it is expected that mixed emotions (both in terms of negative vs. positive valence, but also in terms of the more granular coactivation of specific emotions) will be more common among older adults (Lindquist & Feldman Barrett, 2008).

Recent research has shown that older adults are better affective forecasters than younger adults. Nielsen et al. (2008), for example, compared affective forecasting, experienced affect, and recalled affect in younger and older adults during a task in which participants worked to win and avoid losing small monetary sums. Younger adults reported increased negative arousal during loss anticipation and positive arousal during gain anticipation. In contrast, older adults reported increased positive arousal during gain anticipation, but showed no increase in negative arousal on trials involving loss anticipation (consistent with the positivity bias). Younger, but not older adults exhibited forecasting errors on the arousal dimension, underestimating increases in arousal during anticipation of gains and losses and overestimating increases in arousal in response to gain outcomes. In other research, older adults more accurately predicted future quality of life judgments (Lachman, Röcke, Rosnick, & Ryff, 2008). Building on these recent findings, a reasonable hypothesis is that older adults are better than younger adults at anticipating regret, an important prevention and management strategy. Using the mixed gambles paradigm (with active choices), participants could be probed about anticipated affect (valence and arousal of feelings) and regret/disappointment prior to making each choice. After the choice, they will be asked about experienced affect and regret/disappointment. Regret is a negatively valenced, moderate arousal emotion (Västfjäll & Gärling, 2002; Västfjäll and Gärling, in press) so that, following the findings of Nielsen et al., it is likely that older adults will be more accurate in their forecasts (Larkin et al, 2007).

Previous research has indicated that, while many individuals try to ignore information about other outcomes after selecting, curiosity is a strong motivational impetus for searching for information (Van Dijk & Zeelenberg, 2007). Therefore, using a modified version of the mixed gambles paradigm in which participants can chose to learn about the unobtained outcome is a possible extension. Consistent with the notion that older adults may want to avoid processing emotional taxing information (Kryla-Lighthall & Mather, 2009), it may be expected that older adults will be less likely to opt for counterfactual information.

A recent study by Löckenhoff and Carstensen (2007) examined age differences in information acquisition and recall about health care decisions. Using computer-based decision scenarios, 60 older and 60 younger adults reviewed choice criteria that contained positive, negative, and neutral information about different physicians and health care plans. The results showed that older adults reviewed and recalled a greater proportion of positive than negative information compared with young adults (consistent with the positivity bias; Mather & Carstensen, 2003). The material that Löckenhoff and Carstensen (2007) used consisted of two decision scenarios in which participants chose from among four physicians and four health plans. All choice alternatives were described as average on a global index of quality (i.e., consumer/patient satisfaction). However, on four additional characteristics, each choice alternative was assigned one of the following value labels: very good, good, poor, or very poor. The information was presented in tables with the alternatives (e.g., Plan A) in the rows and the characteristics (e.g., preventive care) in the columns. Initially, only the choice alternatives and characteristics were visible; the specific cell content was concealed. Participants received cues for the emotional valence of the information contained in each cell and were told that the fields were coded such that "white fields = positive information (good or very good), gray fields = neutral information (average), dark fields = negative information (poor or very poor)." This methodology can be modified to test aspects of regret regulation and aging. For instance, relevant feedback about the non-chosen alternatives could be given. In the study by Löckenhoff and Carstensen, regret was not likely a strong influence on choice since the scenario did not involve uncertainty or feedback about the non-chosen alternative. However, a modification with feedback about what would be the "normatively" optimal choice would render regret salient.

Löckenhoff and Carstensen (2007) examined some process measures relevant to regret regulation (e.g., the amount of information viewed and recall of alternatives; the former is a regret prevention strategy whereas the latter is a regret management strategy). It may be expected that older adults, especially in the relevant health choice scenario, to experience more regret, but also to search for less information, especially if it is negative (consistent with the positivity bias). Due to the relevance and complexity of the choice, it may also be expected that older adults will be more prone to delay or prefer having someone else making the decision for them (Luce, 1998; Kryla-Lighthall & Mather, 2009). However, once a choice is made, we expect older adults to remember more positive attributes especially for the chosen alternative (Mather & Johnson, 2000).

## 10.5 Conclusion

Older adults' experience of regret is different from younger adults. Age, as well as the possibility to change and undo the event, as well as what life domain the potentially regret-eliciting event is about will modulate the experience of regret. Age appears to have some specific effects on regret experience: (1) with age, the lesser time to undo regrets is an important factor modulating affective experience (Wrosch et al., 2005, 2007), and (2) an increased focus on positive affect with increasing age can ameliorate the psychological impact of consequences of minor regrets (Carstensen, 2006). This is known for the experience of regret. However, very few studies have examined age differences in the anticipation and regulation of regret. In this chapter we have argued that older adults may regulate (prevent and manage) regret actively and we have outlined a series of way of studying age-related differences in this regulation. We hope that this overview and the framework that we present may stimulate more research in this area. This is important since older adults' quality of life depends to a significant extent on the quality of their decisions. Indirectly, suboptimal decisions may be linked to a wide range of health and financial outcomes that is not only detrimental to the individual, but the whole society. Understanding how older adults' decision making differ from younger adults may help in designing information and decision aids tailored to older adults' abilities.

## References


Anderson, C. J. (2003) The psychology of doing nothing: Forms of decision avoidance result from reason and emotion. *Psychological Bulletin*, *129*, 139–167.

Boninger, D. S., Gleicher, F., & Stratham, A. (1994) Counterfactual thinking: From what might have been to what might be. *Journal of Personality and Social Psychology*, *67*, 297–307.

Brunswik, E. (1956) *Perception and the representative design of experiments*. Berkeley, CA: University of California Press.

Camille, N., Coricelli, G., Sallet, J., Pradat-Diehl, P., Duhamel, J. R., Sirigu, A. (2004) The involvement of the orbitofrontal cortex in the experience of regret. *Science*, *304*, 1167–1170.

Carstensen, L. L. (2006) The influence of a sense of time on human development. *Science*, *312*, 1913–1915.

Carstensen, L. L., Pasupathi, M., Mayr, U., & Nessleroad, J. R. (2000) Emotional experience in everyday life across the adult life span. *Journal of Personality and Social Psychology*, *79*, 644–655.

Charles, S., & Carstensen, L. (2007) Emotion regulation and aging. In J. J. Gross (Ed.), *Handbook of emotion regulation*. New York: Guilford Press.

Clore, G. C. (1994) Why emotions are felt. In P. Ekman & R. J. Davidson (Eds.), *The nature of emotion: Fundamental questions* (pp. 103–111). New York: Oxford University Press.

Cohen, G. (1996) Memory and learning in normal aging. In R. T. Woods (Ed.), *Handbook of the clinical psychology of aging* (pp. 43–58). Chichester: Wiley.

Conner, T., Barrett, L. F., Bliss-Moreau, E., Lebo, K., & Kashub, C. (2003) A practical guide to experience-sampling procedures. *Journal of Happiness Studies*, *4*, 53–78.

Connolly, T., & Zeelenberg, M. (2002) Regret and decision making. *Current Directions in Psychological Science*, *11*, 212–216.

Coricelli, G., Critchley, H. D., Joffily, M., O'Doherty, J. P., Sirigu, A., & Dolan, R. J. (2005) Regret and its avoidance: A neuroimaging study of choice behavior. *Nature Neuroscience*,*8*, 1255–1262.

Ersner-Hershfield, H., Mikels, J. A., Sullivan, S., & Carstensen, L. L. (2008) Poignancy: Mixed emotional experience in the face of meaningful endings. *Journal of Personality and Social Psychology*, *94*, 158–167.

Fredrickson, B. L. (2001) The role of positive emotions in positive psychology: The broaden-and-build theory of positive emotions. *American Psychologist*, *56*, 218–226.

Frijda, N. H. (1986) *The emotions*. Cambridge: Cambridge University Press.

Fung, H., & Carstensen, L. L. (2004) Motivational changes in response to blocked goals and foreshortened time: Testing alternatives to socioemotional selectivity theory. *Psychology and Aging*, *19*, 68–78.

Fung, H. H., & Carstensen, L. L. (2006) Goals change when life's fragility is primed: Lessons learned from older adults, the September 11th attacks and SARS. *Social Cognition*, *24*, 248–278.

Gilovich, T., & Medvec, V. H. (1995) The experience of regret: What, when, and why. *Psychological Review*, *102*, 379–395.

Gleicher, F., Kost, K. A., Baker, S. M., Stratham, A. J., Richman, S. A., & Sherman, S. J. (1990) The role of counterfactual thinking in judgments of affect. *Personality and Social Psychology Bulletin, 16*, 284–295.

Gross, J. J. (2008) Emotion regulation. In M. Lewis, J. M. Haviland-Jones, & L. F. Barrett (Eds.), *Handbook of emotions* (3rd ed.) (pp. 497–512). New York: The Guilford Press.

Hess, T. M. (2000) Aging-related constraints and adaptations in social information processing. In U. Von Hecker, S. Dutke, & G. Sedek (Eds.), *Generative mental processes and cognitive resources: Integrative research on adaptation and control* (pp. 129–155). Dordrecht: Kluwer.

Hess, T. M. (2006) Adaptive aspects of social cognitive functioning in adulthood: Age-related goal and knowledge influences. *Social Cognition, 24*, 279–309.

Hogarth, R. M., Portell, M., & Cuxart, A. (2007) What risks do people perceive in everyday life? A perspective gained from the experience sampling method (ESM). *Risk Analysis, 27*, 1427–1439.

Hogarth, R. M., Portell, M., Cuxart, A., & Kolev, G. I. (2008) *Emotion and reason in everyday risk perception* (2008). UPF working paper.

Kahneman, D. (1992) Reference points, anchors, norms, and mixed feelings. *Organizational Behavior and Human Decision Processes, 51*, 296–312.

Kahneman, D., & Miller, D.T. (1986) Norm theory: Comparing reality to its alternatives. *Psychological Review, 93*, 136–153.

Kennedy, Q., Mather, M., & Carstensen, L. L. (2004) The role of motivation in the age-related positivity effect in autobiographical memory. *Psychological Science, 15*, 208–214.

Kryla-Lighthall, N., & Mather, M. (2009) The role of cognitive control in older adults' emotional well-being. In V. Berngtson, D. Gans, N. Putney, & M. Silverstein (Eds.), *Handbook of theories of aging* (2nd ed.) (pp. 323–344). New York: Springer.

Lachman, M. E., Röcke, C., Rosnick, C., & Ryff, C. D. (2008) Realism and illusion in Americans' temporal views of their life satisfaction: Age differences in reconstructing the past and anticipating the future. *Psychological Science, 19*, 889–897.

Landman, J. (1993) *Regret: The persistence of the possible*. New York: Oxford University Press.

Larkin, G. R. S., Gibbs, S. E. B., Khanna, K., Nielsen, L., Carstensen, L. L, & Knutson, B. (2007) Anticipation of monetary gain but not loss in healthy older adults. *Nature Neuroscience, 10*, 787–791.

Larsen, J. T., McGraw, A. P., Mellers, B. A., & Cacioppo, J. T. (2004) The agony of victory and thrill of defeat: Mixed emotional reactions to disappointing wins and relieving losses. *Psychological Science, 15*, 325–330.

Lindquist, K., & Feldman Barrett, L. (2008) Emotional complexity. In M. Lewis, J. M. Haviland-Jones, & L. F. Barrett (Eds.), *The handbook of emotion* (3rd ed.) (pp. 513–530). New York: Guilford.

Loewenstein, G. F., Weber, E. U., Hsee, C. K., & Welch, E. S. (2001) Risk as feelings. *Psychological Bulletin, 127*, 267–286.

Löckenhoff, C. E., & Carstensen, L. L. (2007) Aging, emotion, and health-related decision strategies: Motivational manipulations can reduce age differences. *Psychology and Aging, 22*, 134–146.

Luce, M. F. (1998) Choosing to avoid: Coping with negatively emotion-laden consumer decisions. *Journal of Consumer Research, 24*, 409–423.

MacPherson, S., Phillips, L. H., & Della Sala, S. (2002) Age, executive function and social decision-making: a dorsolateral prefrontal theory of cognitive aging. *Psychology and Aging, 17*, 598–609.

Magai, C. (2008) Long-lived emotions: A life course perspective. In M. Lewis, J. M. Haviland-Jones, & L. F. Barrett (Eds.), *Handbook of emotions* (3rd ed.) (pp. 376–392). New York: The Guilford Press.

Mather, M., & Carstensen, L. L. (2003) Aging and attentional biases for emotional faces. *Psychological Science, 14*, 409–415.

Mather, M., & Johnson, M. K. (2000) Choice-supportive source monitoring: Do our decisions seem better to us as we age? *Psychology and Aging, 15*, 596–606.

McMullen, M. N. (1997) Affective contrast and assimilation in counterfactual thinking. *Journal of Experimental Social Psychology, 33*, 77–100.

Mellers, B. A., & McGraw, A. P. (2001) Anticipated emotions as guides to choice. *Current Directions in Psychological Science*, *10*, 210–214.

Mellers, B. A., Schwartz, A., Ho, K., & Ritov, I. (1997) Decision affect theory: Emotional reactions to the outcomes of risky options. *Psychological Science*, *8*, 423–429.

Moor, K. A., Connelly, K. H., & Rogers, Y. (2004) *A comparative study of elderly, younger, and chronically ill novice pda users*. Bloomington: Indiana University.

Mroczek, D. K. (2001) Age and emotion in adulthood. *Current Directions in Psychological Science*, *10*, 87–90.

Nielsen, L., Knutson, B., & Carstensen, L. L. (2008) Affect dynamics, affective forecasting, and aging. *Emotion*, *8*, 318–330.

Peters, E. (2006) The functions of affect in the construction of preferences. In S. Lichtenstein & P. Slovic (Eds.), *The construction of preference*. New York: Cambridge University Press.

Peters, E., Hess, T. M., Västfjäll, D., & Auman, C. (2007) Adult age differences in dual information processes: Implications for the role of affective and deliberative processes in older adults' decision making. *Perspectives on Psychological Science*, *2*, 1–23.

Peters, E., Västfjäll, D., Gärling, T., & Slovic, P. (2006) Affect and decision making: A "hot" topic. *Journal of Behavioral Decision Making*, 19, 79–85.

Ready, R. E., Weinberger, M. I., & Jones, K. M. (2007) How happy have you felt lately? Two diary studies of emotion recall in older and younger adults. *Cognition & Emotion*, *21*, 728–757.

Riis, J., Loewenstein, G., Baron, J., Jepson, C., Fagerlin, A., & Ubel, P. A. (2005) Ignorance of hedonic adaptation to hemo-dialysis: A study using ecological momentary assessment. *Journal of Experimental Psychology: General*, *131*, 3–9.

Roese, N. J. (1997) Counterfactual thinking. *Psychological Bulletin*, *121*, 133–148.

Roese, N. J., & Summerville, A. (2005) What we regret most … and why. *Personality and Social Psychology Bulletin*, *31*, 1273–1285.

Russell, J. A. (2003) Core affect and the psychological construction of emotion. *Psychological Review*, *110*, 145–172.

Salthouse, T. A. (1996) The processing-speed theory of adult age differences in cognition. *Psychological Review*, *103*, 403–428.

Sanna, L. J. (1998) Defensive pessimism and optimism: The bitter-sweet influence of mood on performance and prefactual and counterfactual thinking. *Cognition and Emotion*, *12*, 635–665.

Timmers, E., Westerhof, G. J., & Dittmann-Kohli, F. (2005) "When looking back on my past life I regret…": Retrospective regret in the second half of Life. *Death Studies*, *29*, 625–644.

Van Dijk, E., & Zeelenberg, M. (2005) On the psychology of "if only": Regret and the comparison between factual and counterfactual outcomes. *Organizational Behavior and Human Decision Processes*, *97*, 152–160.

Van Dijk, E., & Zeelenberg, M. (2007) When curiosity killed regret: Avoiding or seeking the unknown in decision-making under uncertainty. *Journal of Experimental Social Psychology*, *43*, 656 662.

Västfjäll, D., Friman, M., Gärling, T., & Kleiner, M. (2002) The measurement of core affect: A Swedish self-report measure. *Scandinavian Journal of Psychology*, *43*, 19–31.

Västfjäll, D., & Gärling, T. (2002) Preference for regret, disappointment elation and surprise related to appraisal patterns and core affect. *Göteborg Psychological Reports*, *32*, 5.

Västfjäll, D., & Gärling, T. (in press) Preference for core affect and specific emotions. *Journal of Psychology*.

Västfjäll, D., Peters, E., & Johanson, B. (2009) Regret across the adult lifespan. In review.

Wrosch, C., Bauer, I., Miller, G. E., & Lupien, S. (2007) Regret intensity, diurnial cortisol secretion and physical health in older individuals: Evidence for directional effects and protective factors. *Psychology and Aging*, *22*, 319–330.

Wrosch, C., Bauer, I., & Scheier, M. F. (2005) Regret and quality of life across the adult life span: The influence of disengagement and available future goals. *Psychology and Aging*, *20*, 657–670.

Wrosch, C., & Heckhausen, J. (2002) Perceived control of life regrets: Good for young and bad for old adults. *Psychology and Aging*, *17*, 340–350.

Wurm, L. H., Labouvie-Vief, G., Aycock, J., Rebucal, K. A., & Koch, H. E. (2004) Performance in auditory and emotional Stroop tasks: A comparison of older and younger adults. *Psychology and Aging*, *19*, 523–535.

Zeelenberg, M. (1999) Anticipated regret, expected feedback and behavioral decision-making. *Journal of Behavioral Decision Making*, *12*, 93–106.

Zeelenberg, M., & Pieters, R. (2007) A theory of regret regulation 1.0. *Journal of Consumer Psychology*, *17*, 3–18.

# Chapter 11
# Attachment, Emotion Regulation and Adult Crying

**Joyce Maas, Anja Laan, and Ad Vingerhoets**

## 11.1 Introduction

Emotion regulation refers to "the process by which individuals influence which emotions they have, when they have them, and how they experience and express these emotions" (Gross, 1998, p. 275). Individuals differ considerably in emotion regulation. For example, whereas some people may actively seek emotion stimulation in leisure time, e.g., watching tear jerkers or choose a profession in which they often have to deal with emotions, others, in contrast, may spend much effort to avoid such situations or apply strategies to reduce the emotional impact of situations. Emotion regulation thus both involves the control and inhibition of emotions and their purposeful expression.

Two of the most frequently applied emotion regulation strategies to reduce negative emotions are reappraisal (changing the way one thinks about a potentially emotion-eliciting event) and suppression (changing the way one responds behaviorally to an emotion-eliciting event). Individuals differ considerably in their use of these emotion regulation strategies and there is evidence suggesting that these individual differences have implications for affect, well-being, and social relationships (Gross & John, 2003). Some forms of emotion regulation appear to offer more benefits than others. For example, research findings suggest that in particular reappraisal yields more health benefits in terms of short-term affective, cognitive, and social consequences than suppression (Gross & John, 2003).

Until now, little is known about the factors underlying these individual differences in emotion regulation. It is plausible that both genetic (including stable personality factors) and environmental/socio-cultural influences determine one's emotion regulation. Attachment style has been shown to be an important factor as well. In this chapter we will review the current literature on attachment, emotion regulation, and crying, after having briefly discussed attachment styles and their measurement. More precisely, the focus will be on the role of attachment styles in the expression or inhibition

J. Maas (✉)
Behavioral Science Institute, Radboud University Nijmegen,
P.O. Box 9104, 6500 HE Nijmegen, Netherlands
e-mail: j.maas@psych.ru.nl

I. Nyklíček et al. (eds.), *Emotion Regulation and Well-Being*,
DOI 10.1007/978-1-4419-6953-8_11, 

of emotions, particularly crying. Crying deserves this special attention, because it can be considered as one of the most important attachment behaviors designed to elicit support and help from others (Hendriks, Nelson, Cornelius, & Vingerhoets, 2008).

## 11.2 Primary and Secondary Attachment Strategies

According to Bowlby (1969/1982) all individuals are born with an innate attachment behavioral system. As infants, individuals learn to adopt attachment strategies based on reliable expectations about the people around them and these strategies become part of the child's behavioral repertoire (Mikulincer & Shaver, 2007), which form an important basis for later psychosocial functioning. For normative attachment functioning, it is important that an attachment figure is available, sensitive and responsive to the infant's need of proximity when necessary. In this way a primary attachment strategy develops in which the child learns that it can turn to others in times of need, that others are available and able to alleviate distress, which helps to regulate emotions. When feeling safe and comfortable as a result of the proximity of the caregiver, there is room for other activities, such as the exploration of the world one lives in. Thus, an important postulate of attachment theory is that a healthy dependence on a reliably sensitive and responsive attachment figure is crucial for optimal functioning and one's well-being over the life span. An additional claim is that the attachment system will be activated in stressful and demanding conditions, inducing a desire for proximity to a known and trusted other. When an attachment figure is not available, not sensitive, not responsive, or not able to alleviate distress, the primary goal of attachment, safety, is not attained. Because the primary attachment strategy of proximity seeking has failed, the individual has to resort to so-called secondary attachment strategies (Mikulincer & Shaver, 2007).

Main (1990) distinguished the following two secondary attachment strategies: *hyper*activation and *de*activation. When an attachment figure behaves very inconsistently, that is, sometimes very responsive and at other times not responsive at all, the attachment system is likely to be hyperactivated. The individual desperately tries to attract the attention of the attachment figure, because of the strong need for more support. In contrast, when the attachment figure consistently fails to respond to or punishes proximity seeking, deactivation of the attachment system is more likely to happen. In this case, the individual learns that is it better to "turn off" the attachment system in order to avoid the pain and frustration associated with the non-responsiveness of the attachment figure.

## 11.3 Attachment in Adulthood

Although the basis for attachment functioning lies in childhood, attachment theory emphasizes the relevance of attachment throughout the life span (e.g., Ainsworth, 1991; Bowlby, 1988). An important postulate of attachment theory is that the activation of the attachment system in stressful or taxing situations facilitates the proximity to a known and trusted other. In infancy, the behavioral repertoire to achieve these goals is rather limited and exists mainly of crying and smiling. As children grow older, several developments take place and attachment strategies generally become more diverse, complex, and flexible (Mikulincer & Shaver, 2007).

In infancy, the mother functions as the primary attachment figure. However, with increasing age and interest in romantic engagements, the relationship partner becomes the most important attachment figure. In addition, the number of attachment figures increases in adulthood. In infancy, this number is usually limited, while in adulthood a large number of people can serve as attachment figures, and different people can serve as attachment figures in different contexts, e.g., coworkers, friends, and romantic partners. Even groups or symbolic persons, like God, can be considered as attachment figures (Mikulincer & Shaver, 2007). Bowlby (1969/1982) referred to this as the "hierarchy of attachment figures." Nevertheless, the romantic partner functions as the most important attachment figure in adulthood (Mikulincer & Shaver, 2007).

In adulthood, actual proximity seeking is not always necessary and it is neither the primary aim of attachment behaviors. The adult attachment system is also not activated as quickly as in infancy, because the adult has learned to cope with problems autonomously. When proximity is needed, adults are able to postpone this need until attachment figures are actually available. Moreover, as an alternative to the proximity of one's attachment figure, mental representations of attachment figures can be activated instead (Mikulincer & Shaver, 2004). These mental representations can become symbolic sources of protection.

To achieve autonomy as an adult, it is important to have experienced positive interactions with one's attachment figures early in life. This helps an individual to remember typical interactions with attachment figures. These representations guide the individual in learning how to cope adequately with stressful conditions, such as in the case of self-care or self-soothing (Mikulincer & Shaver, 2007).

Secondary hyperactivating and deactivating strategies still exist in adulthood. These strategies are not only crucial in interpersonal relationships, but they also determine emotional well-being. It is important to realize that these secondary attachment strategies are not only represented in the behavior, but also in the cognitions of individuals. The attachment system is easily activated in the so-called hyperactivating individuals, which often leads to overwhelming, destructive emotions and puts an individual at risk for emotional and adjustment problems. Hypervigilance in terms of constantly searching for possible threats, catastrophizing and ruminating are examples of hyperactivating strategies, although this strategy originally was intended to alleviate distress. In contrast, suppressing threat-related thoughts and distracting attention away from threats are examples of deactivating strategies. Individuals using these strategies typically try, consciously as well as unconsciously, to keep the attachment system deactivated. For these persons it is very difficult to express their emotions, which, however, do exist internally (Mikulincer & Shaver, 2007). This characteristic makes it almost impossible to vent one's feelings. Attachment figures play a vital role in this coping strategy. When the attachment figure is responsive and available, coping with stress and emotions is facilitated. When this is not the case, however, coping is disrupted and this in turn increases distress (Mikulincer & Shaver, 2007).

## 11.4 Categorizing and Assessing Attachment Styles

Ainsworth (1967 Ainsworth, Blehar, Waters, & Wall, 1978) developed the Strange Situation Test to study differences in attachment behavior of young children. She was the first to describe three different attachment styles: secure, avoidant, and anxious. Because not all children fitted in one of these three categories, Main and Solomon (1986) later added a fourth category: disorganized/disoriented. Whereas secure infants are confident that their attachment figures will be available, responsive, and helpful when in need, anxious children, in contrast, lack the confidence that they will receive support when they need it, which results in clinging and dependent behavior. Avoidant children, on the other hand, typically try to resolve their lack of confidence with an attempt to be emotionally self-sufficient and they dismiss the need of emotional support from others. Finally, children with a disorganized-insecure attachment style may experience their caregivers as either frightening or frightened. They lack clear specific attachment behaviors; there is often a mix of behaviors, including avoidance or resistance and anxiety.

Similar to the classification of children in the Strange Situation Test, adults can also be categorized into these attachment styles on the basis of the Adult Attachment Interview (AAI; George, Kaplan, & Main, 1985). The AAI is considered the golden standard to assess adult attachment style. In addition, different self-report measures have been developed, such as the Relationship Questionnaire (RQ; Bartholomew & Horowitz, 1991), the Experiences in Close Relationships Questionnaire (ECR; Brennan, Clark, & Shaver, 1998), and the Experiences in Close Relationships-Revised (ECR-R; Fraley, Waller, & Brennan, 2000). Hazan and Shaver (1987) were the first to develop an assessment method for attachment in romantic relationships, the Adult Attachment Prototypes (AAP), which consisted of brief, multisentence descriptions of each of the three attachment styles.

The AAI and the AAP self-report measure by Hazan and Shaver (1987) have been developed independently of each other and have evolved from different streams of adult attachment research (Bartholomew & Shaver, 1998). The AAI, a semi-structured interview in which personal experiences in primary attachment relationships with parents are described, focuses on the "state of mind" in relation to attachment. Expert coders rate the verbal transcripts of which the coherence is more important than the content (Jacobvitz, Curran, & Moller, 2002). In contrast to the AAI, Hazan and Shaver's AAP measure focuses more on conscious appraisals of adults in romantic relationships (Jacobvitz, Curran, & Moller, 2002).

Over the years, Hazan and Shaver's (1987) original AAP assessment method has undergone several transformations (e.g., Bartholomew & Horowitz, 1991; Brennan, Clark, & Shaver, 1998; Collins & Read, 1990; Feeney, Noller, & Callan, 1994; Fraley, Waller, & Brennan, 2000; Simpson, 1990). In this chapter, the focus will be on one of those refined self-report measures: the Relationship Questionnaire (RQ), developed by Bartholomew and Horowitz. These authors attempted to combine the two research traditions described above into one model. While Hazan and Shaver's AAP measure identifies three different attachment styles, the RQ assesses four attachment styles. It consists of four brief descriptions of the four attachment styles (secure, fearful, preoccupied, and dismissive). Respondents are asked to rate on a 7-point Likert-scale the extent to which the description represents their own experiences in close relationships. Additionally, the respondent is requested to indicate which of the four descriptions best characterizes him or her. This allows researchers to use both categorical and continuous indicators.

Bartholomew and Horowitz (1991) define attachment styles with respect to two dimensions: confidence in oneself and in others. These dimensions are based on Bowlby's ideas about internal working models of self and others (Mikulincer & Shaver, 2007). The self-model reflects the degree of internalized self-worth and the others-model describes the degree to which others are expected to be available and supportive. The four attachment styles can be schematically represented as seen in Fig. 11.1.

The preoccupied category resembles the anxious category of the AAI, while the dismissive attachment style most closely corresponds to the avoidant attachment style. According to Bartholomew and Horowitz (1991), the fearful attachment style is most similar to the disorganized attachment style.

The RQ is a widely used self-report measure of attachment and although the RQ is a very short measure, its validity and reliability estimates are satisfactory (e.g., Scharfe & Bartholomew, 1994; Sibley, Fiher, & Liu, 2005). Furthermore, the RQ is easy to administer and readily scored, which makes it a very feasible measure, also usable in large scale epidemiological investigations.

| | | **Model of self** | |
|---|---|---|---|
| | | + | – |
| **Model of others** | + | **Secure**<br>Comfortable with intimacy and autonomy | **Preoccupied**<br>Overly dependent, preoccupied with relationships |
| | – | **Dismissing**<br>Dismissing of intimacy, counter-dependent | **Fearful**<br>Fearful of intimacy, socially avoidant |

**Fig. 11.1** Four-category model of attachment, adapted from Bartholomew and Horowitz (1991)

## 11.5 Attachment and Emotion Regulation

### *11.5.1 Self-Regulation of Emotions*

The attachment system plays an important role in emotion regulation. Actually, the attachment system may even be considered a kind of emotion regulation device (Mikulincer & Shaver, 2007). When an individual perceives a threat, the attachment system is activated and proximity is sought, which has the function to regulate the negative emotions associated with the threat. The ability to regulate emotions differs substantially between attachment styles. When encountering a negative emotion-eliciting event, securely attached individuals are able to engage in problem-solving behavior, to keep perceiving themselves as self-efficient, and to cognitively reappraise the event, to put things into perspective, or to turn a threat into a challenge. They are also more likely than insecurely attached individuals to seek support from other people or make use of self-caring or self-soothing skills. Securely attached individuals are also more capable of and more comfortable with experiencing and expressing their emotions, because they have learned that activating the attachment system may have beneficial consequences. Individuals who are classified as avoidant attached, in contrast, generally deny and suppress their emotions (Mikulincer & Shaver, 2007) and seem to convert negative stimuli into more positive ones in order to be able to ignore negative emotions (Spangler & Zimmerman, 1999). This can be interpreted as a defense response to the experience of continuous rejection by the attachment figure. As a consequence, they tend to be reluctant to ask for social support.

As said before, reappraisal and suppression are the two most frequently applied emotion regulation strategies (Gross & John, 2003). According to these authors, reappraisers experience more positive emotions and less negative emotions, in contrast to suppressors who show the opposite effect. Reappraisal, in contrast to suppression, is also positively related to better interpersonal functioning and well-being. This is in concordance with the attachment-theory view on emotion regulation. Although negative emotions are viewed as states to be managed or avoided by securely and avoidant attached people, anxiously attached people want to maintain these feelings or even exaggerate them, because they have learned this is the way to receive some attention from their non-responsive attachment figure (Mikulincer & Shaver, 2007). This can be illustrated with the research findings of Pereg and Mikulincer (2004), who examined the role of attachment style as moderator of the effects of induced negative affect. It was found that people with a secure attachment style reacted to negative affect induction with an affect-incongruent pattern. Securely attached individuals possess the ability to control the automatic spread of the activation of one negative cognition to another, because they have easy access to positive information about themselves and the world. Preoccupied attached people, in contrast, have a tendency to hyperactivate the negative emotions, which facilitates the accessibility of negative cognitions. As a consequence, they reacted with an affect-congruent pattern to negative affect induction. The dismissively attached individuals, in contrast, showed no significant reactions to the induction of negative affect, since their deactivating strategy allows them to distance themselves from affectively laden material.

### 11.5.2 Interpersonal Emotion Regulation

Interpersonal emotion regulation is an important skill. In this context, it is interesting to focus on the functions of attachment and empathy. Empathy entails "a positively valenced supportive response to the distress of another creature" (Watt, 2005, p. 187) which is essential for helping others to regulate their negative emotions. Empathy and attachment interact in several ways (Watt, 2005). First, functional imaging studies show a large overlap between brain areas activated in attachment and empathy, although more research is needed to identify shared mechanisms. Second, attachment bonds may be endangered when not enough empathy is shown or when the attachment figure is hurt. Third, empathic abilities seem to be under the influence of earlier and current attachment relationships (see also Britton & Fuendeling, 2005) and it has been suggested by Watt that individuals with an insecure attachment history have poorer empathic skills when compared to individuals with a secure attachment history. More specifically, several studies have found that dismissively attached individuals are the least empathic of all attachment styles (Mikulincer & Shaver, 2007, pp 341–345). Finally, Watt emphasizes that empathy is crucial for the creation and stability of attachment relationships.

Secure individuals are confident that their attachment figures will always be available and willing to help, in that way bolstering self-assurance for exploring one's world. In contrast, anxious individuals lack the confidence that their attachment figures are available and helpful when they need them, which results in a kind of clinging, dependent behavior and little self confidence, which prevents them from exploring the world. Avoidant individuals are also uncertain whether they will receive the needed support when in need; they therefore try to be emotionally self-sufficient and avoid close bonds with others. These so-called working models may be considered as stable personality traits over the whole life span. These different attachment patterns thus are major determinants of how individuals will respond to emotionally demanding situations (Feeney, 2006).

As outlined by Feeney (2006), attachment styles are strongly associated with social support, at least at three levels: (a) the seeking of social support; (b) the provision of social support; and (c) the perception of social support. Taken together, there is convincing evidence that one's attachment style plays an important role in shaping interpersonal behaviors and perceptions. However, avoidant attachment is not associated with less support seeking in general, but only when in stressful conditions. These individuals are reluctant to provide support when it is needed as well, whereas in conditions when no support is needed they do display support behaviors. Avoidant individuals thus cannot be depicted as being cold, distant and neglecting. However, especially when their partner needs it, they fail to provide the necessary support.

Insecure individuals also consider their partners as less willing to provide support. Since these styles are rather stable over the years, this likely may have consequences for the individual's well-being. Indeed, there is evidence that securely attached individuals are generally better adjusted than insecure individuals, which is also reflected in higher social competence and less symptoms of distress. In addition, their relationships may be more satisfying, which also contributes to their well-being.

### *11.5.3 Attachment and the Experience of Emotion*

Above, we already briefly mentioned the conversion of negative emotions into more positive emotions. Securely attached individuals do this by managing their negative emotions, whereas avoidant attached individuals deny their negative emotions and suppress them. We further outlined that securely attached individuals might experience more positive emotions than insecurely attached persons. In other words, it is likely that insecurely attached individuals also show deficits in the regulation of positive emotions. Shiota, Keltner, and John (2006) demonstrated that secure attachment is indeed positively related to the experience of positive emotions including joy, contentment, pride, love and compassion. In contrast, anxious or preoccupied attachment was negatively associated with joy, contentment, and pride but, remarkably, positively with love. However, avoidant or dismissive attachment was associated negatively with love and compassion, but positively with contentment, pride, and amusement. Finally, fearful attachment was negatively correlated with love, contentment, and pride. This study thus highlights the differences between attachment styles with respect to positive emotions: whereas preoccupied attached individuals show deficits in most positive emotions, except love, the opposite seems to be true for dismissively attached individuals, who show striking deficits in love and compassion, while they are still able to experience other positive emotions. Although preoccupied individuals show deficits in other, reward-focused, positive emotions, they nevertheless have the capacity to derive positive emotions from intimate relationships. However, dismissive individuals show the opposite pattern (Shiota et al., 2006). This fits with the notion that positive emotions play an important role in strengthening attachment bonds – something that anxious individuals try to achieve, whereas avoidant individuals do not have that wish (Mikulincer & Shaver, 2007, p. 218).

As for negative emotions, Magai, Distel, and Liker (1995) found attachment styles to be related differently to the experience of various negative feelings. More specifically, preoccupied attachment was found to be associated with fearfulness and shame in adulthood, while dismissive attachment was linked to contempt and disgust.

Recently, there is a growing interest in nostalgia, which is considered a bitter sweet emotion, that may have a facilitating effect on social bonding (Wildschut, Sedikides, Arndt, & Routledge, 2006; see also Chap. 5, this volume). Vingerhoets, Laan, Wildschut, Kalle, & Huis in't Veld (2009) showed that dismissively attached individuals scored considerably lower on two nostalgia measures. In addition, Wildschut's group reported findings suggesting that nostalgia may be helpful to enhance in-the-moment attachment security, by bolstering social bonds and rendering positive relational knowledge structures accessible. In conclusion, nostalgia deserves further research, in particular also in relation to attachment and social bonding.

## 11.6 Attachment and Adult Crying

Human crying in infants may be considered as being an inborn attachment behavior that serves to assure and call for the protective and nurturing presence of caregivers (Mikulincer & Shaver, 2007; Vingerhoets et al., 2009). There is good reason to assume that this important function is maintained during the whole life span. Crying occurs in particular in response to losses, separations, and interpersonal conflicts. It is an important way to express negative, but also maybe positive emotions, and it seems to be especially important for its strong effects in terms of the elicitation of emotional support and the facilitation of social bonding (Walter, 2006). Hendriks, Croon, and Vingerhoets (2008) demonstrated that people report to more readily give emotional support to a crying person, although they judge crying persons less positively than non-crying individuals. Crying can therefore be seen as an attachment behavior that elicits help from others.

Individuals differ considerably in crying frequency. For example, Frey et al. (1983) demonstrated substantial differences between men and women in crying frequency in their 30-day diary study among 286 female and 45 male adults. Women reported a mean emotional crying frequency of 5.3, with a range from 0 to 31, whereas men had an average of just 1.4. Only 6% of the women had no emotional crying episodes in the 30-day recording period, whereas 45% of the male participants had indicated not to have experienced any crying episode.

Individuals may also differ in the kind of stimuli that make them cry. Of course, there are strong emotional situations, like death, romantic break ups, and homesickness that are very strongly associated with tears. However, most of the crying episodes concern rather mundane and everyday events that may have a strong impact on one person in a certain situation, but not on another person or the same person in another situation (Vingerhoets, Boelhouwer, Van Tilburg, & Van Heck, 2001).

Until now, it is not clear which specific factors determine one's crying behavior, although there is substantial evidence that gender, personality (more specifically, neuroticism and empathy), and social learning are involved. In addition, substance abuse (alcohol, cocaine), physical and psychological state, being engaged in a romantic relationship, and having experienced a traumatic event may possibly affect one's crying behavior (Vingerhoets et al., 2009).

Given the associations between attachment styles, emotion regulation, and emotional expression (Kerr, Melley, Travea, & Pole, 2003; Kobak & Sceery, 1988; Mikulincer, 1998; Mikulincer & Shaver, 2007), it is reasonable to expect that attachment style also is associated with the shedding of emotional tears. Indeed, findings point out that different attachment styles, which incorporate different attachment strategies and internal working models of attachment are uniquely related to a pattern of emotional expression in general (Kobak & Sceery, 1998) and crying in particular (Bartholomew & Horowitz, 1991; Nelson, 2008). Assessing crying and non-crying can provide valuable information about the quality of the individual's past and current attachments (Nelson, 2000). Scarce empirical evidence suggests that securely attached individuals cry more often than dismissively attached persons, but less often than preoccupied attached individuals (Bartholomew & Horowitz, 1991).

An infant cries when in need of his or her mother/attachment figure and adults do just the same. Since crying is part of the attachment system (Nelson, 2008), individuals with different attachment styles may be expected to differ in their crying behavior. Securely attached individuals are comfortable activating their attachment system when needed, and they are also comfortable with crying and being soothed when confronted with stressful conditions. Additionally, when others cry, they are capable of providing care and support. Preoccupied attached persons hyperactivate their attachment system, and therefore also hyperactivate crying behavior. According to Nelson, they are difficult to be soothed and are likely to overly care for others too. In contrast, dismissively attached people are not comfortable showing crying behavior, as well as caring for others when they cry. Finally, it is Nelson's expectation that individuals classified as disorganized/disoriented tend to exhibit chaotic and inconsistent crying behavior. Their crying occurs unexpectedly and soothing can at the same time be demanded and resisted. The same holds for caring for others when they cry; sometimes care is excessive and at other times it is withheld.

Until now, there are hardly any empirical data available on the relationship between attachment style and adult crying. As mentioned before, only Bartholomew and Horowitz (1991) have presented data showing that dismissively attached individuals cry less often than securely attached individuals. Laan, Van Assen, and Vingerhoets (in preparation) were among the first to evaluate the above described hypotheses, put forth by Nelson (2008). They conducted two internet studies on the relationship between attachment and crying in general, and crying in response to music, in particular. The respondents' attachment styles were categorized using the RQ. Both studies collected data in two large independent samples and used different operationalizations of crying but yielded very similar and consistent findings. The participants' self-reports on crying and experienced emotions (in general and while listening to various emotion-eliciting songs) as well as questions about their crying tendency when being exposed to different attachment-related songs, yielded a similar pattern of findings. Dismissively attached individuals did not show their emotions easily through crying. Not only did they cry less frequently, shorter, and less intensely, they also reported more inhibition of crying than the other attachment styles. In addition, they reported a lower tendency to cry. Although anxious or preoccupied attachment was related to more crying than secure and dismissive attachment, this was only the case when they indicated to be exposed to negative events or when they reported to experience negative emotions. Finally, securely attached individuals were found to cry more in positive situations. Since gender is an important determinant of crying, it is important to notice that the connection between attachment style and crying behavior was rather similar for both men and women.

The differences were limited in magnitude but very consistent. The fact that the effect sizes were rather small may be related, on the one hand, to the quality of the applied assessment tool to determine the attachment style (the RQ), and, on the other hand, to the influences of several other factors on one's crying behavior, such as social learning, etc. In addition, as Feeney (2006) pointed out, attachment behaviors are hypothesized to be activated in particular when being exposed to stressful conditions. Music at best can be considered as either representations of emotional situations or conditioned stimuli, which are generally weaker than the original stimulus.

Preoccupied and fearfully attached individuals additionally reported more negative emotions when crying while listening to music than the securely and dismissively attached. More specifically, preoccupied and fearful individuals were more likely to experience the negative emotions sadness, helplessness and frustration when compared to the other attachment styles. Fearfully attached individuals were even more likely than preoccupied individuals to experience the emotions disgust, anger, and defeat, while preoccupied individuals were more likely to report feelings of anxiety. Emotional experience while crying thus also seems to differ qualitatively between attachment styles.

Some other recent studies have also investigated the relationship between crying and attachment. For example, Milling and Rowe (2009) demonstrated that the avoidant attachment style was a significant negative predictor of crying frequency, crying through sadness/loss, and crying through threat to self, while the anxious attachment style was a significant positive predictor of crying proneness, crying through threat to self, and crying through sadness/loss. These finding are clearly in line with the just described results, also emphasizing in particular the link between avoidant attachment and emotional inhibition. These authors wonder whether attitude toward crying may mediate the link between attachment style and patterns of crying behavior.

As already indicated above, crying is an attachment behavior designed to elicit help and proximity of significant others. This raises the question, whether the crying response is not only the result of the exposure to an emotional situation, but also of the availability of an attachment figure. In this respect, it is interesting that in former times crying was strongly associated with love and with praying. For example, in the love poems of antique poets like Ovid and Propertius (see Fögen, 2009), the shedding of tears was a common behavior, both in case of unrequited love as well as when the beloved reacted positively. But also famous scholars including Thomas More and the seventeenth century French philosopher René Descartes stressed the association between crying and love. In his treatise "The passions of the soul," Descartes asserts that most tears are not shed because of sadness, but because of the combination of sadness and love. We already mentioned symbolic figures, including God as attachment figures, which might clarify the role of crying when praying (see Lutz, 1999). This raises the question whether the availability of an attachment figure indeed facilitates tears. Preliminary data collected by Vingerhoets (unpublished data) provide support for this idea. This researcher found that students with a romantic partner cried more often than singles, and in two other studies he found a very modest but significant positive associations between self-reported loneliness and the incapacity to weep. In other words, the more lonely people felt, the more likely they reported a general inhibition of their crying. This intriguing aspect of crying certainly deserves further exploration. One obvious research question would be whether lonely people in their crying behavior are comparable to abandoned infants, who also show detached "non-crying."

Finally, one may also wonder about the significance of attachment style for the changes in crying observed in depressed patients or after having been exposed to traumatic events. Vingerhoets, Rottenberg, Cevaal, and Nelson (2007) discuss the relationship between depression and crying. They come to conclude that this relationship is far from clear. They suggest three possible associations, each with very modest empirical evidence at best. First, a linear connection is hypothesized, implying that those who cry more often are more likely to suffer from depression. The second model, in contrast, favors an inverted U-relationship, meaning that only those who suffer from a moderate depression cry more frequently, whereas severely depressed individuals discontinue the shedding of emotional tears. Finally, the authors wonder whether premorbid patient characteristics, including attachment style, might determine the change in crying behavior. A fourth model has been proposed by Keller, Neale, and Kendler (2007). These authors present evidence that the specific symptoms of depression are determined by its causal factors. More precisely, if the depression is triggered by a significant loss or separation (death or romantic breakup, and homesickness is another nice example in this respect), sadness and crying will be among the main symptoms, whereas in case of a depression caused by other life events such as conflicts, health problems, etc., other symptoms such as loss or gain of appetite, fatigue, or sleep problems prevail. This finding supports the idea that there is a link between attachment and crying, also in these patients with mood disorders. Further research is needed to reveal whether attachment style is additionally associated with how depression manifests itself.

## 11.7 Conclusion

Attachment plays an important role throughout the life span and may be considered as a determinant of emotion regulation. As infants, individuals already learn how to regulate their emotions. While securely attached individuals learn how to reappraise events, dismissively attached individuals develop a strong tendency to suppress or deactivate negative affect. In contrast, preoccupied attached individuals hyperactivate negative affect to get attention from their attachment figure. These findings are replicated in different studies.

The four attachment styles also display different crying behavior. Dismissively attached individuals – the deactivators, cry less frequently, less intensely, shorter and are more inhibited when experiencing negative emotions or events. Anxious or preoccupied attached individuals – the hyperactivators, cry more often in negative circumstances. Securely attached individuals also cry when experiencing positive events or emotions. In anxiously attached individuals' "negative" crying is more frequent because it is their way to get attention from their attachment figures. They do not feel the need to manage or avoid negative feelings and hyperactivate their attachment system.

Nelson's (2008) theory on crying may need some refinement and further elaboration with respect to the experience and expression of positive emotions, and with respect to the role of crying in depression and loneliness. People not only cry in negative circumstances but also in more positive situations (e.g., marriage, birth, celebrations), although it has been argued that also in such seeming positive situations, the tears may occur because of negative reasons (Vingerhoets et al., 2009). Crying related to positive emotions only seems to be freely expressed by securely attached individuals. Apparently, they are the only ones who feel comfortable to ventilate their positive emotions through crying and thus cry more in these situations than individuals who are not securely attached.

There can be little doubt that early attachment experiences have a lasting effect on our adult life, in particular how we regulate our emotions. Although other factors are probably involved, attachment could be an important etiological factor for deficits in affect regulation disorders and, as a consequence, of psychopathology.

More research is needed to investigate this link in more detail. There are currently several issues that need to be explored. Not much is known yet about the various qualitatively different positive and negative emotions. For instance, does attachment also affect feelings of guilt, shame, and pride, to mention some examples?

Results of such research can possibly help to design innovative therapeutic interventions. Interventions targeting attachment-related issues, such as schema focus therapy and emotion-focused therapy already exist (Dozier & Tyrrell, 1998), but deeper insight into the role of attachment style may result in more tailor-made approaches. This might improve the clients' quality of life in several ways; it could lead to improved affect, well-being, as well as improved social relationships.

## References


Ainsworth, M. D. S. (1967) *Infancy in Uganda*. Baltimore, MD: Johns Hopkins University Press.

Ainsworth, M. D. S. (1991) Attachments and other affectional bonds across the life-span. *Bulletin of the New York Academy of Medicine*, *61*, 792–811.

Ainsworth, M. D. S., Blehar, M. C., Waters, E. & Wall, S. (1978) *Patterns of attachment: A psychological study of the strange situation*. Hillsdale, NJ: Erbaum.

Anderson, C., John, O. P., Keltner, D., & Kring, A. (2001) Who attains social status effects of personality and physical attractiveness in social groups. *Journal of Personality and Social Psychology*, *81*, 116–132.

Bartholomew, K. & Horowitz, L. M. (1991) Attachment styles among young adults: A test of a four-category model. *Journal of Personality and Social Psychology*, *61*, 226–244.

Bartholomew, K. & Shaver, P. R. (1998) Methods of assessing adult attachment: Do they converge? In J. A. Simpson & W. S. Rholes (Eds.), *Attachment theory and close relationships* (pp. 25–45). New York: Guilford Press.

Bowlby, J. (1969/1982) *Attachment and loss, Vol. 1: Attachment*. New York: Basic Books.

Bowlby, J. (1988) Developmental psychiatry comes of age. *American Journal of Psychiatry, 145*, 1–10.
Brennan, K. A., Clark, C. L., & Shaver, P. R. (1998) Self-report measurement of adult romantic attachment: An integrative overview. In J. A. Simpson & W. S. Rholes (Eds.), *Attachment theory and close relationships* (pp. 46–76). New York: Guilford Press.
Britton, C. P., & Fuendeling, J. M. (2005). The relations among varieties of adult attachment and the components of empathy. *The Journal of Social Psychology, 145*, 519–530.
Collins, N. & Read, S. (1990) Adult attachment relationships, working models and relationship quality in dating couples. *Journal of Personality and Social Psychology, 58*, 644–683.
Dozier, M. & Tyrrell, C. (1998) The role of attachment in therapeutic relationships. In J. A. Simpson, & W. S. Rholes (Eds.), *Attachment theory and close relationships* (pp. 221–248). New York: Guilford Press.
Feeney, B. C. (2006) An attachment theory perspective on the interplay between intrapersonal and interpersonal processes. In K. D. Vohs & E. J. Finkel (Eds.), *Self and relationships: Connecting intrapersonal and interpersonal processes* (pp. 133–159). New York: Guilford.
Feeney, J. A., Noller, P., & Callan, V. J. (1994) Attachment style, communication and satisfaction in the early years of marriage. *Advances in Personal Relationships, 5*, 269–308.
Fögen, T. (2009) Tears in Propertius, Ovid and Greek epistolographers. In T. Fögen (Ed.), *Tears in the Graeco-Roman world* (pp. 179–208). New York: Walter de Gruyter.
Fraley, R. C., Waller, N. G., & Brennan, K. A. (2000) An item-response theory analysis of self-report measures of adult attachment. *Journal of Personality and Social Psychology, 78*, 350–365.
Frey, W. H., Hoffman-Ahern, C., Johnson, R. A., Lykken, D. T., & Tuason, V. B. (1983) Crying behavior in the human adult. *Integrative Psychiatry, 1*, 94–100.
George, C., Kaplan, N., & Main, M. (1985) *The Adult Attachment Interview*. Unpublished protocol, Department of Psychology, University of California, Berkeley.
Gross, J. J. (1998) The emerging field of emotion regulation: An integrative review. *Review of General Psychology, 2*, 271–299.
Gross, J. J. & John, O. P. (2003) Individual differences in two emotion regulation processes: implications for affect, relationships and well-being. *Journal of Personality and Social Psychology, 85*, 348–362.
Hazan, C. & Shaver, P. R. (1987) Romantic love conceptualized as an attachment process. *Journal of Personality and Social Psychology, 59*, 511–524.
Hendriks, M. C. P., Croon, M. A., & Vingerhoets, A. J. J. M. (2008) Social reactions to adult crying: The help-soliciting function of tears. *Journal of Social Psychology, 148*, 22–41.
Hendriks, M. C. P., Nelson, J. K., Cornelius, R. R., & Vingerhoets, A. J. J. M. (2008) Why crying improves our well-being: An attachment-theory perspective on the functions of adult crying. In A. J. J. M. Vingerhoets, I. Nyklícek, & J. Denollet (Eds.), *Emotion regulation: Conceptual and clinical issues*, (pp. 87–96). New York: Springer.
Jacobvitz, D., Curran, M., & Moller, N. (2002) Measurement of adult attachment: The place of self-report and interview methodologies. *Attachment and Human Development, 4*, 207–215.
Keller, M. C., Neale, M. C, & Kendler, K. S. (2007) Association of different adverse life events with distinct patterns of depressive symptoms. *American Journal of Psychiatry, 164*, 1521–1529.
Kerr, S. L., Melley, A. M., Travea, L., & Pole, M. (2003) The relationship of emotional expression and experience to adult attachment style. *Individual Differences Research, 1*, 108–123.
Kobak, R. & Sceery, A. (1988) Attachment in late adolescence: Working models, affect regulation, and representations of self and others. *Child Development, 59*, 135–146.
Lutz, T. (1999) *Crying. The natural and cultural history of tears*. New York: Norton.
Magai, C., Distel, N., & Liker, R. (1995) Emotion socialization, attachment, and patterns of adult emotional traits. *Cognition and Emotion, 9*, 461–481.
Main, M. (1990) Cross-cultural studies of attachment organization: Recent studies, changing methodologies and the concept of conditional strategies. *Human Development, 33*, 48–61.
Main, M. & Solomon, J. (1986) Discovery of an insecure disorganized/ disoriented attachment pattern: Procedures, findings, and implications for classification of behaviour. In T. B. Brazelton & M. W. Yogman (Eds.), *Affective development in infancy* (pp. 95–124). Norwood, NJ: Ablex.

Milling, A. & Rowe, A. (2009) *Attachment styles and adult crying behaviour*. International Society for Research on Emotion, Leuven, Belgium, August 2009, Conference Proceedings.

Mikulincer, M. (1998) Adult attachment style and individual differences in functional versus dysfunctional experiences of anger. *Journal of Personality and Social Psychology, 74*, 513–524.

Mikulincer, M. & Shaver, P. R. (2004) Security-based self-representations in adulthood: Contents and processes. In W. S. Rholes & J. A. Simpson (Eds.), *Adult attachment: Theory, research, and clinical implications* (pp. 159–195). New York: Guilford Press.

Mikulincer, M. & Shaver, P. R. (2007) *Attachment in adulthood: Structure, dynamics, and change*. New York: Guilford Press.

Nelson, J. K. (2000) Clinical assessment of crying and crying inhibition based on attachment theory. *Bulletin of the Menninger Clinic, 64*, 509–529.

Nelson, J. K. (2008) Crying in psychotherapy: Its meaning, assessment, and management based on attachment theory. In A. J. J. M. Vingerhoets, I. Nyklícek, & J. Denollet (Eds.), *Emotion regulation: Conceptual and clinical issues*, (pp. 202–214). New York: Springer.

Pereg, D. & Mikulincer, M. (2004) Attachment style and the regulation of negative affect: Exploring individual differences in mood congruency effects on memory and judgment. *Personality and Social Psychology Bulletin, 30*, 67–80.

Scharfe, E. & Bartholomew, K. (1994) Reliability and stability of adult attachment patterns. *Personal Relationships, 1*, 23–43.

Shiota M.N., Keltner D., John O.P. (2006). Positive emotion dispositions differentially associated with Big Five Personality and attachment style. *Journal of Positive Psychology*, 61–71.

Sibley, C. G., Fischer, R., & Liu, J. H. (2005) Reliability and validity of the revised experiences in close relationships (ECR-R) self-report measure of adult romantic attachment. *Personality and Social Psychology Bulletin, 31*, 1524–1536.

Simpson, J. A. (1990) Influence of attachment styles on romantic relationships. *Journal of Personality and Social Psychology, 59*, 971–980.

Spangler, G. & Zimmerman, P. (1999) Attachment representation and emotion regulation in adolescents: A psychobiological perspective on internal working models. *Attachment and Human Development, 1*, 270–290.

Vingerhoets, A. J. J. M. & van Assen, M. A. L. M. (2009) *Love and tears*. International Society for Research on Emotion, Leuven, Belgium, August 2009, Conference Proceedings.

Vingerhoets, A. J. J. M., Bylsma, L., & Rottenberg, J. (2009) Crying: A biopsychosocial phenomenon. In T. Fögen (Ed.), *Tears in the Graeco-Roman world* (pp. 439–475). New York: Walter de Gruyter

Vingerhoets, A. J. J. M., Boelhouwer, A. J. W., Van Tilburg, M. A. L. & Van Heck, G. L. (2001) The situational and emotional context of adult crying. In A. J. J. M. Vingerhoets & R. R. Cornelius (Eds.), *Adult crying: A biopsychosocial approach* (pp. 71–89). Hove, United Kingdom: Brunner-Routledge

Vingerhoets, A. J. J. M., Laan, A. J., Wildschut, R. T., Kalle, M. J. C., & Huis in't Veld, L. (2009) *Attachment style and nostalgia in adults*. International Attachment Conference, Barcelona, Spain, October 2009.

Vingerhoets, A. J. J. M., Rottenberg, J., Cevaal, A., & Nelson, J. K. (2007) Is there a relationship between depression and crying? A review. *Acta Psychiatrica Scandinavica, 115*, 340–351.

Walter, C. (2006) *Thumbs, toes, and tears and other traits that make us human*. New York: Walker & Company.

Watt, D. F. (2005) Social bonds and the nature of empathy. *Journal of Consciousness Studies, 12*, 185–209.

Wildschut, T., Sedikides, C., Arndt, J., & Routledge, C. (2006) Nostalgia: Content, triggers, functions. *Journal of Personality and Social Psychology, 91*, 975–993.

# Chapter 12
# Self-Conscious Emotions and Social Functioning

**Ilona E. de Hooge, Marcel Zeelenberg, and Seger M. Breugelmans**

## 12.1 Introduction

Have you ever felt guilty about hurting a loved one, or been proud after achieving something that you always dreamed of? These emotions, but also embarrassment, shame, and hubris, are called self-conscious emotions. They are a special kind of emotions that cannot be described solely by examining facial movements (Darwin, 1872/1965) and that do not have clear, distinct elicitors (Lewis, 2000). Self-conscious emotions are cognitively complex and play a central role in the motivation and regulation of thoughts, feelings, and behaviors (Baumeister, Stillwell, & Heatherton, 1994; Leith & Baumeister, 1998; Tangney & Fischer, 1995). Until now, most research concerning the relationship between self-conscious emotions and social behavior has focused on their anticipation affects of what people do (e.g., Gruenewald, Dickerson, & Kemeny, 2007; Keltner & Buswell, 1997; Tracy & Robins, 2004). The anticipation of negative self-conscious emotions such as shame or guilt can motivate avoidance of immoral or asocial behavior (I will not do that, otherwise I will feel ashamed), and the anticipation of positive self-conscious emotions such as pride can stimulate compliance with social and moral norms (If I do that, I will be proud of myself).

Also, actual experiences of self-conscious emotions may exert an influence. For example, when people feel ashamed, they do certain things because of that (e.g., hide or try to appease). The aim of the present chapter is to shed some light on how experiences of self-conscious emotions are regulated and as such influence social behavior. We will start with a discussion concerning the definition of self-conscious emotions and how they differ from so-called basic emotions. Then the focus shifts to existing research concerning the influences of self-conscious emotions on moral and social behavior. We will discuss how these often-contrasting findings can be interpreted using an emotion-specific approach. Finally, two self-conscious emotions, namely

I.E. de Hooge (✉)
Rotterdam School of Management, Erasmus University, Burgemeester Oudlaan 50, 3062 PA Rotterdam, Netherlands
e-mail: IHooge@rsm.nl

I. Nyklíček et al. (eds.), *Emotion Regulation and Well-Being*,
DOI 10.1007/978-1-4419-6953-8_12, © Springer Science+Business Media, LLC 2011

shame and guilt will be highlighted. We will explain how our approach can clarify the contrasting, empirical findings concerning the influences of shame and guilt on behavior (e.g., Gilbert & Andrews, 1998; Lewis, 1971, 1992; Tangney & Dearing, 2002; Tangney & Fischer, 1995).

## 12.2 What Are Self-Conscious Emotions?

The central feature of self-conscious emotions involves self-recognition and self-evaluation (Tangney, 1999). Self-conscious emotions arise when people reflect upon themselves and compare their behavior with a set of rules or social norms that determine whether their actions are right or wrong (Beer, 2007; Tangney, Stuewig, & Mashek, 2007b). The comparison gives rise to both an evaluation of the ethics of the behavior and of *what* the behavior reveals about the self. Dependent on the results of those evaluations, people experience shame, guilt, embarrassment, pride, envy, jealousy, or hubris. In other words, self-conscious emotions rely on having a sense of self and involve injury to or enhancement of the sense of self (Niedenthal, Krauth-Gruber, & Ric, 2006). Basic emotions may involve these self-evaluative processes, but self-conscious emotions need self-awareness and self-representations in order to arise (Tangney & Dearing, 2002; Tracy & Robins, 2007).

Because self-conscious emotions need an awareness of the self, awareness that others are judging that self, and an awareness that there are a set of rules or social norms that determine whether the actions of the self are right or wrong, they arise later in life than most basic emotions (Beer, 2007; Izard, 1977). While most basic emotions emerge within the first 9 months of life, self-conscious emotions emerge around the third year of life (Izard, Ackerman, & Schultz, 1999). Even generalized feelings of self-consciousness do not develop until around 18–24 months (Lewis, 2000). The reason is that all self-conscious emotions require that the individual is able to have a sense of self distinct from others, which begins to develop around the age of 2 (Niedenthal et al., 2006).

Self-conscious emotions and basic emotions also differ in that self-conscious emotions are cognitively complex emotions (Tracy & Robins, 2004). Self-conscious emotions arise after the self is evaluated against some standard. Cognitive processes are thus the elicitors of these emotions, and the emotion arising from the cognitive processes is dependent on the situation and on the individual (Lewis, 2000). For example, different emotions arise when people evaluate themselves to be responsible for the behavior being evaluated, or when they evaluate themselves to be not responsible. In addition, the evaluation of people's behavior as being successful or unsuccessful depends on the social standards they use in the comparison. In that way, the same behavior can be perceived as a failure and give rise to shame in one person, or be perceived as a success and give rise to pride in another. The set of standards, rules, or goals against which people's behavior is compared, is provided by culture and transmitted to children, who then incorporate them as their own (Lewis, 2000). This means that there is more cultural variation in self-conscious emotions on their subjective experiences and on display rules than in basic emotions (Kitayama, Rose Markus, & Matsumoto, 1995).

## 12.3 Self-Conscious Emotions as Moral Emotions

Self-conscious emotions are based on an ability to evaluate the self, in which the self is viewed as an object of scrutiny and matched with standards that are taught by society or by the immediate social context. Because these standards are often standards for moral behavior, self-conscious emotions are regularly perceived as moral emotions (Niedenthal et al., 2006).

Moral emotions are emotions that are linked to the well-being of others and of society as a whole (Haidt, 2003). Already in 1759, the founder of modern economics Adam Smith suggested that moral sentiments stimulate people to focus on other people and on how their own behavior affects these others' well-being. When there is a conflict between people's own interests and others' interests (i.e., a social dilemma), moral sentiments motivate people to take into account others' interests. In other words, these emotions motivate people to act in a morally appropriate way (to do well and to avoid doing bad), even though this can be contrary to their immediate economic self-interest (Kroll & Egan, 2004; Tangney, Stuewig, & Mashek, 2007a). Frank (1988, 2004) added to this that moral emotions can be understood as commitment devices. When people find themselves to be in a social dilemma situation, a choice for self-interest (or an imaginary choice for self-interest) immediately gives rise to negative moral emotions, such as guilt. As a consequence, the self-interest option becomes less attractive, stimulating people to choose the prosocial, long-term option. The prosocial option is not only beneficial for others and for society, it also benefits people themselves by making future collaborations more probable, by avoiding punishments from others for acting selfishly, and more generally by creating trust among people. In summary, moral emotions act as commitment devices, stimulating prosocial behavior and committing people to options that are best for the society and for *themselves* in the long run.

The effects of moral emotions on prosocial behavior may depend on person characteristics. Some people, called prosocials, have a natural tendency to act prosocially, whereas others, called proselfs, have a natural tendency to act more selfishly (Messick & McClintock, 1968). Moral emotions act as a situational activation of a prosocial goal by making immediate selfish options less attractive. Ample research has shown that situational activation of a goal only affects behavior of people for whom that goal is not already chronically activated (Higgins, 1996). Because acting prosocially can be seen as a chronically activated goal for prosocials (Nelissen, Dijker, & De Vries, 2007), moral emotions have little effect on their level of prosocial behavior. In contrast, because acting selfishly is a chronically activated goal for proself, moral emotions especially have a large effect on their level of prosocial behavior. Indeed, recent empirical research has shown that negative moral emotions such as guilt and shame especially motivate prosocial behavior in proselfs and not in prosocials (De Hooge, Zeelenberg, & Breugelmans, 2007; De Hooge, Breugelmans, & Zeelenberg, 2008; Ketelaar & Au, 2003; Nelissen et al., 2007).

## 12.4 Specific Self-Conscious Emotions and Behavior

One possible way to study the influence of emotions on behavior is to make predictions on the basis of their valence (i.e., whether the emotions are positive or negative). However, this approach overlooks the fact that different self-conscious emotions of the same valence may motivate quite different behaviors. Recent empirical research has already shown that a specific-emotions approach gives more insights into the effects of basic emotions on behavior. For example, the two negative emotions anger and fear have been found to generate contrasting risk-taking behaviors (Lerner & Keltner, 2001). Similarly, regret and disappointment had different effects on behavior (Zeelenberg & Pieters, 1999). Thus it seems that a focus on specific emotions will give more insight into the influences of self-conscious emotions on behavior than a mere valence approach. For this reason, we will adopt an approach based on specific emotions, namely the feeling-is-for-doing approach (Zeelenberg & Pieters, 2006).

In general, emotions are thought to arise after an evaluation (an appraisal) of an event as positively or negatively relevant to one's goals or concerns (Frijda, 1986). Emotions concern an object or a person, and are acute and relatively momentary experiences. The appraisal, the process of judging the significance of an event for personal well-being, determines whether an emotion is felt, and which specific emotion is experienced. A specific pattern of cognitive appraisals of the emotion-eliciting situation gives rise to a specific emotion (Ortony, Clore, & Collins, 1988; Smith & Lazarus, 1993). In a situation, people may have different patterns of cognitive appraisals, but the same pattern of appraisals always gives rise to the same emotion. As we will show later on, the appraisal pattern tells us why a specific emotion arises and thus what behaviors it will motivate. Importantly, the appraisal process results in the experience of emotion which is a conglomerate of motivational goals, action tendencies, and actions. Discrete emotions contain goals, such as avoiding danger when feeling fear, or taking revenge when feeling angry (Roseman, Wiest, & Swartz, 1994). These general goals are labeled emotivational goals by Roseman et al. and patterns of action readiness by Frijda (1986, 2006). The emotivational goal translates into an inclination to respond with a particular action (the action tendency), and finally, when it is possible in the situation, an action will follow.

Emotions can therefore be understood as motivational processes that are instrumental to the goal one is striving for (Zeelenberg, Nelissen, & Pieters, 2007). Negative emotions arise when a concern of a person is threatened, and then motivate behavior to close the gap between the present situation and the goal. Our approach also explains why it is important to focus on the effects of different emotions and not on the mere valence of emotions. Different problems may arise in relation to a person's concerns. Because these different problems require different solutions, different emotions exist. They signal a specific problem, and motivate behaviors concentrated on that specific problem. The specific behavior that is motivated to solve a problem depends on the accessibility and acceptability in the situation, and on the instrumentality to the overarching goal.

Importantly, the feeling-is-for-doing approach not only makes a distinction between different emotions, but also between endogenous and exogenous influences of emotions (Zeelenberg et al., 2008; Zeelenberg & Pieters, 2006). These terms capture whether the emotional influence comes from within (endogenous) or outside (exogenous) the goal striving process. Emotions can influence behavior in situations that are related to the emotion-causing event. In this case, the influence of the emotion is relevant for and part of current goal pursuit, and is labeled an endogenous influence. For example, the influence of anger with banks because of the 2009 financial crisis on the decision to open a bank-account, or the experience of fear when moving to an unknown country for a year. Influences of emotions are labeled exogenous when they influence behaviors in situations that are unrelated to the emotion-causing event. These influences are irrelevant for and external to current goal-pursuit, and can be found in examples of spill-over effects of emotions resulting from a prior experience, such as hearing happy or sad music, on subsequent, unrelated decisions, such as deciding to buy a car.

The distinction between exogenous and endogenous influences of emotions can play an important role in the study of self-conscious emotions. Research on exogenous influences of self-conscious emotions may give us insights in spill-over effects and show us how self-conscious emotions influence behaviors in ways that should logically not occur. However, the results of exogenous influences cannot always be used to interpret the function of an emotion, because these effects may be influenced by the changing surrounding. Endogenous influences of emotions show us what the emotion signals to the decision maker and therefore do give insights in the functioning of self-conscious emotions. Importantly, exogenous and endogenous influences of a single emotion may give rise to completely different behaviors. As we will show with the self-conscious emotions shame and guilt, not taking into account these distinct influences may result in diverse understandings of the same emotion.

## 12.5 Not So Ugly After All: The Case of Shame

Perhaps the most complicated self-conscious emotion is shame. This self-conscious emotion is by many scholars described as "one of the most powerful, painful, and potentially destructive experiences known to humans" (Gilbert, 1997, p. 113). It arises after a moral transgression or incompetence, in which people appraise the situation as having violated a moral or social standard (Fessler, 2004; Keltner & Buswell, 1996). The behavior generalizes to the whole self-image, and as *a* consequence, people have a heightened degree of self-awareness and think the whole self is fundamentally flawed (Izard, 1977; Lewis, 1971; Sabini & Silver, 1997). In addition, shame heightens the awareness of others around and stimulates a focus on others' actual or imagined negative evaluations (Fessler, 2004; Haidt, 2003; Tangney & Dearing, 2002). During a shame experience, people often feel small, alone, powerless, helpless, and inferior to others (Fontaine et al., 2006; Nathanson, 1992; Tangney, 1995, 1999). The feeling can express itself in bodily posture: after a shame experience the body is often collapsed with the shoulders falling in, and the eyes are lowered with the gaze downwards (Keltner & Buswell, 1996; Lewis, 2003).

It has often been stated that shame has a negative influence on behavior. It would make speech, movement, and action more difficult and less likely (Gilbert, 1997), and would be related to submission, social avoidance, withdrawal, rejection, and disengagement from others (Dickerson & Gruenewald, 2004; Lewis, 2003; Probyn, 2004; Tangney, 1991, 1995; Tangney et al., 2007a). According to Tangney (1999), shame motivates behaviors that "are likely to sever or interfere with interpersonal relationships." The thought behind these submissive and withdrawal behaviors is that they function as a form of appeasement, signaling to others that people are aware of their norm-violating behavior and will not fight back but will conform to the group standards (Gilbert, 1997; Izard, 1977; Mills, 2005; Nathanson, 1987).

In contrast with the fair amount of theoretical research on shame, there is hardly any empirical research on the behaviors elicited in attempts to regulate current experiences of shame. Even more, the few existing empirical studies on shame-induced behaviors produced contradicting results. Often, participants were asked to recall a situation in which they had experienced shame, and subsequently they rated what they felt, what they thought, and what they wanted to do after the described situation. On the one hand, findings of these studies suggest that shame promotes withdrawal and avoidance behaviors. For example, shame was found to be characterized by withdrawal tendencies compared to other emotions such as joy, anger, disgust, sadness, and fear (Scherer & Wallbott, 1994). On the other hand, some studies suggest that shame can promote approach behaviors. For example, Tangney, Miller, Flicker, and Barlow (1996) showed that shame activated a higher willingness to make amends than to hide. In addition, some scholars such as Wicker, Payne, and Morgan (1983) showed that shame experiences were rated neutral on items ranging from wanting to hide to making restitutions, while others such as Frijda, Kuipers, and ter Schure (1989) even found that shame activated *both* a desire to disappear from view and a desire to undo the situation compared to guilt and regret.

We believe that, by applying the feeling-is-for-doing approach and focusing on the emotion elements and the situation, we can explain how shame can motivate seemingly contradictory behaviors. When we think back of the definition of shame, the central theme appears to be a negative or hurt self-image (Lewis, 1971). One of the most important fundamental human motives is the desire to have a positive self view (e.g., Alexander & Knight, 1971; Schlenker & Leary, 1982; Taylor & Brown, 1988). People compare themselves to others, make self-serving attributions, and they react defensively or act assertively to achieve and maintain such a positive view (Gibbons, 1990). Exactly this positive view of the self is threatened during a shame experience (Lewis, 1971), and this gives rise to feelings of inferiority and worthlessness, and to negative thoughts about the self and about what others would think about the self. When applying the feeling-is-for doing approach, it appears that the emotivational goal of shame is to deal with the threatened self.

First, based on the emotion elements of shame, we suggest that shame motivates approach behaviors to restore the self, and when this is not possible and to too risky, it motivates avoidance behaviors to protect the self. In other words, the behaviors following from shame are first and foremost approach behaviors. Because having a positive self view is a fundamental motive, people experiencing shame will be motivated to restore that positive self view. This restore motivation will elicit approach behaviors such as entering achievement situations, performing new challenges, and undertaking reparative actions. But when for any reason it is impossible or too risky to restore the self, we suggest that shame will motivate withdrawal behaviors instead of approach behaviors to protect the threatened self from more possible harm. Thus, shame "can prompt behaviors to protect the self from additional scrutiny or self-threatening exposure" (Ferguson, 2005, p. 378).This was recently supported by findings showing that shame activates both a restore motive and a protect motive, which then motivate approach behavior (De Hooge, Zeelenberg, & Breugelmans, 2010). In addition, recent follow-up studies (De Hooge, Zeelenberg, & Breugelmans, in press) revealed that when repair after a shame event is risky, the restore motive lowers and the protect motive stimulates avoidance behavior.

Second, we suggest that the approach behavior motivated by shame depends on the situation and on whether the emotion is endogenous or exogenous. One important form of approach behavior discussed above is prosocial behavior. Prosocial behavior not only deals with the threatened self after a shame event, it also improves the image the audience has of the actor. In addition, the prosocial behavior corresponds with what moral emotions theory would predict (Frank, 1988). When taking a close look at the emotivational goal of shame, namely restoring the self-image and the image the audience has of the actor, prosocial effects are expected to appear only in situations related to the shame event. In other words, approach behavior, and especially prosocial behavior, is expected when studying endogenous influences of shame. We do not expect approach behaviors following from shame when studying exogenous influences, because the situation in which the self was threatened is already different from the decision situation at hand. By being in a situation unrelated to shame, the emotivational goal to deal with the threatened self underlying shame has already been (partially) satisfied because one has already left the threatening situation (i.e., the protect motive is fulfilled). As a consequence, people will not act upon their shame feelings. The absence of effects for exogenous influences of shame corresponds with what shame theories would predict (Lewis, 2003; Tangney, 1999). In summary, according to the feeling-is-for-doing approach, endogenous shame does motivate prosocial behavior, while exogenous shame does not. Indeed, in previous studies, we found no effects of shame on prosocial behavior in situations unrelated to the induction procedure (De Hooge et al., 2007). Recent findings of De Hooge et al. (2008) revealed that shame does motivate prosocial behavior in situations related to the shame event, but does not motivate prosocial behavior in situations unrelated to the shame event.

## 12.6 Not So Social After All: The Case of Guilt

The picture that emerges from emotion literature for guilt is much more positive than that for shame. Guilt mainly arises after a moral transgression in which people have hurt, intentionally or unintentionally, another person (Fessler & Haley, 2003;

Izard, 1977; Tangney, 1991, Zeelenberg & Breugelmans, 2008). The most common category of causes of guilt are neglecting partners in close relationships and failing to live up to commitments or obligations to others (Baumeister, Reis, & Delespaul, 1995). While shame involves perceiving the entire self as bad and worthless, guilt only involves perceiving a self-produced specific behavior as bad, hurtful, or immoral (Lewis, 1971). As a consequence, people are completely focused on the harm and distress that they have caused to the other person (Baumeister et al., 1994; Lewis, 1987). After the transgression, people often feel tense, remorseful, worried, and less competent (Ferguson, Stegge, & Damhuis, 1991; Lewis, 1971).

Most emotion theories perceive guilt to exert positive influences on behavior. Guilt would be linked to better perspective taking and feelings of empathy (Leith & Baumeister, 1998; Tangney & Dearing, 2002). It motivates a desire to compensate the victim, and actions to repair the hurt caused, to make amends, or to apologize (Caplovitz Barrett, 1995; Lindsay-Hartz, 1984; Thrane, 1979). The function of guilt is to preserve and strengthen the hurt relationship by making up past transgression and stimulating more appropriate behavior in the future (Amodio, Devine, & Harmon-Jones, 2007; Baumeister et al., 1994).

The theoretical perspective of guilt as a self-conscious emotion with positive, adaptive influences is empirically supported. For example, guilt has been found to motivate a heightened sense of personal responsibility, compliance, and forgiveness, and to generate more constructive strategies to cope with anger (Freedman, Wallington, & Bless, 1967; Izard, 1977; McCullough, Worthington, & Rachal, 1997; Strelan, 2007; Tangney et al., 1992). Several studies have also shown that guilt is strongly related to reparative intentions (Schmader & Lickel, 2006; Tangney, 1993). For example, when studying the phenomenology, action tendencies, and emotivational goals of ten different emotions, Roseman et al. (1994) found that after a guilt experience participants felt like undoing their actions, punishing themselves, apologizing, and wanting to make up for their transgression and to be forgiven. Importantly, cross-cultural studies have shown that these characteristics of guilt are quite similar across a wide array of cultures (Breugelmans & Poortinga, 2006; Fontaine et al., 2006), which is testimony to the universal moral character of guilt. Perhaps the most direct evidence for moral effects of guilt has been given by a recent series of studies on the effects of emotions on prosocial behavior in dyadic relationships. These studies found that, after experiencing guilt, people acted more prosocially in social dilemma games towards an unknown other (De Hooge et al., 2007; Ketelaar & Au, 2003; Nelissen et al., 2007). To summarize, guilt appears to be a good, moral self-conscious emotion that produces beneficial consequences for people in one's social surrounding.

However, when paying attention to the emotion elements of guilt and applying our feeling-is-for-doing approach, it appears that guilt may not have such positive effects overall. Taking a closer look at guilt, it becomes clear that this emotion revolves around a threatened relationship that needs to be dealt with. People are focused on what they have done wrong and on the person that has been hurt by their actions (Lewis, 1971). It follows that guilt has the goal to improve the violated or threatened relationship. This means that the action tendencies ensuing from guilt are mainly aimed at restoring this dyadic relationship. In the words of Baumeister et al. (1994): “After doing something bad to another person, people are motivated *to help that person* or comply with that person’s wishes, apparently to rectify any inequity and to repair any damage to the relationship” (p. 260, italics added). Similar to shame, we suggest that the following action tendencies of guilt depend on the situation and on the whether the emotion is endogenous or exogenous to current goal striving.

First, when the hurt person is present (and hence the guilt is endogenous to the situation), it is possible to repair the damage and guilt will motivate prosocial behavior towards the hurt person. This suggestion is supported by the findings that guilt motivates prosocial behavior in dyadic relationships (De Hooge et al., 2007; Ketelaar & Au, 2003; Nelissen et al., 2007). However, in daily life, people interact with multiple others at the same time. Taking this broader perspective on moral behavior, looking beyond dyadic relationships, it becomes clear that guilt can also have negative interpersonal consequences. More specifically, we argue that the dyadic preoccupation that is central to experiences of guilt can lead to behavior that is negative for the outcomes of others around us. When focusing on repairing the hurt relationship, people temporarily pay less attention to other social partners and generally compensate at the expense of the resources allocated to other people rather than those allocated to themselves. In other words, guilt may lead to an extra investment in the relationship with the victim, but someone else will have to pay the bill. Indeed, recent studies showed that in three-person situations, guilt motivated prosocial behavior towards the hurt other at the expense of the third one around and not at the expense of oneself (De Hooge, Nelissen, Breugelmans, & Zeelenberg, 2009).

Second, in situations where the hurt person is not present (and hence the guilt is exogenous), guilt will have other behavioral effects. In those situations, it is not possible to restore the damage. The emotivational goal of improving the hurt relationship will then translate into improving relationships in general, stimulating actions to avoid damaging other relationships. In other words, exogenous influences of guilt do motivate prosocial behavior towards others in people’s surrounding.

## 12.7 Conclusion

The present chapter constitutes a first step toward an understanding of the ways in which self-conscious emotions regulate behavior and how behavior may regulate the experience of the emotions. Self-conscious emotions are cognitively complex emotions that have not been studied much over the years. Now it appears that it is possible to understand the effects of self-conscious emotions, but that certain aspects must be taken into account.

First of all, this chapter showed us that a focus on the experiential contents of discrete self-conscious emotions is necessary for a complete understanding.

Different self-conscious emotions can have different effects on decision making and behavior, even when they are such resembling as shame and guilt. Only when making a distinction between different self-conscious emotions and taking a closer look at the experiential elements of an emotion, it is possible to fully understand how self-conscious emotions regulate behavior.

Second, the present chapter shows that a distinction between exogenous and endogenous influences of self-conscious emotions is essential in emotion research. Previous research has made this distinction theoretically (Zeelenberg & Pieters, 2006), but most scholars do not take this distinction into account when empirically studying the effects of self-conscious emotions. As a consequence, they may find different or even contrasting results depending on the used methods, and subsequently may draw incorrect conclusions about the effects, goal, or function of a self-conscious emotion.

A third and last implication of this chapter is the extension of focus towards multiple-person situations. In the last couple of years, more and more scholars have focused on interpersonal effects of emotions. Because many decisions and behaviors take place in situations with other people present, this is an important development in emotion research. However, most, if not all, of these studies have concentrated on situations in which the person is alone or together with one other person (e.g., Lerner & Keltner, 2001; Van Kleef et al., 2004), while in daily life people often interact with multiple persons at the same time. Especially for self-conscious emotions, the study of dyadic situations may give only a limited perspective on effects of self-conscious emotions and may not capture the full picture. The conclusion is that the role of self-conscious emotions in decision making and behavior can only be fully understood when taking a broader approach using multiple-person situations.

Additionally, we have also learned something about the specific self-conscious emotions shame and guilt. Apparently, shame is not such an ugly and complicated emotion as was thought previously. It signals a negative evaluation about the whole self and activates the emotional goal of dealing with this negative self. As a consequence, people restore their positive self by approaching performance and achievement opportunities, and when they interact with audience from the shame event, they act prosocially towards those people. Only when it is too risky or not possible to restore their self, people revert to withdrawal or avoidance behaviors in order to protect themselves from further possible damage. The conclusion that can be drawn concerning guilt is that it is indeed often an adaptive, social emotion, but can also have its negative side effects. Guilt signals having hurt another person and activate the emotivational goal to repair this hurt. If people find themselves subsequently in situations where the hurt other is not present, they act prosocially towards every person they encounter. But if they find themselves in situations together with that hurt person, they act prosocially towards the hurt person at the expense of others they encounter, and avoid as much as possible costs for themselves.

## References

Alexander, C. N., & Knight, G. W. (1971) Situates identities and social psychological experimentation. *Sociometry*, *34*, 65–82.

Amodio, D. M., Devine, P. G., & Harmon-Jones, E. (2007) A dynamic model of guilt: Implications for motivation and self-regulation in the context of prejudice. *Psychological Science*, *18*, 524–530.

Baumeister, R. F., Reis, H. T., & Delespaul, P. A. E. G. (1995) Subjective and experiential correlates of guilt in daily life. *Personality and Social Psychology Bulletin*, *21*, 1256–1268.

Baumeister, R. F., Stillwell, A. M., & Heatherton, T. F. (1994) Guilt: An interpersonal approach. *Psychological Bulletin*, *115*, 243–267.

Beer, J. S. (2007) Neural systems for self-conscious emotions and their underlying appraisals. In J. L. Tracy, R. W. Robins, & J. P. Tangney (Eds.), *The self-conscious emotions: Theory and research* (pp. 53–67). New York: Guilford.

Breugelmans, S. M., & Poortinga, Y. H. (2006) Emotion without a word: Shame and guilt with Rarámuri Indians and rural Javanese. *Journal of Personality and Social Psychology*, *91*, 1111–1122.

Caplovitz Barrett, K. (1995) A functionalist approach to shame and guilt. In J. P. Tangney & K. W. Fischer (Eds.), *Self-conscious emotions: The psychology of shame, guilt, embarrassment, and pride* (pp. 25–63). New York: Guilford.

Darwin, C. (1872/1965) *The expression of the emotions in man and animals*. Chicago, IL: University of Chicago Press.

De Hooge, I. E., Zeelenberg, M., & Breugelmans, S. M. (2007) Moral sentiments and cooperation: Differential effects of guilt and shame. *Cognition and Emotion*, *21*, 1025–1042.

De Hooge, I. E., Nelissen, R. M. A., Breugelmans, S. M., & Zeelenberg, M. (in press). What is moral about guilt? Acting "prosocially" at the disadvantage of others. Journal of Personality and Social Psychology.

De Hooge, I. E., Zeelenberg, M., & Breugelmans, S. M. (2010) Restore and protect motivations following shame. *Cognition and Emotion*, *24*, 111–127.

De Hooge, I. E., Zeelenberg, M., & Breugelmans, S. M. (in press). A functionalist account of shame induced behaviour. *Cognition and Emotion*

De Hooge, I. E., Breugelmans, S. M., & Zeelenberg, M. (2008) Not so ugly after all: When shame acts as a commitment device. *Journal of Personality and Social Psychology*, *95*, 933–943.

De Hooge, I. E., Nelissen, R. M. A., Breugelmans, S. M., & Zeelenberg, M. (2009) The dark side of guilt. *Manuscript under review.*

Dickerson, S. S., & Gruenewald, T. L. (2004) When the social self is threatened: Shame, physiology, and health. *Journal of Personality*, *72*, 1191–1216.

Ferguson, T. J. (2005) Mapping shame and its functions in relationships. *Child Maltreatment*, *10*, 377–386.

Ferguson, T. J., Stegge, H., & Damhuis, I. (1991) Children's understanding of guilt and shame. *Child Development*, *62*, 827–839.

Fessler, D. M. T. (2004) Shame in two cultures: Implications for evolutionary approaches. *Journal of Cognition and Culture*, *4*, 207–262.

Fessler, D. M. T., & Haley, K. J. (2003) The strategy of affect: Emotions in human cooperation. In P. Hammerstein (Ed.), *The genetic and cultural evolution of cooperation* (pp. 7–36). Cambridge, MA: MIT Press.

Fontaine, J. R. J., Luyten, P., De Boeck, P., Corveleyn, J., Fernandez, M., Herrera, D., et al. (2006) Untying the Gordian knot of guilt and shame: The structure of guilt and shame reactions based on situation and person variation in Belgium, Hungary, and Peru. *Journal of Cross-Cultural Psychology*, *37*, 273–292.

Frank, R. H. (1988) *Passions within reason: The strategic role of the emotions*. New York: Norton.

Frank, R. H. (2004) Introducing moral emotions into models of rational choice. In A. S. R. Manstead, N. Frijda, & A. Fischer (Eds.), *Feelings and emotions: The Amsterdam symposium* (pp. 422–440). Cambridge, MA: Cambridge University Press.

Freedman, J. L., Wallington, S. A., & Bless, E. (1967) Compliance without pressure: The effects of guilt. *Journal of Personality and Social Psychology*, *7*, 117–124.

Frijda, N. H. (1986) *The emotions*. New York: Cambridge University Press.

Frijda, N. H. (2006) *The laws of emotion*. Nawwah, NJ: Erlbaum.

Frijda, N. H., Kuipers, P., & ter Schure, E. (1989) Relations among emotion, appraisal, and emotional action readiness. *Journal of Personality and Social Psychology*, *57*, 212–228.

Garg, et al. (2005) N., Inman, J. J., & Mittal, V. (2005) Incidental and task-related affect: A re-inquiry and extension of the influence of affect on choice. *Journal of Consumer Research*, *32*, 154–159.

Gibbons, F. X. (1990) The impact of focus of attention and affect on social behavior. In W. R. Crozier (Ed.), *Shyness and embarrassment: Perspectives from social psychology* (pp. 119–143). Cambridge, MA: Cambridge University Press.

Gilbert, P. (1997) The evolution of social attractiveness and its role in shame, humiliation, guilt, and therapy. *British Journal of Medical Psychology*, *70*, 113–147.

Gilbert, P., & Andrews, B. (1998) *Shame: Interpersonal behavior, psychopathology, and culture*. Oxford: Oxford University Press.

Gruenewald, T. L., Dickerson, S. S., & Kemeny, M. E. (2007) A social function for self-conscious emotions: The social self preservation theory. In J. L. Tracy, R. W. Robins, & J. P. Tangney (Eds.), *The self-conscious emotions: Theory and research*. New York: Guilford.

Haidt, J. (2003) The moral emotions. In R. J. Davidson, K. R. Scherer, & H. H. Goldsmith (Eds.), *Handbook of affective sciences* (pp. 852–870). Oxford: Oxford University Press.

Higgins, E. T. (1996) Knowledge activation: Accessibility, applicability, and salience. In E. T. Higgins & A. W. Kruglanski (Eds.), *Social psychology: Handbook of basic principles* (pp. 133–168). New York: Guilford.

Izard, C. E. (1977) *Human emotions*. New York: Plenum.

Izard, C. E., Ackerman, B. P., & Schultz, D. (1999) Independent emotions and consciousness: Self-consciousness and dependent emotions. In J. A. Singer & P. Singer (Eds.), *At play in the fields of consciousness: Essays in the honor of Jerome L. Singer* (pp. 83–102). Mahwah, NJ: Erlbaum.

Keltner, D., & Buswell, B. N. (1996) Evidence for the distinctness of embarrassment, shame and guilt: A study of recalled antecedents and facial expressions of emotion. *Cognition and Emotion*, *10*, 155–171.

Keltner, D., & Buswell, B. N. (1997) Embarrassment: Its distinct form and appeasement functions. *Psychological Bulletin*, *122*, 250–270.

Ketelaar, T., & Au, W. T. (2003) The effects of guilt on the behavior of uncooperative individuals in repeated social bargaining games: An affect-as-information interpretation of the role of emotion in social interaction. *Cognition and Emotion*, *17*, 429–453.

Kitayama, S., Rose Markus, H., & Matsumoto, H. (1995) Culture, self, and emotion: A cultural perspective on "self-conscious" emotions. In J. P. Tangney & A. H. Fischer (Eds.), *Self-conscious emotions: The psychology of shame, guilt, embarrassment, and pride* (pp. 439–465). New York: Guilford.

Kroll, J., & Egan, E. (2004) Psychiatry, moral worry, and moral emotions. *Journal of Psychiatric Practice*, *10*, 352–360.

Leith, K. P., & Baumeister, R. F. (1998) Empathy, shame, guilt, and narratives of interpersonal conflicts: Guilt-prone people are better at perspective taking. *Journal of Personality*, *66*, 1–38.

Lerner, J. S., & Keltner, D. (2001) Fear, anger, and risk. *Journal of Personality and Social Psychology*, *81*, 146–159.

Lewis, H. B. (1971) *Shame and guilt in neurosis*. New York: International Universities Press.

Lewis, H. B. (1987) Shame and the narcissistic personality. In D. L. Nathanson (Ed.), *The many faces of shame* (pp. 93–124). New York: Guilford.

Lewis, M. (1992) *Shame: The exposed self*. New York: The Free Press.

Lewis, M. (2000) Self-conscious emotions: Embarrassment, pride, shame, and guilt. In M. Lewis & J. M. Haviland-Jones (Eds.), *Handbook of emotions* (pp. 623–636). New York: Guilford.

Lewis, M. (2003) The role of the self in shame. *Social Research, 70*, 1181–1204.

Lindsay-Hartz, J. (1984) Contrasting experiences of shame and guilt. *American Behavioral Scientist, 27*, 689–704.

McCullough, M. E., Worthington, E. L. J., & Rachal, K. C. (1997) Interpersonal forgiving in close relationships. *Journal of Personality and Social Psychology, 73*, 321–336.

Messick, D. M., & McClintock, C. G. (1968) Motivational basis for choice in experimental games. *Journal of Experimental Social Psychology, 4*, 1–25.

Mills, R. S. L. (2005) Taking stock of the developmental literature on shame. *Developmental Review, 25*, 26–63.

Nathanson, D. L. (1987) *The many faces of shame*. New York: Guilford.

Nathanson, D. L. (1992) *Shame and pride*. New York: Norton.

Nelissen, R. M. A., Dijker, A. J., & De Vries, N. K. (2007) How to turn a hawk into a dove and vice versa: Interactions between emotions and goals in a give-some dilemma game. *Journal of Experimental Social Psychology, 43*, 280–286.

Niedenthal, P., Krauth-Gruber, S., & Ric, F. (2006) Self-conscious emotions. In P. Niedenthal, S. Krauth-Gruber, & F. Ric (Eds.), *Psychology of emotion: Interpersonal, experiential, and cognitive approaches* (pp. 77–114). New York: Psychology Press.

Ortony, A., Clore, G. L., & Collins, A. (1988) *The cognitive structure of emotions*. New York: Cambridge University Press.

Probyn, E. (2004) Everyday shame. *Cultural Studies, 18*, 328–349.

Roseman, I. J., Wiest, C., & Swartz, T. S. (1994) Phenomenology, behaviors, and goals differentiate discrete emotions. *Journal of Personality and Social Psychology, 67*, 206–221.

Sabini, J., & Silver, M. (1997) In defense of shame: Shame in the context of guilt and embarrassment. *Journal for the Theory of Social Behaviour, 27*, 1–15.

Scherer, K. R., & Wallbott, H. G. (1994) Evidence for universality and cultural variation of differential emotion response patterning. *Journal of Personality and Social Psychology, 66*, 310-328.

Schlenker, B. R., & Leary, M. R. (1982) Social anxiety and self-presentation: A conceptualization and model. *Psychological Bulletin, 92*, 641–669.

Schmader, T., & Lickel, B. (2006) The approach and avoidance function of guilt and shame emotions: Comparing reactions to self-caused and other-caused wrongdoing. *Motivation and Emotion, 30*, 43–56.

Smith, C. A., & Lazarus, R. S. (1993) Appraisal components, core relational themes, and the emotions. *Cognition and Emotion, 7*, 295–323.

Strelan, P. (2007) Who forgives others, themselves, and situations? The roles of narcissism, guilt, self-esteem, and adreeableness. *Personality and Individual Differences, 42*, 259–269.

Tangney, J. P. (1991) Moral affect: The good, the bad, and the ugly. *Journal of Personality and Social Psychology, 61*, 598–607.

Tangney, J. P., Miller, R. S., Flicker, L., & Barlow, D. H. (1996) Are shame, guilt and embarrassment distinct emotions? *Journal of Personality and Social Psychology, 70*, 1256-1269.

Tangney, J. P. (1993) Shame and guilt. In C. G. Costello (Ed.), *Symptoms of depression* (pp. 161–180). New York: Wiley.

Tangney, J. P. (1995) Recent advances in the empirical study of shame and guilt. *American Behavioral Scientist, 38*, 1132–1145.

Tangney, J. P. (1999) The self-conscious emotions: Shame, guilt, embarrassment, and pride. In T. Dalgleish & M. Power (Eds.), *Handbook of cognition and emotion* (pp. 541–568). Chichester, West Sussex: Wiley.

Tangney, J. P., & Dearing, R. L. (2002) *Shame and guilt*. New York: Guilford.

Tangney, J. P., & Fischer, K. W. (1995) *Self-conscious emotions: The psychology of shame, guilt, embarrassment, and pride*. New York: Guilford.

Tangney, J. P., Stuewig, J., & Mashek, D. J. (2007a) Moral emotions and moral behavior. *Annual Review of Psychology, 58*, 345–372.

Tangney, J. P., Stuewig, J., & Mashek, D. J. (2007b) What's moral about the self-conscious emotions? In J. L. Tracy, R. W. Robins, & J. P. Tangney (Eds.), *The self-conscious emotions: Theory and research* (pp. 21–37). New York: Guilford.

Tangney, J. P., Wagner, P. E., Fletcher, C., & Gramzow, R. (1992) Shamed into anger? The relation of shame and guilt to anger and self-reported aggression. *Journal of Personality and Social Psychology, 62*, 669–675.

Taylor, S. E., & Brown, J. D. (1988) Illusion and well-being: A social psychological perspective on mental health. *Psychological Bulletin, 103*, 193–210.

Thrane, G. (1979) Shame. *Journal for the Theory of Social Behaviour, 9*, 139–166.

Tracy, J. L., & Robins, R. W. (2004) Putting the self into self-conscious emotions: A theoretical model. *Psychological Inquiry, 15*, 103–125.

Tracy, J. L., & Robins, R. W. (2007) The self in self-conscious emotions: A cognitive appraisal approach. In J. L. Tracy, R. W. Robins, & J. P. Tangney (Eds.), *The self-conscious emotions: Theory and research* (pp. 3–20). New York: Guilford.

Van Kleef, G. A., De Dreu, K. W., & Manstead, S. R. (2004) The interpersonal effects of anger and happiness in negotiations. *Journal of Personality and Social Psychology, 86*, 57-76.

Wicker, F. W., Payne, G. C., & Morgan, R. D. (1983) Participant descriptions of guilt and shame. *Motivation and Emotion, 7*, 25-39.

Zeelenberg, M., & Breugelmans, S. M. (2008) The role of interpersonal harm in regret and guilt. *Emotion, 8*, 589–596.

Zeelenberg, M., Nelissen, R., & Pieters, R. (2007) Emotion, motivation and decision making: A feeling is for doing approach. In H. Plessner, C. Betsch, & T. Betsch (Eds.), *A new look on intuition in judgment and decision making*. Mahwah, NJ: Erlbaum.

Zeelenberg, M., Nelissen, R. M. A., Breugelmans, S. M., & Pieters, R. (2008) On emotion specificity in decision making: Why feeling is for doing. *Journal of Judgment and Decision Making, 3*, 18–27.

Zeelenberg, M., & Pieters, R. (1999) Comparing service delivery to what might have been: Behavioral responses to regret and disappointment. *Journal of Service Research, 2*, 86–97.

Zeelenberg, M., & Pieters, R. (2006) Feeling is for doing: A pragmatic approach to the study of emotions in economic behavior. In D. De Cremer, M. Zeelenberg, & K. Murnighan (Eds.), *Social psychology and economics* (pp. 117–137). Mahwah, NJ: Erlbaum.

# Chapter 13
# Gender and Emotion Regulation: A Social Appraisal Perspective on Anger

**Catharine Evers, Agneta H. Fischer, and Antony S.R. Manstead**

## 13.1 Common Beliefs Regarding Gender and Emotion

There is a prevailing belief in our society that women are emotionally different from men. According to this commonly held belief, emotionality is typically connected to women, given that women seem to experience their emotions more intensely and express them more overtly than men do, and because women talk more frequently about their emotional life than their male counterparts (Shields, 1991). Men, on the other hand, are believed to typically bury and deny their emotions. These perceptions of gender differences in emotional responding compose one of the most robust elements of gender stereotypes (Fabes & Martin, 1991; Fischer, 1993; Grossman & Wood, 1993; Hess et al., 2000; Plant, Hyde, Keltner, & Devine, 2000; Timmers, Fischer, & Manstead, 2003) and has even been labeled a "master stereotype" (Shields, 2003) that generalizes across a wide range of positive and negative emotions (Briton & Hall, 1995; Grossman & Wood, 1993; Kelly & Hutson-Comeaux, 1999; Shields, 2003).

These lay convictions put aside, it seems more important how they relate to the actual emotionality of men and women in everyday life. In accordance with popular views, empirical evidence seems to indicate – at first sight – that women are indeed more emotionally responsive than men (e.g., Bradley, Codispoti, Sabatinelli, & Lang, 2001; Lucas & Gohm, 2000; Seidlitz & Diener, 1998). However, studies confirming those beliefs mainly relied on retrospective reports on emotions (Grossman & Wood, 1993; Hess et al., 2000). When people report on emotions that they are not currently experiencing, they shift to a semantic retrieval strategy (Robinson & Clore, 2002). Such strategy entails that people access generalized beliefs about emotions rather than actual experiential emotion knowledge. Consequently, retrospective reports on emotions are especially

C. Evers (✉)
Department of Clinical and Health Psychology, Utrecht University, P.O. Box 80140, 3508 TC Utrecht, Netherlands
e-mail: c.evers@uu.nl

I. Nyklíček et al. (eds.), *Emotion Regulation and Well-Being*,
DOI 10.1007/978-1-4419-6953-8_13, © Springer Science+Business Media, LLC 2011

vulnerable to the effect of gender stereotypes. When retrospective and stereotypical biases are prevented, gender differences in emotional responding tend to disappear (Barrett, Robin, Pietromonaco, & Eyssell, 1998; Robinson, Johnson, & Shields, 1998). Thus, altogether female emotionality may tell us more about gender stereotypes than about women's actual emotions (Fischer, 1993).

There is one important exception to this stereotypical view of women's emotions; however, women's supposed emotionality does not apply to anger. For this emotion, men are thought to be more emotionally responsive than women (Brody & Hall, 1993; Fabes & Martin, 1991; Kring, 2000). In the present chapter, we provide a review of the empirical evidence relating to gender differences in anger and anger regulation. Rather than the idea of the "angry male and the passive female," we argue that this is a simplified view of male and female anger (see also Shields, 2003). Gender *is* assumed to be relevant, however, but only in interaction with the social context.

## 13.2 Empirical Evidence Regarding Gender and Anger

In certain areas of the USA, there are more female than male perpetrators of homicide against one's spouse (Wilson & Daly, 1992). Although the reason for this gender disparity is not entirely clear and may not be driven by anger, this empirical finding compellingly illustrates the weakness of the straightforward belief that anger-related expressions, like severe aggressive acts such as homicide, are typically male. In more detail, empirical evidence on actual gender differences in anger can be specified for separate emotion components.

Firstly, most studies concerning *anger experience* showed an absence of gender differences (e.g., Harris, 1994; Kring, 2000; Kring & Gordon, 1998; Wagner, Buck, & Winterbotham, 1993). For example, studies comparing men and women on trait anger (Deffenbacher et al., 1996; Kopper, 1991; Kopper & Epperson, 1991, 1996) did not find any gender differences in the likelihood to experience anger across a variety of situations. Studies drawing on self-reported anger intensity did not reveal any gender differences either (Allen & Haccoun, 1976; Averill, 1983; Fischer & Roseman, 2007; Harris, 1994; Kring & Gordon, 1998; Oatley, 1998; Wagner et al., 1993). This is supported by a meta-analysis on daily aggressive incidents, including anger measures, revealing no significant differences between men and women (Archer, 2004).

If gender differences were found, however, these were in contrast to the prevailing stereotype, as women reported more rather than less anger in comparison to men (Brody, Lovas, & Hay, 1995; Fischer, Rodriguez-Mosquera, Van Vianen, & Manstead, 2004; Fischer & Roseman, 2007; Strachan & Dutton, 1992). Interestingly, the more intense anger on the part of women seems to be more prevalent in reaction to men than to women (Brody et al., 1995; Harris, 1994), in reaction to condescending behavior by men in intimate settings (Buss, 1989; Frodi, 1977; Harris, 1994), or in Western cultures (Fischer et al., 2004; Strachan & Dutton, 1992). Such findings illustrate the importance of incorporating contextual factors.

Secondly, anger also has a profound physiological component. Surprisingly, little is known about *physiological responses* in relation to gender and anger. Kring and Gordon (1998) found that men, in comparison to women, demonstrated more arousal (as measured with skin conductance responding) in response to film excerpts intended to induce anger although they experienced anger to the same degree. Another study (Labouvie-Vief, Lumley, Jain, & Heinze, 2003) showed that during anger experience, young women showed more arousal, as measured with heart rate variability, than young men did although at older ages the two sexes were nearly identical in their physiological reactions. Thus, the few studies present on gender and physiological responding do not point toward any consistent gender differences.

The stereotype of anger as a typical male emotion is also not consistently supported regarding *anger expression*. The extent to which gender differences in anger expression appear across studies, however, is largely dependent on how anger expression is operationalized. For example, studies using self-reports on the incidence of anger expressions did not result in any gender differences (e.g., Allen & Haccoun, 1976; Balswick & Avertt, 1977; Campbell & Muncer, 1987; King & Emmons, 1990; Kopper & Epperson, 1991). Studies using scenarios, however, have shown some gender differences, but again opposite from the prevailing stereotype (e.g., Dosser, Balswick, & Halverson, 1983; Gross & John, 1995; Timmers, Fischer, & Manstead, 1998; Fischer & Roseman, 2007). Thus, if differences were found, women reported to express anger more regularly than men.

Gender differences seem larger in the case of *direct anger expressions*, for example, forms of physical or verbal aggression. For example, meta-analyses on aggression have concluded that men engage more in physical aggression, though only slightly more in verbal aggression (Archer, 2004; Bettencourt & Miller, 1996; Hyde, 1984; Eagly & Steffen, 1986). When focusing on *indirect anger expressions*, such as gossiping, ignoring, or stonewalling, however, the direction of the gender difference reverts: Women show more indirect anger expressions than men (Archer, 2004; Fischer & Roseman, 2007; Hess & Hagen, 2006). Further, women typically show more powerless anger expressions than men. That is, women more often cry when angry, compared to men (e.g., Eagly & Steffen, 1986; Frost & Averill, 1982; Lombardo, Cretser, Lombardo, & Mathis, 1983; Timmers et al., 1998).

It seems important, however, to take into account the social contexts in which anger expressions occur. For example, a meta-analysis of aggression in heterosexual relations (Archer, 2000) showed that women more frequently use physical aggression against their partners than men, although they are not more likely to inflict an actual injury on their partner. In other words, they aggress slightly more frequently toward their partners, but their aggression has less severe effects than that of their male counterparts. Interestingly, these gender differences in aggression were not related to gender differences in anger experience. Thus, the finding that men more often use physical and verbal aggression is modified when contextual factors are considered. In addition, several studies have shown that women engage in more direct anger expression when their position is more powerful, which is the case in more egalitarian relationships – compared to traditional relationships, or in countries where women have higher status and power positions (Fischer et al., 2004; Fischer & Evers, 2010).

Altogether, these studies do not support the stereotype of the angry male and the passive female. First of all, gender differences in the subjective experience and physiological responding component are generally absent. If differences in the experience of anger are found, they are in contrast with the stereotype. Second, men often use more physical and verbal aggression and women often use more indirect ways of anger expression; however, this is not the case in specific social contexts. To frame it differently, these findings suggest that men and women differ, especially with respect to the regulation of their anger expressions. Because the regulation of anger expressions often occurs in social interactions, where the pressure for emotion regulation is greatest (Barrett, Gross, Christensen, & Benvenuto, 2001), we assume that the social context is important in explaining why gender differences in the regulation of anger expressions occur.

However, "the social context" is a broad concept, and entails countless factors that may be crucial. An important question is therefore how gender differences in anger regulation can be explained by a contextual framework. We propose that *Social Appraisal Theory* (Manstead & Fischer, 2001) entails such a framework. Social Appraisal Theory explains how one's emotional reaction to a situation is partly shaped by one's expectancies and subsequent appraisals of others present in the social context.

## 13.3 Social Appraisal Theory and Anger Regulation

The essence of appraisal models is that a stimulus situation has a particular meaning for a particular person, and this meaning drives emotion elicitation and a set of emotional outputs, including expressions (Scherer, 1984). Social Appraisal Theory assumes that the anticipated effect of one's own emotional behavior is important in the appraisal process. We appraise the interpersonal consequences of our emotional expression. As a consequence, these *social appraisals* can influence the regulation of emotion expressions.

Two types of social appraisal may be distinguished. On the one hand, social appraisals should play a significant role in shaping the *experience* of an emotion, that is, the way in which we evaluate an emotional event can be affected by the way in which others (apparently) evaluate that same event (see Parkinson, 2001; Fischer, Rotteveel, Evers, & Manstead, 2004). This type of social appraisal would especially operate in conditions, where the emotional stimulus is ambiguous or low in intensity. In such situations, others' appraisals are more diagnostic and more likely to shape one's own feelings. For example, when someone insults you, your friend's enraged reaction toward the person who makes the insult may make you feel very angry as well. Second, social appraisals can also play a significant role in the *expression* of emotion, that is, the way in which people express their emotions is influenced by the expected social implications of these expressions. Imagining the negative effect of your anger with respect to your friendship with the other person, for example, may inhibit overt anger expressions, whereas considering the positive effects of one's anger may reinforce the intensity and directness of an anger expression. In sum, social appraisals refer to the appraisal of others' reactions on an emotional event, including others' reaction to one's own emotional reaction.

Social appraisals are thus by definition highly sensitive to variations in social context and may therefore play an important role in explaining different anger reactions by men and women. First of all, men and women may be differently sensitive to other persons' reactions toward their anger because of gender-specific role concerns (Eagly, 1987). Men, for example, may be less concerned with how others evaluate their anger because anger does not negatively affect their masculine identity. Second, the expected social implications may be different for men and women depending on the social context. If one expects negative social implications of one's anger expression, it seems likely that one suppresses the anger, whereas the absence of such negative social appraisals may result in the overt expression of one's anger.

Various lines of evidence suggest that men and women indeed expect different social implications of their anger expressions and that negative social consequences of anger are more salient for women than for men. For example, various meta-analyses on gender differences in aggression have shown that perceptions of danger for retaliation (Bettencourt & Miller, 1996), perceived harm to the target of one's anger (Eagly & Steffen, 1986), or the anxiety about the possible negative consequences for others (Eagly & Steffen, 1986) are important predictors of gender differences in aggression. This is also apparent from a study involving autobiographical incidents of anger (Fischer & Roseman, 2007) that showed that women reported more verbal aggression than did men, but also more reconciliation. This may indicate that women more quickly feel regret about the negative effects of their anger, and therefore try to make up. Possible negative consequences that have been found to be especially important for women include negative social sanctions (Graham, Gentry, & Green, 1981; Stoppard & Gruchy, 1993), such as threat to the future of the relationship of the parties involved or the loss of control (Campbell & Muncer, 1987; Timmers et al., 1998). Men tend to anticipate such negative reactions to a lesser extent, and may in some situations even expect positive outcomes of their anger expression, such as admiration (Campbell & Muncer, 1987). Women may also be more likely to empathize with the victim (Frodi, Macaulay, & Thome, 1977), and such an empathic motive may result in a greater tendency by women to suppress their anger (Timmers et al., 1998).

We tested the assumption that men and women expect different social implications of their intended anger reactions in a series of studies (Evers, Fischer, Rodriguez-Mosquera, & Manstead, 2005; Evers, Fischer, Manstead, & Rodriguez Mosquera, 2010). Participants were first asked to recall an autobiographical event in which they had experienced and expressed their anger (express condition) or a situation in which they had experienced, but suppressed their anger (suppress condition). Next, we asked various questions about the incident. As hypothesized, men and women differed in their social appraisals: When anger was suppressed, women reported stronger negative social appraisal than men, and when anger was expressed, women reported weaker negative social appraisals than men. This pattern of results suggests that women are more sensitive to the negative social consequences of their anger, resulting in stronger regulation of their anger. Interestingly, the results also showed that women had a more intimate relationship with their provoker than men, but only in the express condition. This may suggest that women expect fewer negative implications of their anger expressed toward their partner.

We therefore manipulated intimacy in a second scenario study. Because a pilot study showed that many participants mentioned a no-show at an appointment as the reason why they would become angry with both intimates and nonintimates, participants were asked to read a vignette describing a situation in which they are waiting in a restaurant for a person who is not there at the agreed time. Then, a text message arrives on their phone, saying that the other is not going to show up because he or she is out with other people. Immediately after this message, they try to call the other person, but the phone is not answered. Participants had to imagine that the provoker in this scenario was either a partner or a colleague. The results showed that women indeed reported to express their anger more directly than men in the intimate condition. However, this gender difference in direct or overt anger expression was not related to gender differences in negative social appraisal. We assumed that this was due to the fact that negative expectations are more closely associated with the suppression of anger and thus should be more salient when suppressing one's overt and direct anger, resulting in more indirect anger expressions, such as powerless expressions (e.g., disclosing your anger about the provoker to someone else or crying). This was confirmed in another scenario study, in which powerless expressions were included. Women expected more negative social implications of their initial anger than men and reported to express their anger in a more powerless way than men did. Negative social appraisals explained this gender difference in powerless anger expressions. In a final scenario study with a different social situation, this effect was exactly replicated.

Together these studies support the general idea of Social Appraisal Theory that the anticipated effect of one's own emotional behavior is important for the regulation of anger expressions. The finding that women reported stronger negative social appraisals and that these appraisals entailed stronger effects, suggests that women are more focused than men on the negative social implications of their anger expressions. This difference in social appraisal is responsible for at least some of the gender differences in anger expressions.

Because these studies are based on self-reports, which have the danger of retrospective interpretations by subjects, we also conducted an experiment in which anger was evoked in vivo in the laboratory, in different social contexts. In this experiment (Evers et al., 2005), participants were made angry because a bogus fellow-student judged their writing abilities very negatively. As a consequence of this negative false feedback, participants did not receive a financial reward. Moreover, the feedback also contained a note indicating that participants were naïve and had an immature point of view. The participants had not actually met the fellow student. Participants were then randomly assigned to either a *social* condition, in which they expected to meet the fellow-student who provided the negative feedback, or to a *nonsocial* condition, in which they had no such expectation. Subsequently, participants were instructed to allocate hot sauce to the fellow-student, which he or she had to taste in an ostensible unrelated study. This "hot sauce paradigm" is a method that has proven to be effective as a way of implicitly measuring anger-related expressions (e.g., Bushman, Baumeister, & Philips, 2001; Lieberman, Solomon, Greenberg, & McGregor, 1999).

Results indicated that men and women experienced anger equally intense; however, they differed in their anger expression. Women expressed anger to a lesser extent than men, but only in the social condition. In other words, when women expected to meet the fellow-student, they allocated less hot sauce than men. Moreover, women again focused more strongly on the negative social implications of their anger. These negative social appraisals partly accounted for the gender difference in anger expression.

Together the findings of these studies on social appraisal enhance our understanding of how social processes affect anger and the regulation of one's anger expression. Men and women are both sensitive to others' reactions, yet women seem to be especially sensitive to the negative implications of their anger displays, resulting in either more indirect anger expressions or more reconciliation after direct expressions.

## 13.4 Discussion

On some occasions, people may explode when angry, whereas on other occasions they may become speechless, despite feeling equally angry in both cases. Emotion expressions are obviously influenced by the social context in which they emerge and develop (Fischer & Manstead, 2008; Keltner & Haidt, 1999; Parkinson, Fischer, & Manstead, 2005). In particular, social factors arc thought to influence whether and how emotions are expressed in order to meet one's goals in a social context (Mackie, Silver, & Smith, 2004; Kitayama, Mesquita, & Karasawi, 2006; Parrott & Smith, 1993). In the present chapter, we discussed the association between the social context and the regulation of anger expression for men and women, and focused on expectations about others' reactions, that is, social appraisals. More precisely, we argued that men and women regulate their anger differently because they expect different social implications of their anger expressions. A series of studies replicated previous findings showing that men and women express their anger differently. Women seem to regulate their anger into less antagonistic anger expressions, especially when they appraise others' reactions as negative. A question that follows is why women would more strongly fear for these negative social consequences.

According to the tend-and-befriend theory (Taylor et al., 2000), men react upon stress with the well-known fight-or-flight reaction. Women, however, react with tending-and-befriending: Tending involves the activities to protect the self, and befriending is the creation and maintenance of social networks that may help in this process. For women, negative social appraisals and the resulting downplaying of overt and direct anger expressions may reflect the safeguarding of their social networks, because direct anger could harm their relations with others. On the other hand, these relations with others are used as a way of indirectly expressing anger, by excluding others from their social networks. It thus seems that men and women regulate their anger in ways that fit their social styles.

Research on individual differences in the self indirectly supports this idea. Cross and colleagues (Cross, Gore, & Morris, 2003; Cross & Morris, 2007) showed that individuals with a "relational self" think and behave in ways that nurture important or close relationships. These individuals also take the implications of their own anger expression more strongly into account. Because women generally have a more relational self than men, this research suggests that women are more focused on the social consequences of their anger.

Women's more relational self and their tendency to affiliate rather than compete, is also dependent on their social role. According to the Social Role Theory (Eagly, 1987) men and women occupy different roles, originally based on the different physical capacities of men (protecting family against enemies) and women (bearing and feeding children). As these roles have evolved in roles that are related to these capacities, women are more likely than men to engage in domestic roles of primary caretaker of children, whereas men are more likely than women to occupy roles in the paid economy and to be primary family provider. These different roles do not only comprise different activities, but are also associated with different status and power positions. Such differences in power and status are likely to play a role in the expected social implications of one's anger expression. Female leaders, for example, are perceived as less effective when expressing either sadness or anger, while for men this is only the case when expressing sadness (Lewis, 2000). Another compelling example is provided by a recent study (Brescoll & Uhlmann, 2008) showing that both men and women conferred lower status on angry female professionals than on angry male professionals. Moreover, women's anger reactions were attributed to internal characteristics, like "she is an angry person" or "she is out of control," while men's anger reactions were attributed to external circumstances. That social roles are also directly related to social appraisals was found in one of our recent studies (Fischer & Evers, 2010): Women in egalitarian relationships were more likely to express their anger because they did not fear revenge or social disapproval compared to women in more traditional relationships. Another motive for women's more direct anger expression toward their male partners is that relationship concerns and the protection of children may be more important for women as part of their care-taker role. As a consequence, they may believe that they are entitled to express their anger in more intimate settings.

## 13.5 Concluding Remark

Angry males and passive females? We tried to show that such a phrase is popular, but incorrect. However, although there is no male or female anger, this does not mean that gender is irrelevant. Men and women make different social appraisals, depending on their social role, their goals in the social context, and the target of their anger. Thus, gender typically affects the regulation of anger expressions in interaction with the social context, such that gender differences occur when men and women have different expectations about other persons' feelings and reactions with respect to one's own anger behavior and act in accordance with these expectations.

## References

Allen, J. G., & Haccoun, D. M. (1976) Sex differences in emotionality: A multi-dimensional approach. *Human Relations*, *29*, 711–722.

Archer, J. (2000) Sex differences in aggression between heterosexual partners: A meta-analytic review. *Psychological Bulletin*, *126*, 651–680.

Archer, J. (2004) Sex differences in aggression in real-world settings: A meta-analytic review. *Review of General Psychology*, *8*, 291–322.

Averill, J. R. (1983) Studies on anger and aggression: Implications for theories of emotion. *American Psychologist*, *38*, 1145–1160.

Balswick, J., & Avertt, C. (1977) Differences in expressiveness: Gender, interpersonal orientation, and perceived parental expressiveness as contributing factors. *Journal of Marriage and Family*, *39*, 121–127.

Barrett, L., Gross, J., Christensen, T. C., & Benvenuto, M. (2001) Knowing what you're feeling and knowing what to do about it: Mapping the relation between emotion differentiation and emotion regulation. *Cognition and Emotion*, *15*, 713–724.

Barrett, L., Robin, L., Pietromonaco, P. R., & Eyssell, K. M. (1998) Are women the "more emotional" sex? Evidence from emotional experiences in social context. *Cognition and Emotion*, *12*, 555–578.

Bettencourt, B. A., & Miller, N. (1996) Gender differences in aggression as a function of provocation: A meta-analysis. *Psychological Bulletin*, *119*, 422–447.

Bradley, M. M., Codispoti, M., Sabatinelli, D., & Lang, P. J. (2001) Emotion and motivation. II: Sex differences in picture processing. *Emotion*, *1*, 300–319.

Brescoll, V. L., & Uhlmann, E. L. (2008) Can an angry woman get ahead? Status conferral, gender, and expression of emotion in the workplace. *Psychological Science*, *19*, 268–275.

Briton, N., & Hall, J. (1995) Beliefs about female and male nonverbal communication. *Sex Roles*, *32*, 79–90.

Brody, L. R., & Hall, J. (1993) Gender and emotion. In M. Lewis & J. Haviland (Eds.), *Handbook of emotion*. New York: Guilford Press

Brody, L. R., Lovas, G. S., & Hay, D. H. (1995) Gender differences in anger and fear as a function of situational context. *Sex Roles*, *32*, 47–78.

Bushman, B. J., Baumeister, R. F., & Philips, C. P. (2001) Do people aggress to improve their mood? Catharsis beliefs, affect regulation opportunity, and aggressive responding. *Journal of Personality and Social Psychology*, *81*, 17–32.

Buss, D. M. (1989) Conflict between the sexes: Strategic interference and the evocation of anger and upset. *Journal of Personality and Social Psychology*, *5*, 735–747.

Campbell, A., & Muncer, S. (1987) Models of anger and aggression in the social talk of women and men. *Journal for the Theory of Social Behaviour*, *17*, 489–511.

Cross, S. E., Gore, J. S., & Morris, M. L. (2003) The relational-interdependent self-construal, self-concept consistency, and well-being. *Journal of Personality and Social Psychology*, *85*, 933–944.

Cross, S. E., & Morris, M. L. (2007) Getting to know you: The relational self-construal, relational cognition, and well-being. *Personality and Psychological Bulletin*, *29*, 512–523.

Deffenbacher, J. L., Oetting, E. R., Thwaites, G. A., Lynch, R. S., Baker, D. A., Stark, R. S., Thacker, S., & Eiswerth-Cox, L. (1996) State-trait anger theory and the utility of the trait anger scale. *Journal of Counseling Psychology*, *43*, 131–148.

Dosser, D., Balswick, J., & Halverson, C. (1983) Situational context of emotional expressiveness. *Journal of Counseling Psychology, 30*, 375–387.

Eagly, A. H. (1987) *Sex differences in social behavior: A social-role interpretation*. Hillsdale, NJ: Erlbaum.

Eagly, A. H., & Steffen, V. J. (1986) Gender and aggressive behavior: A meta-analytic review of the social psychological literature. *Psychological Bulletin, 100*, 309–330.

Evers, C., Fischer, A. H., Manstead, A. S. R., & Rodriguez Mosquera, P. M. (2010) *Beware of my anger! The social appraisal of anger at the interpersonal level.*

Evers, C., Fischer, A. H., Rodriguez Mosquera, P. M., & Manstead, A. S. R. (2005) Anger and social appraisal: A "spicy" sex difference? *Emotion, 5*, 258–266.

Fabes, R. A., & Martin, C. L. (1991) Gender and age stereotypes of emotionality. *Personality and Social Psychology Bulletin, 17*, 532–540.

Fischer, A. H. (1993) Sex differences in emotionality: Fact or stereotype. *Feminism and Psychology, 3*, 303–318.

Fischer, A. H., & Evers, C. (2010) Angry men, angry bitches, and silent wives: Sex differences in anger in different relationship contexts. Manuscript submitted for publication.

Fischer, A. H., & Manstead, A. S. R. (2008) Social functions of emotion. In M. Lewis, J. Haviland, & L. Feldman Barrett (Eds.), *The handbook of emotion* (3rd ed.). New York: Guilford.

Fischer, A. H., Rodriguez-Mosquera, P. M., Van Vianen, A. E. M., & Manstead, A. S. R. (2004) Gender and culture differences in emotion. *Emotion, 4*, 87–94.

Fischer, A. H., & Roseman, I. J. (2007) Beat them or ban them: The characteristics and social functions of anger and contempt. *Journal of Personality and Social Psychology, 93*, 103–115.

Fischer, A. H., Rotteveel, M., Evers, C., & Manstead, A. S. R. (2004) Emotional assimilation: How we are influenced by others' emotions. *Cahier de Psychologie Cognitive, 22*, 223–245.

Frodi, A. (1977) Sex differences in the perception of a provocation: A survey. *Perceptual and Motor Skills, 44*, 113–114.

Frodi, A., Macaulay, J., & Thome, P. R. (1977) Are women always less aggressive than men? A review of the experimental literature. *Psychological Bulletin, 84*, 634–660.

Frost, W. D., & Averill, J. R. (1982) Differences between men and women in the everyday experience of anger. In J. R. Averill (Ed.), *Anger and aggression: An essay on emotion* (pp. 281–317). New York: Springer.

Graham, J. W., Gentry, K. W., & Green, J. (1981) The self-presentational nature of emotional expression: Some evidence. *Personality and Social Psychology Bulletin, 7*, 467–474.

Gross, J. J, & John, O. P. (1995) Facets of emotional expressivity: Three self-report factors and their correlates. *Personality and Individual Differences, 19*, 555–568.

Grossman, M., & Wood, W. (1993) Sex differences in intensity of emotional experience: A social role interpretation. *Journal of Personality and Social Psychology, 65*, 1010–1022.

Harris, M. B. (1994) Gender of subject and target as mediators of aggression. *Journal of Applied Social Psychology, 24*, 453–471.

Hess, N. H., & Hagen, E. H. (2006) Sex differences in indirect aggression: Psychological evidence from young adults. *Evolution and Human Behavior, 27*, 231–245.

Hess, U., Senécal, S., Kirouac, G., Herrera, P., Philippot, P., & Kleck, R. E. (2000) Emotional expressivity in men and women: Stereotypes and self-perceptions. *Cognition & Emotion, 14*, 609–642.

Hyde, J. S. (1984) How large are gender differences in aggression? A developmental meta-analysis. *Developmental Psychology, 20*, 722–736.

Kelly, J. R., & Hutson-Comeaux, S. L. (1999) Gender-emotion stereotypes are context specific. *Sex Roles, 40*, 107–140.

Keltner, D., & Haidt, J. (1999) Social functions of emotions at four levels of analysis. *Cognition and Emotion, 13*, 505–521.

King, L., & Emmons, R. A. (1990) Conflict over emotional expression: Psychological and physical correlates. *Journal of Personality and Social Psychology, 58*, 864–877.

Kitayama, S., Mesquita, B., & Karasawi, M. (2006) Cultural affordances and emotional experience: Socially engaging and disengaging emotions in Japan and the United States. *Journal of Personality and Social Psychology, 91*, 890–903.

Kopper, B. A. (1991) Role of gender, sex role identity, and Type A behavior in anger expression and mental health functioning. *Journal of Counseling Psychology*, *40*, 232–237.

Kopper, B. A., & Epperson, D. L. (1991) Women and anger. Sex and sex role comparisons in the expression of anger. *Psychology of Women Quarterly*, *15*, 7–14.

Kopper, B. A., & Epperson, D. L. (1996) The experience and expression of anger: Relationships with gender, gender role socialization, depression, and mental health functioning. *Journal of Counseling Psychology*, *43*, 158–165.

Kring, A. M. (2000) Gender and anger. In A. H. Fischer (Ed.), *Gender and emotion: Social psychological perspectives* (pp. 211–231). Cambridge: Cambridge University Press.

Kring, A. M., & Gordon, A. H. (1998) Sex differences in emotion: Expression, experience, and physiology. *Journal of Personality and Social Psychology*, *74*, 686–703.

Labouvie-Vief, G., Lumley, M. A., Jain, E., & Heinze, H. (2003) Agen and gender differences in cardiac reactivity and subjective emotion responses to emotional autobiographical memories. *Emotion*, *3*, 115–126.

Lewis, K. M. (2000) When leaders display emotion: How followers respond to negative emotional expression of male and female leaders. *Journal of Organizational Behavior*, *21*, 221–234.

Lieberman, J. D., Solomon, S., Greenberg, J., & McGregor, H. A. (1999) A "hot" new way to measure aggression: Hot sauce allocation. *Aggressive Behavior*, *25*, 331–348.

Lombardo, W. K., Cretser, G. A., Lombardo, B., & Mathis, S. L. (1983) Fer cryin' out loud – There is a sex difference. *Sex Roles*, *9*, 987–995.

Lucas, R. E., & Gohm, C. L. (2000) Age and sex differences in subjective well-being across cultures. In E. Diener & E. M. Suh (Eds.), *Culture and subjective well-being* (pp. 291–318). Cambridge, MA: MIT Press.

Mackie, D. M, Silver, L. A., & Smith, E. R. (2004) Intergroup emotions: Emotion as an intergroup phenomenon. In C. W. Leach & L. Z. Tiedens (Eds.), *The social life of emotions* (pp. 227–245). New York: Cambridge University Press.

Manstead, A. S. R., & Fischer, A. H. (2001) Social appraisal: The social world as object of and influence on appraisal processes. In K. R. Scherer, A. Schorr, & T. Johnstone (Eds.), *Appraisal processes in emotion: Theory, method, research* (pp. 221–232). Oxford: Oxford University Press.

Oatley, K. (1998) State of the art: Emotion. *The Psychologist*, *11*, 286–288.

Parkinson, B. (2001) Putting appraisal in context. In K. R. Scherer, A. Schorr, & T. Johnstone (Eds.), *Appraisal processes in emotion: Theory, method, research* (pp. 173–186). New York: Oxford University Press.

Parkinson, B., Fischer, A. H., & Manstead, A. S. R. (2005) Emotion in social relations: Cultural, group, and interpersonal processes. New York: Psychology Press.

Parrott, W. G., & Smith, R. H. (1993) Distinguishing the experiences of envy and jealousy. *Journal of Personality and Social Psychology*, *64*, 906–920.

Plant, E. A., Hyde, J. S., Keltner, D., & Devine, P. G. (2000) The gender stereotyping of emotions. *Psychology of Women Quarterly*, *24*, 81–92.

Robinson, M. D., & Clore, G. L. (2002) Episodic and semantic knowledge in emotional self-report: Evidence for two judgment processes. *Journal of Personality and Social Psychology*, *83*, 198–215.

Robinson, M. D., Johnson, J. T., & Shields, S. A. (1998) The gender heuristic and the database: Factors affecting the perception of gender-related differences in the experience and display of emotions. *Basic and Applied Social Psychology*, *20*, 206–219.

Scherer, K. R. (1984) On the nature and function of emotion: A component process approach. In K. R. Scherer & P. Ekman (Eds.), *Approaches to emotion* (pp. 293–317). Hillsdale, NJ: Erlbaum.

Seidlitz, L., & Diener, E. (1998) Sex differences in the recall of affective experiences. *Journal of Personality and Social Psychology*, *74*, 262–271.

Shields, S. A. (1991) Gender in the psychology of emotion: A selective research review. In K. T. Strongman (Ed.), *International review of studies on emotion* (pp. 227–245). New York: Wiley.

Shields, S. A. (2003) *Speaking from the heart: Gender and the social meaning of emotion*. New York: Cambridge University Press.
Strachan, C. E., & Dutton, D. G. (1992) The role of power and gender in anger responses to sexual jealousy. *Journal of Applied Social Psychology, 22*, 1721–1740.
Stoppard, J. M., & Gruchy, C. G. (1993) Gender, context, and expression of positive emotion. *Personality and Social Psychology Bulletin, 19*, 143–150.
Taylor, S. E., Klein, L. C., Lewis, B. P., Gruenewald, T. L., Gurung, R. A. R., & Updegraff, J. A. (2000) Biobehavioral responses to stress in females: Tend-and-befriend, not fight-or-flight. *Psychological Review, 107*, 411–429.
Timmers, M., Fischer, A. H., & Manstead, A. S. R. (1998) Gender differences in motives for regulating emotions. *Personality and Social Psychology Bulletin, 9*, 974–985.
Timmers, M., Fischer, A. H., & Manstead, A. S. R. (2003) Ability versus vulnerability: Beliefs about mens's and women's emotional behavior. *Cognition and Emotion, 17*, 41–63.
Wagner, H. L., Buck, R., & Winterbotham, M. (1993) Communication of specific emotions: Gender differences in sending accuracy and communication measures. *Journal of Nonverbal Behavior, 17*, 29–53.
Wilson, M., & Daly, M. (1992) Who kills whom in spouse killings? On the exceptional sex ratio of spousal homicides in the United States. *Criminology, 30*, 189–215.

# Part III
# Clinical Perspective

# Chapter 14
# Uncovering the Dynamics of Emotion Regulation and Dysfunction in Daily Life with Ecological Momentary Assessment

**Lauren M. Bylsma and Jonathan Rottenberg**

## 14.1 Introduction

Psychological research and clinical practice traditionally relies on self-report questionnaires, which ask people to retrospect and to report on their feelings, behaviors, and experiences. Recalling this information involves a reconstructive process that is prone to systematic biases and errors (e.g., current mood states and contextual cues bias retrieval; for review, see Schwarz & Oyserman, 2001). The temporal resolution of the obtained data is typically limited, precluding a fine-grained analysis of how variables and relationships between variables change over time. Although obtaining online self-reports in a laboratory setting avoids some of these problems, laboratory contexts are artificial and do not reproduce what an individual experiences in daily life. Fortunately, Ecological Momentary Assessment (EMA), also known as the Experience Sampling Method (ESM), permits researchers to overcome some of the limitations of typical self-report methods and enable study of the dynamics of experiences and behaviors as they occur over time and across settings in daily life. Since Myin-Germeys and colleagues (2009) recently published an excellent overview of applications to EMA in psychopathology research, we focus this chapter specifically on EMA applications for understanding *emotion* in psychopathology. We briefly survey EMA methods developed over the past 30 years. Next, we explain the utility of using EMA to study emotional functioning, highlighting selected areas in emotion research where the potential of EMA modalities for clinical description, assessment, and clinical interventions are beginning to be realized. Our discussion of applications draws upon our own work with mood and anxiety disorders. Finally, we discuss the promise of EMA for improving the assessment and treatment of emotional disorders, as well as highlighting several priority areas for future investigation.

L.M. Bylsma (✉)
Mood and Emotion Laboratory, University of South Florida, 4202 E. Fowler Avenue, PCD4118G, Tampa, FL 33620, USA
e-mail: lmbylsma@gmail.com

I. Nyklíček et al. (eds.), *Emotion Regulation and Well-Being*,
DOI 10.1007/978-1-4419-6953-8_14, 

## 14.2 What Is Ecological Momentary Assessment?

Before considering applications of EMA to psychopathology, we first provide a brief description of the method (and note key resources for learning more about EMA). In EMA, individuals typically describe thoughts, feelings, and behaviors across a range of situations encountered in their daily lives. In this respect, EMA reduces the methodological disadvantages of standard self-report procedures. EMA minimizes biases in retrieval or memory reconstruction, and potentially increases the accuracy of reported information. Utilizing repeated assessments over time, EMA allows researchers to examine the temporal sequence of complex interactions of emotion, thoughts, behavior, and contexts unfolding (over minutes, hours, days, or weeks) in participants' natural environments.

EMA encompasses a diverse collection of related methodologies employing different designs and technologies with the common feature being repeated assessments in real life settings. EMA modalities include diaries in paper-and-pencil form, palmtop computers, online questionnaires, telephone reports, and even ambulatory physiological monitoring (often combined with self-report assessments; e.g., Fahrenberg & Myrtek, 2001). EMA with palmtop computers has become increasingly popular as costs of the equipment and software packages have decreased (for a practical guide to computerized EMA methods, see Barrett & Barrett, 2001; or Christensen, Barrett, Bliss-Moreau, Lebo, & Kaschub, 2003).

The flexibility of EMA allows a large variety of assessment targets, including individual-level and time-level variables. Experience sampling can occur at regular pre-programmed intervals or at random times (i.e., designated by a stopwatch or computer), or in response to events of interest (e.g., social interaction). In the case of physiology (e.g., heart rate or blood pressure monitoring, salivary cortisol), recordings can be continuous or combined with event or time based self-report assessments. Different levels of time resolution are also used, from daily reports to reports many times a day. Protocol duration is also flexible, ranging from 1 day to many months. Most EMA studies use a sampling strategy that inquires about the present moment; however, others employ a coverage strategy that asks individuals to retrospect about a recent time interval to obtain more complete coverage of the day. One example of this broader method is the Day Reconstruction Method (Kahneman, Krueger, Schkade, Schwarz, & Stone, 2004), which creates a systematic reconstruction of the events of the previous day. For a more detailed discussion of the variety of EMA methodologies, see recent reviews by Christensen and colleagues (2003), Scollon, Kim-Prieto, and Diener (2003), or Shiffman, Stone, and Hufford (2008).

The flexibility of EMA affords unique methodological advantages. EMA researchers can capitalize on naturally occurring events to study emotional responses to potent real-life triggers that may be difficult or unethical to induce in a laboratory setting. EMA data can be aggregated across trials to characterize an individual's general patterns of emotion, thoughts, or behaviors (e.g., overall affect), which permits the flexibility to examine a variety of between-person differences as they relate to emotion (e.g., gender; Barrett, Robin, Pietromonaco, & Eyssell, 1998; age, Carstensen, Pasupathi, Mayr, & Nesselroad, 2000).

One of the most significant advantages of EMA over global recall data is that EMA can be used to characterize within-individual variations in variables over time (for review of correspondence between global recall data and aggregated EMA data, see Shiffman et al., 2008). EMA studies typically capitalize on the excellent sampling resolution of the multi-point assessments afforded by the method to examine within-subject changes in thoughts, emotion experience, or behavior over time, across contexts, as well as the predictors and antecedents of specific events. Further, by including time as a predictor, temporal changes in variables can be modeled. By extension, the ability to analyze within-person changes over time with EMA allows testing of whether individual-level patterns of experiences and behaviors generalize to a group of individuals within a population (by modeling person-specific variables over time and providing estimates of slope and intercept variability in random effects models). In designs examining within-individual effects such as these, statistical procedures involving random coefficient multilevel modeling (Bryk & Raudenbush, 1992) are typically used, because these methods can simultaneously model both within-individual and between-individual factors on a dependent variable. Strengths of these procedures include their ability to account for missing data or unequal numbers of data points across individuals, which occur frequently in EMA studies. Larson and Delespaul (1992) provide a good review of multilevel modeling techniques for use with EMA data.

## 14.3 Application of EMA to Research in Emotion and Psychopathology

Despite the advantages of EMA, as well as evidence that EMA is feasible and valid with individuals with major psychopathology (i.e., hospitalized schizophrenics with active psychotic experiences, Kimhy et al., 2006), the potential for EMA to illuminate emotion processes in psychopathology remains largely untapped. In this section, we discuss how the methodological advantages unique to EMA, not only suit it for elucidating the dynamics of emotional processes in the heterogeneous contexts of daily life, but also for elucidating characteristics of psychopathology, particularly those that vary between, (e.g., gender, age, personality, diagnostic status) or within (e.g., mood state, environmental setting, social context) individuals. At both the group and individual level, psychopathology varies over time and with differing contexts (i.e., symptom severity may vary with time and with environmental changes). Collapsing observations over time periods and averaging over groups – often necessary in global retrospective self-report measures – obscures important information about variability. In sum, EMA may help reveal the nature of emotional disturbances underlying psychopathology through its ability to simultaneously examine changes in emotion over time, emotion regulation processes, antecedents and consequences of emotional reactions, and predictors of emotional disturbance. We will illustrate how the growing database of EMA research in normative samples is answering key questions about emotional experience and regulation, which can be readily applied to psychopathology research.

### *14.3.1 How Do Individual Differences and Environmental Contexts Influence Emotional Responses in Daily Life?*

The ability of EMA to assess interactions among aspects of the immediate environmental context, individual-level characteristics, and their influence on experiences, thoughts, and behaviors, make it ideal for examining individual and contextual factors that constitute the heterogeneity of emotional reactivity. Behavior and experience are greatly influenced by characteristics of the immediate context, and a growing corpus of research in unselected samples examines how emotional reactions interact with environmental contexts, including how contextual appraisal, or evaluation impacts emotional experience. For example, research on predictors of positive affect in daily life found that time spent in school and social activities was directly related to the experience of positive affect in school children (Csikszentmihalyi & Hunter, 2003), and engaging in eudaimonic behaviors aimed at increasing one's potential has been shown to predict greater increases in positive affect relative to hedonic behaviors aimed at increasing pleasure (Steger, Kashdan, & Oishi, 2008). Similar studies of negative affect have revealed that even minor daily stressors are followed by reliable increases in negative affect (e.g., van Eck, Nicolson, & Berkhof, 1998). Specifically, high perceived stress was positively associated with negative reactivity, while situation controllability predicted reduced negative emotional reactivity. Interestingly, future events had an even greater impact on current mood, which was interpreted as anticipation effects (van Eck et al., 1998).

Initial work in unselected samples also examines the full-time course of emotional responding, capitalizing on EMA's multi-point assessments. For example, event importance ratings and the initial emotion response intensity predict duration of positive and negative emotional experience in daily life (Verduyn et al., 2009). Intensity of negative emotional reactivity has also been found to be more intense for individuals for whom the prior time period was problem free (Marco & Suls, 1993). Interestingly, individuals high on trait negative affect were more distressed by current problems and recovered more slowly from problems the preceding day relative to individuals low on trait negative affect. These studies illustrate that our understanding of emotional functioning becomes richer when the interconnections between assessment periods are taken into account.

In addition to the impact of the immediate context, the influence of person characteristics – such as gender (e.g., Barrett et al., 1998) and age (e.g., Carstensen et al., 2000), on emotional responding in daily life has also been examined. As discussed by Shiffman and colleagues (2008), the influence of context (e.g., environmental factors, internal states) is demonstrated not only for highly variable constructs, such as affect, but also for more stable trait-like constructs, including personality (Fleeson, 2001; Bolger & Schilling, 1991), self-esteem (Kernis, 2005), self-efficacy (Gwaltney, Shiffman, & Sayette, 2005), and coping styles (Schwartz, Neale, Marco, Shiffman, & Stone, 1999). In one EMA study with potential applicability to psychopathology, van Eck and colleagues (1998) found that self-reported trait anxiety was associated with greater experiences of agitation to minor negative events. Similarly, Gable, Reis, and Elliot (2000) examined the relationship between dispositional sensitivities of the appetitive (Behavioral Activation System, BAS) and aversive motivational systems (Behavioral Inhibition System, BIS) on emotional reactivity. Here, higher BIS sensitivity (a characteristic that is associated with anxiety) amplified negative emotional reactivity, while BAS increased positive emotional responses. In another applicable study that tested the helplessness-hopelessness theory of depression, Swendsen (1997) demonstrated with EMA, in sample of individuals with attributional styles at high or low risk for depression that causal attributions of stability and globality predicted increases in depressed mood in reaction to negative events. These studies illustrate the potential utility of obtaining multiple time point assessments of trait measures to understand emotional dysfunction in daily life in disordered individuals, as well as the potential for testing theories of the etiology of emotional dysfunction.

EMA studies are also helpful for disentangling whether differences in emotion are due to environmental vs. individual differences. For example, Bolger and Schilling (1991) sought to determine whether individuals high on neuroticism were more distressed due to greater exposure to negative events, problematic situation selection, or overly intense emotional reactions. It was found that while both stressful events exposure and stress reactivity predicted distress, stress reactivity accounted for more variance. This type of design could also be used to elucidate the origin of emotional dysfunctions in psychopathology.

### *14.3.2 What Can EMA Reveal About Emotional Experience and Dysfunction in Mood and Anxiety Disorders?*

EMA studies of emotion in normative samples serve as a platform for EMA studies of emotional dysfunction among persons with psychiatric disorders. Mood and anxiety disorders are an especially promising target for EMA, given that these disorders are characterized by emotional dysfunction (Rottenberg & Johnson, 2007). Thus, describing the interaction of emotional functioning with person characteristics and environmental contexts is likely to improve the description and the conceptualization of the disorders and provide information that would otherwise be unattainable.

A few studies have begun to capitalize on the advantages of EMA to examine the factors that influence emotional reactivity in everyday life settings among individuals with major depression. Peeters, Nicolson, Berkhof, Delespaul, and de Vries (2003) examined emotional reactivity to daily life events among individuals with major depression and healthy controls using EMA. In this sample, participants diagnosed with major depressive disorder (MDD) reported blunted positive and negative emotional responses to negative life events, and negative emotional responses persisted longer in depressed individuals. Unexpectedly, depressed individuals reported greater reductions in negative affect and larger increases in positive affect when responding to positive events relative to controls. We recently replicated this effect in a sample of individuals with major and minor depression (Bylsma, Clift, & Rottenberg, in press), and we further examined individual characteristics and contextual factors that predicted the intensity of emotional reactivity. Further, depressed individuals have also been found to exhibit greater increases in negative affect in response to minor daily stressors in comparison to healthy controls and bipolar individuals (Myin-Germeys et al., 2003). Similar to findings for unipolar depression, individuals with bipolar disorder currently experiencing depressive symptoms experienced greater stress reactivity to negative events (daily hassles; Havermans, Nicolson, & de Vries, 2007). These findings are in contrast to laboratory studies of emotional reactivity which typically find blunted positive and negative emotional reactivity in major depression across self-report, behavioral, and physiological measures (for review, see Bylsma, Morris, & Rottenberg, 2008), possibly because naturalistic contexts are more heterogeneous and have greater idiographic meaning than laboratory contexts.

Self-report and psychophysiological EMA methods have begun to be combined in mood-disordered samples, providing revealing information about the interaction between experience and physiology in daily life. For example, Peeters, Nicolson, and Berkhof (2003) examined cortisol response to daily events and demonstrated that individuals with major depression experienced more blunted increases in cortisol following negative events relative to healthy individuals, particularly in depressed individuals who also had a family history of mood disorders, and the effects of negative events on cortisol appeared to be mediated by changes in mood. Further, Peeters, Nicolson, and Berkhof (2004) found that MDD individuals exhibited no baseline differences in cortisol levels overall and more intra-individual variability in cortisol in the MDD individuals; however, cortisol patterns were more erratic in more severe or recurrent MDD individuals. In another study using combined methods, Conrad, Wilhelm, Roth, Spiegel, and Taylor (2008) examined heart rate variability, cortisol, and electronic diary reports of positive and negative affect in depressed individuals at risk for cardiovascular disease over the course of day. Diurnal negative and positive affect were predictive of depression status. Negative affect was inversely related to heart rate variability in nondepressed individuals, though overall heart rate variability and cortisol did not distinguish the groups. The authors suggest that these findings may indicate that the pervasive negative affect present in major depression may disrupt the normal circadian connection between mood state and autonomic nervous system control.

Some studies have also begun to employ EMA to examine the dynamics of emotional dysfunction in individuals with anxiety symptoms in the context of daily life. For example, researchers have found that social anxiety symptoms and engaging in emotion suppression were associated with the experience of fewer positive events and less positive affect over the course of a day (Kashdan & Steger, 2006; Kashdan & Collins, 2010) as well as higher ratings of negative affect and self-consciousness (Brown, Silvia, Myin-Germeys, & Kwapil, 2007). These studies have not yet been applied to diagnosed anxious samples, but they do provide important clues about the interplay between anxiety, emotion, and behavior.

### 14.3.3 What Is the Structure of Affect in an Ecologically Relevant Context?

Examining the temporal dynamics of emotion can also shed light on theories of affective structure. For example, researchers have used EMA to examine the relationship between pleasant and unpleasant affect (Scollon, Diener, Oishi, & Biswas-Diener, 2005), and mood factor structure and reliability (Wilhelm & Schoebi, 2007). Emotion models have also been tested with EMA; for example, Zelenski and Larsen (2000) found that a discrete emotions model best fit their EMA data for emotions states, while a dimensional model fit best for emotion traits. Barrett (1998) found that EMA combined with structural analyses revealed that individuals vary greatly in their tendency to represent their emotional experience in highly differentiated, or discrete, emotional responses. Specifically, individuals high in valence-focus (i.e., the degree to which individuals attend to the hedonic component of their affective experience) and low in arousal-focus (i.e., the degree to which individual attend to the arousal component of their affective experience) fit a dimensional model of affect better, whereas those lower in valence focus and higher in arousal focus fit a discrete model better. Therefore, Barrett (1998) concludes from these findings that one static, nomothetic theory may not accurately describe the subjective affective experience of a group of individuals. These findings are also relevant for psychopathology, in that the representation of emotion may be heterogeneous even within a particular diagnostic group.

### 14.3.4 How Does Mood Vary Over the Course of the Day, and How Is It Dysregulated in Mood and Anxiety Disorders?

Another important application of EMA to understanding emotional dysfunction is examination of diurnal mood variation. Given that EMA can assess each individual at multiple time points each day, it is particularly well suited to measure patterns in diurnal mood change and daily mood variability. In healthy individuals, positive affect has consistently been shown to exhibit a quadratic waveform across the day (lowest in the morning, peaking in the afternoon, and falling throughout the evening that mirror circadian rhythms in body temperature and sleep-wake timing; e.g., Clark, Watson, & Leeka, 1989; Watson, Wiese, Vaidya, & Tellegen, 1999), while negative affect typically does not demonstrate consistent diurnal rhythms (e.g., Clark et al., 1989). A number of EMA studies have compared diurnal mood patterns in depressed and healthy individuals. Typically, depressed individuals are found to have diurnal mood patterns, such that mood is worse upon waking and better in the evening (e.g., Murray, 2007; Peeters, Berkhof, Delespaul, Rottenberg, & Nicolson, 2006); although studies with subthreshold depression symptoms or individuals scoring high on measures of negative emotion are shown to have the opposite pattern, with worse mood in the evening (e.g., Rusting & Larsen, 1998). This positive linear trend found in depression is thought to reflect an attenuated circadian rhythm, which is normally expressed as a quadratic waveform of diurnal variation in positive affect (e.g., Murray, 2007; Murray, Allen, & Trinder, 2002). Decreased circadian amplitudes also observed in physiological variables in depression, such as body temperature and cortisol levels (e.g., Daimon, Yamada, Tsujimoto, & Takahashi, 1992; von Zerssen et al., 1985), suggest that decreased circadian amplitudes are an aspect of pathogenesis in depression (Murray, 2007). Further, studies have shown that depressed individuals tend to have more variable negative effect across the day (e.g., Hall, Sing, & Romanoski, 1991; Peeters et al., 2006). In sum, EMA studies have demonstrated utility for describing diurnal variations in mood in depression, and may reveal circadian rhythm disturbances that are fundamental to the development and maintenance of mood disorders.

### *14.3.5 What Are the Characteristics of Emotion Regulation in Daily Life?*

Given that emotion is continuously subject to regulatory processes, the examination of emotion regulatory processes is critical to understanding emotional reactions. Emotion regulation includes a wide variety of multi-componential processes (i.e., including cognitive, behavioral, and physiological; conscious and non-conscious; controlled and automatic) that impact the trajectory of emotional experience and behaviors over time (e.g., Gross, 1998). Indeed, understanding the dynamics of these regulatory processes is challenging, given the vast number of processes involved. To gain traction on this problem, EMA can be implemented to measure predictors of emotional changes over time to examine the impact of specific emotion regulation processes on the experience of emotion in everyday life.

Research on emotion regulation using EMA designs has begun to accumulate in unselected samples. For example, use of distraction, acceptance, and relaxation coping strategies in response to stress has been related to greater daily positive affect (Stone, Kennedy-Moore, & Neale, 1995). Strategies such as repressive coping or seeking positive social support are associated with lower levels of daily negative affect (Cutler, Larsen, & Bunce, 1996; de Vries & Delespaul, 1989). Further, self-regulation strategies of disengagement or rumination have been found to be ineffective in regulating negative affect in daily life, leading to depression symptoms and behavioral problems in adolescents (Silk, Steinberg, & Morris, 2003).

EMA can also be used to test theories of emotion regulation. Along these lines, Barrett, Gross, Christensen, and Benvenuto (2001) tested the hypothesis that emotion differentiation (i.e., ability to experience and distinguish among many discrete emotions) would be related to better emotion regulation abilities, because discrete emotion concepts are related to more specific knowledge about how to effectively, cognitively, and behaviorally cope with a particular emotion and the situation that elicited it. Indeed, they found that individuals with highly differentiated negative emotions (i.e., as evaluated with EMA) were found to experience greater levels of negative emotion regulation (i.e., using a retrospective self-report measure of self-regulation behaviors), particularly for more intense negative emotions.

More recently, Gross, Richards, and John (2006) measured individual differences in the frequency of reported self-regulation strategies in daily life and found evidence that the type of emotion regulation strategies (e.g., reappraisal, suppression, enhancement) that individuals report using in daily life is related to effectiveness at implementing these strategies in the lab in response to emotional film stimuli when instructed, as evidence by their self-report. Given that physiological laboratory studies have found specific effects of emotional regulation strategies on physiological responses to emotional stimuli (e.g., Gross, 1998), a clear, next step would be to examine ambulatory physiological responses concurrently with EMA reports of emotional experience following specific emotional regulation strategies. In sum, the existence of several lines of research about normative emotion regulation, coupled with the assumption that many forms of psychopathology are likely to be characterized by emotion regulation deficits, suggests that the time is ripe to apply EMA to study emotion regulation in clinical populations.

### *14.3.6 Does Variation in Emotion in Daily Life Predict the Development and Course of Psychopathology?*

Basic research and theory has shown that emotional reactions often have functional value (e.g., Nesse, 2000), suggesting that emotions may retain functional value in individuals experiencing psychopathology. Thus, variations in emotional experience in the context of daily life (as assessed by EMA) may prove valuable as predictors of the development and course of mental disorders. For example, Schneiders and colleagues (2006) examined predictors of the development of psychopathology in an adolescent sample. Adolescents at high risk for developing psychopathology exhibited greater momentary emotional reactivity to daily events relative to low-risk peers. Further, high risk individuals with greater levels of stress over the past 3 months demonstrated additional increases in negative emotional reactivity. In another prospective study, Peeters, Berkhof, Rottenberg, and Nicolson (2010) examined the relationship between daily emotional reactivity and the course of MDD: Blunted emotional reactivity to daily events, particularly for negative events, predicted a failure to recover from the disorder over 18 months, independent of depression severity at baseline. These studies demonstrate that sampling emotion in everyday life settings with EMA may have important predictive value for understanding the course of mental disorders.

EMA has also been used to examine the interplay between variables that may confer vulnerability for the first onset of a disorder. Wichers and colleagues (2007a) examined the hypothesis that negative emotional reactivity to daily life stressors may represent a depression endophenotype in the development of the disorder. The researchers examined stress reactivity and negative affect in 279 female twin pairs and revealed that probands with co-twins diagnosed with a lifetime history of depression exhibited a stronger negative emotional response to stress in comparison to co-twins without such a diagnosis, independent of probands' current depressive symptoms. Therefore, the authors concluded that genetic vulnerability to depression may be expressed as an endophenotype defined as a tendency for increased negative emotional reactivity to minor daily stressors. Similarly, Wichers and colleagues (2007b) demonstrated that positive affect buffers the genetic predisposition to negative emotional reactivity in individuals at risk for depression. Indeed, EMA has clear utility in uncovering gene-environment interactions in depression and anxiety (for detailed discussion of EMA studies examining gene-environment interactions, see Myin-Germeys et al., 2009).

## 14.4 Applications of EMA for Clinical Assessment and Treatment

### *14.4.1 Clinical Assessment Applications*

Clinical assessment has also traditionally relied on self-report measures and clinical interviewing about past symptoms, which are prone to retrospective biases and memory failures (e.g., Schwarz and Oyserman, 2001). When what individuals' report in daily life diverges from what is reported in retrospective self-reports or during clinical interviews, EMA opens a key window on clinical assessment of symptoms and symptom change. EMA studies have demonstrated significant discrepancies between daily life assessment and traditional clinical assessment of symptoms, even for relatively discrete symptoms that should be relatively easy to recall, such as smoking lapses (Shiffman et al., 1997), alcohol use (Hammersley, 1994), symptoms of physical pain (Stone, Broderick, Shiffman, & Schwartz, 2004), and incidence of panic attacks (De Beurs et al., 1992). Even for basic recall questions, such as reporting on frequency of behavior, which should be relatively straightforward, a complicated set of cognitive processes is involved which can result in recall errors (for review, see Schwarz & Oyserman, 2001). Specifically, the most accurate approach would be for respondents to identify the behavior of interest, scan the reference period, retrieve all instances that match the target behavior, and count these instances to determine its overall frequency. However, as reviewed by Schwarz and Oyserman (2001), respondents are unlikely to follow such a strategy, unless the events in question are highly salient and small in number, instead, they rely on heuristic strategies. Clearly, requiring respondents to recall more ambiguous non-discrete phenomena such as mood would be even more difficulty to accomplish accurately, since it requires an individual to parse, then weight, and integrate a stream of experience (see Piasecki, Hufford, Solhan, & Trull 2007). Indeed, Horan, Green, Kring, and Nuechterlein (2006) reveal that while schizophrenics retrospectively report significant anhedonia, they do not differ from healthy controls in their reported experience of pleasure during immediate or short-term delayed laboratory assessments, suggesting that schizophrenics may significantly underestimate their ability to experience pleasure when making omnibus retrospective reports of pleasure.

Given the divergence between retrospective vs. on-line reports of emotion, EMA also has clear applications for clinical assessment of symptoms (Piasecki et al., 2007). Although researchers have begun to use EMA to examine symptoms of attention-deficit hyperactivity disorder (ADHD), substance abuse, and depression, much the work to date has been done in schizophrenia patients, including examination of psychotic symptoms, affect, stress sensitivity, cognitive symptoms, and daily life functioning. For example, Delespaul, de Vries, and van Os (2002), and Myin-Germeys, Nicolson, and Delespaul (2001) both examined predictors (triggers and protective factors) and consequences of psychotic symptoms in daily life in schizophrenia patients. Delespaul and colleagues (2002) also compared psychotic experiences in schizophrenia and severe depression and found that while schizophrenics had a higher frequency of psychotic symptoms, the quality and context of the symptoms were comparable for the two groups.

EMA has also been used in schizophrenia research to examine the interplay between different types of symptoms. Specifically, Myin-Germeys, Krabbendam, Jolles, Delespaul, and van Os (2002) examined the relationship between cognitive impairments and abnormal sensitivity to stress in the daily lives of schizophrenics. It was found that in some contexts, cognitive functioning (as measured by a neuropsychological tests before the EMA protocol) was unrelated to emotional reactivity to stress in daily life, while in other contexts better cognitive performance was related to greater emotional reactivity to stress. The relationship between symptoms in daily life has also been examined in ADHD. For example, Knouse and colleagues (2008) found that symptoms of inattention and hyperactivity-impulsivity symptoms were differentially related to daily life experiences, with higher inattentive symptoms being associated with more distress and worse affect and hyperactive-impulsive symptoms with reduced sensitivity to contextual factors in perceptions of situations. Clearly, these types of designs can also be applied to the symptoms of mood and anxiety disorders to better understand their everyday life triggers.

EMA methods have also identified important discrepancies between laboratory assessments and what the individual reports in daily life about emotional experience. Although flat affect is a core symptom of schizophrenia, Myin-Germeys, Delespaul, and de Vries (2000) found that schizophrenics experienced more intense and variable negative emotions and less intensity and variability in positive emotions compared to healthy individuals. Surprisingly, schizophrenics identified as blunted or non-blunted did not differ on these measures of emotion when assessed in daily life. Similar discrepancies have been found in applications of EMA to depression. For example, Peeters, Nicolson, Berkhof, Delespaul, and de Vries (2003) found that individuals with major depression did not report more negative events than healthy individuals in their EMA reports. Further, depressed individuals also reported smaller reactions to negative events and larger reactions to positive events (greater reductions in negative affect) compared to health individuals. Similarly, Bylsma, Clift, and Rottenberg (in press) also found that individuals with major and minor depression experienced greater reductions in negative affect in response to positive events.

It is clear that EMA can often provide incremental information for clinical assessment. EMA can be used to collect important information about the daily experiences of individuals with psychopathology that is germane to diagnosis, treatment planning, treatment implementation, and treatment evaluation. EMA has received limited use in the assessment of the emotional symptoms present in mood and anxiety disorders. However, current research is encouraging. For example, in work on anxiety disorders, Hibbert and Pilsbury (1988, 1989) investigated the role of hyperventilation during panic attacks by combining ambulatory transcutaneous carbon dioxide monitoring with self-report event sampling to examine whether hyperventilation is a cause or consequence of a panic attack. Their results did not demonstrate that hyperventilation caused panic attacks, but was likely a consequence of them. Studies of this nature can be used to examine the causal relationship between other features of these disorders. By identifying the triggers of symptoms, interventions can be tailored more effectively.

### *14.4.2 Clinical Intervention Applications*

Given EMA's utility for examining emotional dysfunction in research and clinical assessment, EMA can also be extended to clinical interventions applications and evaluations of treatment outcomes. The use of EMA in clinical interventions began with the development of computer-assisted cognitive-behavioral therapy (CCBT) in the 1980s on desktop computer platforms, a precursor to its implementation in an EMA format. A variety of software programs are now available that can implement many therapeutic tasks involved in traditional cognitive-behavioral treatments (for review, see Proudfoot, 2004), and several clinical trials examining the effectiveness of CCBT for anxiety and depression have been conducted, with all demonstrating efficacy of CCBT programs in significantly reducing symptoms that did not differ from traditional psychotherapy treatments (Selmi, Klein, Greist, Sorrell, & Erdman, 1990; Proudfoot et al., 2004; Wright et al., 2005).

However, desktop applications are limited in that patients are unable to take the technology with them into their daily lives. Further, current CCBT technologies are criticized as being rigid, lacking flexibility to tailor the program to the client or context. EMA technology with palmtop computers would be a useful extension of CCBT to bring therapy into the daily lives of individuals. Given that CCBT has already demonstrated effectiveness, it is likely that EMA-based interventions derived from desktop applications would be at least as effective, with the added advantage of their mobility. In addition to recording individual's experiences, EMA technology can be implemented to therapeutic messages tailored to the individuals' needs and the context. Further, due to its mobility, the use of EMA may facilitate generalization of skills learned in therapy beyond sessions into the context of daily life.

CCBT with palmtops has begun to be implemented for treatment of anxiety disorders (for review, see Anderson, Jacobs, & Rothbaum, 2004). Several palmtop computer programs have been developed for various anxiety disorders including obsessive-compulsive disorder (Baer, Minichiello, & Jenike, 1987; Baer, Minichiello, Jenike, & Holland, 1988), social phobia (Gruber, Moran, Roth, & Taylor, 2001), generalized anxiety disorder (Newman, 1999; Newman, Consoli, & Taylor, 1999), panic disorder (Newman, Kenardy, Herman, & Taylor, 1996, 1997), and specific phobia (Kenardy & Adams, 1993) that have been designed within a CBT framework. These programs typically employ several modules that include both assessment of client's symptoms and treatment strategies. Based on the assessment information, the treatment modules used are modified to provide only the modules relevant to the individual's symptom presentation. CCBT treatments for anxiety disorders have included modules aimed at recognizing and putting into perspective anxiety-inducing thoughts, reduction of black and white thinking, coping statements, relaxation training, and guided exposures (Anderson et al., 2004). CCBT could also be extended to add additional focus on symptoms of emotional dysfunction by targeting variables associated with emotional disturbance. Assessment data collected before and after treatment are used to evaluate outcome. While these studies have suggested that CCBT using computerized EMA technology is effective, this research is still in its infancy due to the small sample sizes and inconsistent programs used across studies.

To our knowledge, there have been no studies evaluating the effectiveness of CCBT using EMA for mood disorders or any studies specifically examining treatment for emotional dysfunction. In the assessment phase, EMA modules could identify triggers of negative thoughts and emotions more effectively than retrospective measures. In the treatment phase, similar modules as those used in prior studies with anxiety disorders could also be used to target negative cognitions. In addition, programs providing emotion regulation instructions could be valuable in reducing emotional symptoms of depression, as emotion regulation instructions have been shown to be effective in reducing emotional reactivity in laboratory studies (e.g., Gross, 2002). Although it has not yet been implemented, EMA technologies also have the ability to be programmed to respond to a given input (e.g., an emotion eliciting situation) with more specific strategies tailored to the current context.

CCBT with mobile computing technology may be a means of providing cost-effective psychotherapy to individuals experiencing barriers to treatment by improving treatment access. Further, the introduction of computer technology into psychotherapy offers the significant advantages that could make psychotherapy more effective. The continued proliferation of mobile electronic devices will promote their wider use in clinical and research settings, and with their wider availability, clinicians and patients will become increasingly comfortable with the technologies. Further, the convergence of other technologies with mobile computers (e.g., phone capability, web access, wireless technology) will continue to increase the potential applications of CCBT.

### *14.4.3 Evaluating Treatment Outcomes*

Given that EMA methods are useful in providing detailed and accurate assessments of symptoms in psychopathology, EMA could also be extended to the evaluation of treatment outcomes. Surprisingly, use in this context has been limited thus far. For example, Barge-Schaapveld, Nicolson, van der Hoop, and de Vries (1995) examined depressed outpatients experience of daily activities after 6 weeks of antidepressant treatment. It was found that treatment responders showed greater increases in positive affect and decreases in negative affect during all activities examined. More recently, Barge-Schaapveld and Nicolson (2002) examined the effect of antidepressant treatment on measures of quality of life and daily activities in MDD individuals during and after antidepressant treatment. During treatment, it was found that physical side effects of the medication were associated with lower quality of life ratings, particularly in dropouts, and EMA identified more physical complaints that were not specifically identified as side effects in other measures. Further, medicated individuals demonstrated greater clinical improvement according to conventional measures after treatment, but they did not exhibit higher quality of life ratings as measured by EMA. However, they did show more stable quality of life ratings, with less fluctuation as well as less time spent "doing nothing." Individuals that were still remitted at an 18-week follow-up continued to show deficits in quality of life measures relative to controls even though they had returned to levels comparable to controls on retrospective measures of quality of life. Finally, Cohen and colleagues (2008) found that emotional reactivity to daily stressors predicted rate of improvement in response to cognitive-behavioral therapy, such that next-day negative reactivity (i.e., elevated negative affect resulting from a reaction to a stressor the previous day) predicted a slower rate of symptom change during the first four sessions, but was not related to later response to therapy. These studies demonstrate that EMA can provide useful information for treatment studies that may not be available in traditional outcome measures that are based on global retrospective self-reports.

These methods could also be extended to examine psychotherapy treatment outcomes as well as other disorders and outcome variables. EMA could also be useful to examine treatment progress in clinical settings on a case-by-case basis. Specifically, additional information obtained from EMA could help tailor treatments to individuals more effectively to have the greatest impact in their daily life functioning and may provide information that is more accurate than that obtained from conventional retrospective self-report measures. For example, instead of using a Beck Depression Inventory (BDI-II; Beck, Steer, & Brown, 1996) that asks individuals to report changes in depressive symptoms over the past 2 weeks, EMA could measure changes in these symptoms over time more accurately, with the added ability of examining potential contextual influences on those changes.

## 14.5 Limitations of EMA

Although EMA has many clear advantages, it has some limitations. Like other self-report methods, EMA methods rely on reports of experience, and still require self-reflection and may still be subject to reporting biases or expectations. Further, there is some evidence that retrospective impressions can be more predictive of subsequent behavior compared to momentary assessments, since retrospective reports represent the information that people use to make subsequent decisions (for review, see Shiffman et al., 2008). Clearly, which methods are prioritized depends on the research question and what the researcher is interested in predicting.

EMA methods can also be expensive with a high participant burden relative to traditional retrospective self-report measures, and they require technological expertise on the part of the clinician or researcher. However, with continued improvements in technology and feasibility, these limitations may diminish with time.

## 14.6 Summary and Future Directions

EMA has recently developed as an important tool for examining dynamic experiences and behaviors in the daily lives of individuals as they unfold and interact over time. Despite the advantages of EMA, research and clinical applications utilizing EMA are still in their infancy. EMA may be particularly useful for elucidating the dynamics of emotional processes in the heterogeneous contexts of daily life. As reviewed in this chapter, initial progress has been made towards understanding emotional functioning in daily life in healthy and disordered samples. Although many important questions remain that EMA could be used to address, we prioritize four questions. First, what is the specific nature of the interplay between individual differences (e.g., personality, genetics, affect) and contextual variables (e.g., appraisals, environmental features) on emotional functioning in healthy and disordered individuals? Examination of the interactions of these components may lead to a better understanding of the developing of emotional dysfunction and psychopathology. Second, how does emotional functioning in daily life correspond to physiological variables? The correspondence between physiological variables and emotional experience has been examined in the laboratory; however, little research has extended examination of this correspondence to daily life. Examination of the correspondence between physiology, emotional experience, and behavioral, can reveal important information about the time course of emotional experience (i.e., how emotion, behavior, and physiology interact over time). Third, what is the specific relationship between maladaptive thoughts, emotions, and behaviors, thought to underlie psychopathology? Cognitive-behavioral therapy is based on the idea that negative maladaptive conditions lead to the emotional disturbance in depression; however, the specific nature of this relationship has not been systematically demonstrated in daily life. And fourth, is it possible to combine the advantages of EMA and experimental designs in the same study to examine causal effects in daily life (for discussion, see Barrett et al., 2001). For example, EMA technology could be used to give participants instructions to engage in particular behaviors or cognitions, such as emotion regulation strategies, and examine the self-reported effects on emotional experience and engagement in daily activities.

In closing, as technology improves and becomes more widely available, the use of EMA is likely to expand and be applied to more research questions and clinical applications. With its ability to explore the interplay between emotions, cognitions, behaviors, and contexts over time, EMA has the potential to elucidate the dynamic processes of emotion and its regulation in both normative and clinical samples, providing a number of applications that can be used to augment the assessment and treatment of emotion disorders.

# References


Anderson, P., Jacobs, C., & Rothbaum, B. O. (2004). Computer-supported cognitive behavioral treatment of anxiety disorders. *Journal of Clinical Psychology, 60*, 253–267.

Baer, L., Minichiello, W. E., & Jenike, M. A. (1987). Use of a portable-computer program in behavioral treatment of obsessive-compulsive disorder. *The American Journal of Psychiatry, 144*, 1101.

Baer, L., Minichiello W. E., Jenike M. A. & Holland A. (1988). Use of a portable computer program to assist behavioral tratement in a case of obsessive-compulsive disorder. *Journal of Behavior Research and Therapy*, 19, 237–240.

Barge-Schaapveld, D. Q., & Nicolson, N. A. (2002). Effects of antidepressant treatment on the quality of daily life: An experience sampling study. *The Journal of Clinical Psychiatry, 63*, 477–485.

Barge-Schaapveld, D. Q., Nicolson, N. A., van der Hoop, R. G., & de Vries, M. W. (1995). Changes in daily life experience associated with clinical improvement in depression. *Journal of Affective Disorders, 34*, 139–154.

Barrett, L. F. (1998). Discrete emotions or dimensions? The role of valence focus and arousal focus. *Cognition & Emotion, 12*, 579–599.

Barrett, L. F., & Barrett, D. J. (2001). An introduction to computerized experience sampling in psychology. *Social Science Computer Review, 19*, 175–185.

Barrett, L. F., Gross, J., Christensen, T. C., & Benvenuto, M. (2001). Knowing what you're feeling and knowing what to do about it: Mapping the relation between emotion differentiation and emotion regulation. *Cognition & Emotion, 15*, 713–724.

Barrett, L. F., Robin, L., Pietromonaco, P. R., & Eyssell, K. M. (1998). Are women the "more emotional" sex? Evidence from emotional experiences in social context. *Cognition & Emotion, 12*, 555–578.

Beck, A. T., Steer, R. A., & Brown, G. K. (1996). *BDI-II manual*. San Antonio: The Psychological Corporation.

Bolger, N., & Schilling, E. A. (1991). Personality and the problems of everyday life: The role of neuroticism in exposure and reactivity to daily stressors. *Journal of Personality, 59*, 355–386.

Brown, L. H., Silvia, P. J., Myin-Germeys, I., & Kwapil, T. R. (2007). When the need to belong goes wrong: The expression of social anhedonia and social anxiety in daily life. *Psychological Science: A Journal of the American Psychological Society/APS, 18*, 778–782.

Bryk, A. S., & Raudenbush, S. W. (1992). Hierarchical linear models: Applications and data analysis methods. Newbury Park, CA: Sage Publications.

Bylsma, L. M., Clift, A., & Rottenberg, R. (in press). Emotional reactivity to daily events in major and minor depression. *Journal of Abnormal Psychology*.

Bylsma, L. M., Morris, B. H., & Rottenberg, J. (2008). A meta-analysis of emotional reactivity in major depressive disorder. *Clinical Psychology Review, 28*, 676–691.

Carstensen, L. L., Pasupathi, M., Mayr, U., & Nesselroade, J. R. (2000). Emotional experience in everyday life across the adult life span. *Journal of Personality and Social Psychology, 79*, 644–655.

Christensen, T. C., Barrett, L. F., BlissMoreau, E., Lebo, K., & Kaschub, C. (2003). A practical guide to experience-sampling procedures. *Journal of Happiness Studies, 4*, 53–78.

Clark, L. A., Watson, D., & Leeka, J. (1989). Diurnal variation in the positive affects. *Motivation and Emotion, 13*, 205–234.

Cohen, L. H., Gunthert, K. C., Butler, A. C., Parrish, B. P., Wenze, S. J., & Beck, J. S. (2008). Negative affective spillover from daily events predicts early response to cognitive therapy for depression. *Journal of Consulting and Clinical Psychology, 76*, 955–965.

Conrad, A., Wilhelm, F. H., Roth, W. T., Spiegel, D., & Taylor, C. B. (2008). Circadian affective, cardiopulmonary, and cortisol variability in depressed and nondepressed individuals at risk for cardiovascular disease. *Journal of Psychiatric Research, 42*, 769–777.

Csikszentmihalyi, M., & Hunter, J. (2003). Happiness in everyday life: The uses of experience sampling. *Journal of Happiness Studies, 4*, 185–199.

Cutler, S. E., Larsen, R. J., & Bunce, S. C. (1996). Repressive coping style and the experience and recall of emotion: A naturalistic study of daily affect. *Journal of Personality*, *64*, 379–405.

Daimon, K., Yamada, N., Tsujimoto, T., & Takahashi, S. (1992). Circadian rhythm abnormalities of deep body temperature in depressive disorders. *Journal of Affective Disorders*, *26*, 191–198.

Delespaul, P., deVries, M., & van Os, J. (2002). Determinants of occurrences and recovery from hallucinations in daily life. *Social Psychiatry and Psychiatric Epidemiology, 39*, 97–104.

de Vries, M. W., & Delespaul, P. A. (1989). Time, context, and subjective experiences in schizophrenia. *Schizophrenia Bulletin, 15*, 233–244.

Fahrenberg, J., & Myrtek, M. (2001). *Progress in ambulatory assessment: Computer-assisted psychological and psychophysiological methods in monitoring and field studies*. Kirkland, WA: Hogrefe and Huber.

Fleeson, W. (2001). Toward a structure- and process-integrated view of personality: Traits as density distributions of states. *Journal of Personality and Social Psychology*, *80*, 1011–1027.

Gable, S. L., Reis, H. T., & Elliot, A. J. (2000). Behavioral activation and inhibition in everyday life. *Journal of Personality and Social Psychology*, *78*, 1135–1149.

Gross, J. J., Richards, J. M., & John, O. P. (2006). Emotion regulation in everyday life. In D. K. Snyder, J. A. Simpson, & J. N. Hughes (Eds.), *Emotion regulation in families: Pathways to dysfunction and health*. Washington, DC: American Psychological Association.

Gross, J. J. (1998). The emerging field of emotion regulation: An integrative review. *Review of General Psychology*, *2*, 271–299.

Gross, J. J. (2002). Emotion regulation: Affective, cognitive, and social consequences. *Psychophysiology*, *39*, 281–291.

Gruber, K., Moran, P. J., Roth, W. T., & Taylor, C. B. (2001). Computer-assisted cognitive behavioral group therapy for social phobia. *Behavior Therapy*, *32*, 155–165.

Gwaltney, C. J., Shiffman, S., & Sayette, M. A. (2005). Situational correlates of abstinence self-efficacy. *Journal of Abnormal Psychology*, *114*, 649–660.

Hall, D. P. Jr, Sing, H. C., & Romanoski, A. J. (1991). Identification and characterization of greater mood variance in depression. *The American Journal of Psychiatry*, *148*, 1341–1345.

Hammersley, R. (1994). A digest of memory phenomena for addiction research. *Addiction*, *89*, 283–293.

Havermans, R., Nicolson, N. A., & deVries, M. W. (2007). Daily hassles, uplifts, and time use in individuals with bipolar disorder in remission. *The Journal of Nervous and Mental Disease, 195*, 745–751.

Hibbert, G., & Pilsbury, D. (1988). Hyperventilation in panic attacks. Ambulant monitoring of transcutaneous carbon dioxide. *The British Journal of Psychiatry: The Journal of Mental Science*, *153*, 76–80.

Hibbert, G., & Pilsbury, D. (1989). Hyperventilation: Is it a cause of panic attacks? *The British Journal of Psychiatry: The Journal of Mental Science*, *155*, 805–809.

Horan, W. P., Green, M. F., Kring, A. M., & Nuechterlein, K. H. (2006). Does anhedonia in schizophrenia reflect faulty memory for subjectively experienced emotions? *Journal of Abnormal Psychology*, *115*, 496–508.

Kahneman, D., Krueger, A. B., Schkade, D. A., Schwarz, N., & Stone, A. A. (2004). A survey method for characterizing daily life experience: The day reconstruction method. *Science*, *306*, 1776–1780.

Kashdan, T. B., & Collins, R. L. (2010). Social anxiety and the experience of positive emotions and anger in everyday life: An ecological momentary assessment approach. *Anxiety, Stress, and Coping, 23*, 259–272.

Kashdan, T. B., & Steger, M. F. (2006). Expanding the topography of social anxiety: An experience-sampling assessment of positive emotions, positive events, and emotion suppression. *Psychological Science*, *17*, 120–128.

Kenardy, J., & Adams, C. (1993). Computers in cognitive-behavior therapy. *Australian Psychologist, 28*, 189–194.

Kernis, M. H. (2005). Measuring self-esteem in context: The importance of stability of self-esteem in psychological functioning. *Journal of Personality*, *73*, 1569–1605.

Kimhy, D., Delespaul, P., Corcoran, C., Ahn, H., Yale, S., & Malaspina, D. (2006). Computerized experience sampling method (ESMc): Assessing feasibility and validity among individuals with schizophrenia. *Journal of Psychiatric Research, 40*, 221–230.

Knouse, L. E., Mitchell, J. T., Brown, L. H., Silvia, P. J., Kane, M. J., Myin-Germeys, I., et al. (2008). The expression of adult ADHD symptoms in daily life: An application of experience sampling methodology. *Journal of Attention Disorders, 11*, 652–663.

Larson, R., & Delespaul, P. (1992). Analyzing experience sampling data: A guidebook for the perplexed. In M. V. de Vries (Ed.), *The experience of psychopathology: Investigating mental disorders in their natural settings* (pp. 58–78). Cambridge: Cambridge University Press.

Marco, C. A., & Suls, J. (1993). Daily stress and the trajectory of mood: Spillover, response assimilation, contrast, and chronic negative affectivity. *Journal of Personality and Social Psychology, 64*, 1053–1063.

Murray, G., Allen, N. B., & Trinder, J. (2002). Mood and the circadian system: Investigation of a circadian component in positive affect. *Chronobiology International, 19*, 1151–1169.

Murray, G. (2007). Diurnal mood variation in depression: A signal of disturbed circadian function? *Journal of Affective Disorders, 102*, 47–53.

Myin-Germeys, I., Delespaul, P.A.E.G., deVries, M. W. (2000). Schizopherenia patients are more emotionally active than is assumed on their behavior. *Schizophrenia Bulletin, 26*, 847–854.

Myin-Germeys, I., Nicolson, N. A. & Delespaul, P.A.E.G.. (2001). The context of delusional experiences in the daily life of patients with schizophreina. *Psychological Medicine, 31*, 489–498.

Myin-Germeys, I., Oorschot, M., Collip, D., Lataster, J., Delespaul, P., & van Os, J. (2009). Experience sampling research in psychopathology: Opening the black box of daily life. *Psychological Medicine, 39*, 1533–1547.

Myin-Germeys, I., Krabbendam, L., Jolles, J., Delespaul, P. A., & van Os, J. (2002). Are cognitive impairments associated with sensitivity to stress in schizophrenia? An experience sampling study. *American Journal of Psychiatry, 159*, 443–449.

Myin-Germeys, I., Peeters, F., Havermans, R., Nicolson, N. A., de Vries, M. W., Delespaul, P., et al. (2003). Emotional reactivity to daily life stress in psychosis and affective disorder: An experience sampling study. *Acta Psychiatrica Scandinavica, 107*, 124–131.

Nesse, R. M. (2000). Is depression an adaptation? *Archives of General Psychiatry, 57*, 14–20.

Newman, M. G., Kenardy, J., Herman, S., & Taylor, C. B. (1996). The use of hand-held computers as an adjunct to congntive-behavior therapy. *Computes in Human Behavior, 12*, 135–143.

Newman, M. G., Kenardy, J., Herman, S., & Taylor, C. B. (1997). Comparison of palmtop-computer-assisted brief cognitive-behavioral treatment to cognitive-behavioral treatment for panic disorder. *Journal of Consulting and Clinical Psychology, 65*, 178–183.

Newman, M. G., Consoli, A. J., & Taylor, C. B. (1999). A palmtop computer program for the treatment of generalized anxiety disorder. *Behavior Modification, 23*, 597–619.

Newman, M. G. (1999). The clinical use of palmtop computers in the treatment of generalized anxiety disorder. *Congnitive and Behavioral Practice, 6*, 222–234.

Peeters, F., Berkhof, J., Rottenberg, J., & Nicolson, N. A. Ambulatory emotional reactivity to daily life events predicts the eighteen-month course of major depressive disorder.

Peeters, F., Berkhof, J., Rottenberg, J., & Nicolson, N. A. (2010). Ambulatory emotional reactivity to negative daily life events predicts remission from major depressive disorder. Behaviour Research and Therapy, 48, 754-760.

Peeters, F., Nicholson, N. A., & Berkhof, J. (2003). Cortisol responses to daily events in major depressive disorder. *Psychosomatic Medicine, 65*, 836–841.

Peeters, F., Nicolson, N. A., & Berkhof, J. (2004). Levels and variability of daily life cortisol secretion in major depression. *Psychiatry Research, 126*, 1–13.

Peeters, F., Nicolson, N. A., Berkhof, J., Delespaul, P., & de Vries, M. (2003). Effects of daily events on mood states in major depressive disorder. *Journal of Abnormal Psychology, 112*, 203–211.

Peeters, F., Berkhof, J., Delespaul, P., Rottenberg, J., & Nicolson, N. A. (2006). Diurnal mood variation in major depressive disorder. *Emotion, 6*, 383–391.

Piasecki, T. M., Hufford, M. R., Solhan, M., & Trull, T. J. (2007). Assessing clients in their natural environments with electronic diaries: Rationale, benefits, limitations, and barriers. *Psychological Assessment*, *19*, 25–43.

Proudfoot, J. G. (2004). Computer-based treatment for anxiety and depression: Is it feasible? Is it effective? *Neuroscience and Biobehavioral Reviews*, *28*, 353–363.

Proudfoot, J., Ryden, C., Everitt, B., Shapiro, D. A., Goldberg, D., Mann, A., et al. (2004). Clinical efficacy of computerised cognitive-behavioural therapy for anxiety and depression in primary care: Randomised controlled trial. *British Journal of Psychiatry*, *185*, 46–54.

Rottenberg, J., & Johnson, S. L. (Eds.) (2007). *Emotion and psychopathology: Bridging affective and clinical science*. Washington, DC: APA Books.

Rusting, C. L., & Larsen, R. J. (1998). Diurnal patterns of unpleasant mood: Associations with neuroticism, depression, and anxiety. *Journal of Personality*, *66*, 85–103.

Schneiders, J., Nicolson, N. A., Berkhof, J., Feron, F. J., van Os, J., & de Vries, M. W. (2006). Mood reactivity to daily negative events in early adolescence: Relationship to risk for psychopathology. *Developmental Psychology*, *42*, 543–554.

Schwartz, J. E., Neale, J., Marco, C., Shiffman, S. S., & Stone, A. A. (1999). Does trait coping exist? A momentary assessment approach to the evaluation of traits. *Journal of Personality and Social Psychology*, *77*, 360–369.

Schwarz, N., & Oyserman, D. (2001). Asking questions about behavior: Cognition, communication, and questionnaire construction. *American Journal of Evaluation*, *22*, 127–160.

Scollon, C. N., Diener, E., Oishi, S., & Biswas-Diener, R. (2005). An experience sampling and cross-cultural investigation of the relation between pleasant and unpleasant affect. *Cognition & Emotion*, *19*, 27–52.

Scollon, C. N., Kim-Prieto, C., & Diener, E. (2003). Experience sampling: Promises and pitfalls, strengths and weaknesses. *Journal of Happiness Studies*, *4*, 5–34.

Selmi, P. M., Klein, M. H., Greist, J. H., Sorrell, S. P., & Erdman, H. P. (1990). Computer-administered cognitive-behavioral therapy for depression. *The American Journal of Psychiatry*, *147*, 51–56.

Shiffman, S., Stone, A. A., & Hufford, M. R. (2008). Ecological momentary assessment. *Annual Review of Clinical Psychology*, *4*, 1–32.

Shiffman, S., Hufford, M., Hickcox, M., Paty, J. A., Gnys, M., & Kassel, J. D. (1997). Remember that? A comparison of real-time versus retrospective recall of smoking lapses. *Journal of Consulting and Clinical Psychology*, *65*, 292–300.

Silk, J. S., Steinberg, L., & Morris, A. S. (2003). Adolescents' emotion regulation in daily life: Links to depressive symptoms and problem behavior. *Child Development, 37*, 97–104.

Steger, M. F., Kashdan, T. B., & Oishi, S. (2008). Being good by doing good: Daily eudaimonic activity and well-being. *Journal of Research in Personality*, *42*, 22–42.

Stone, A. A., Broderick, J. E., Shiffman, S. S., & Schwartz, J. E. (2004). Understanding recall of weekly pain from a momentary assessment perspective: Absolute agreement, between- and within-person consistency, and judged change in weekly pain. *Pain*, *107*, 61–69.

Stone, A. A., Kennedy-Moore, E., & Neale, J. M. (1995). Association between daily coping and end-of-day mood. *Health Psychology*, *14*, 341–349.

Swendsen, J. D. (1997). Anxiety, depression, and their comorbidity: An experience sampling test of the helplessness-hopelessness theory. *Cognitive Therapy and Research*, *21*, 97–114.

van Eck, M., Nicolson, N. A., & Berkhof, J. (1998). Effects of stressful daily events on mood states: Relationship to global perceived stress. *Journal of Personality and Social Psychology*, *75*, 1572–1585.

Verduyn, P., Delvaux, E., Van Coillie, H., Tuerlinckx, F., & Van Mechelen, I. (2009). Predicting the duration of emotional experience: Two experience sampling studies. *Emotion*, *9*, 83–91.

von Zerssen, D., Barthelmes, H., Dirlich, G., Doerr, P., Emrich, H. M., von Lindern, L., et al. (1985). Circadian rhythms in endogenous depression. *Psychiatry Research*, *16*, 51–63.

Watson, D., Wiese, D., Vaidya, J., & Tellegen, A. (1999). The two general activation systems of affect: Structural findings, evolutionary considerations, and psychobiological evidence. *Journal of Personality and Social Psychology*, *76*, 820–838.

Wichers, M., Myin-Germeys, I., Jacobs, N., Peeters, F., Kenis, G., Derom, C., et al. (2007a). Genetic risk of depression and stress-induced negative affect in daily life. *The British Journal of Psychiatry: The Journal of Mental Science*, *191*, 218–223.

Wichers, M. C., Myin-Germeys, I., Jacobs, N., Peeters, F., Kenis, G., Derom, C., et al. (2007b). Evidence that moment-to-moment variation in positive emotions buffer genetic risk for depression: A momentary assessment twin study. *Acta Psychiatrica Scandinavica*, *115*, 451–457.

Wilhelm, P., & Schoebi, D. (2007). Assessing mood in daily life: Structural validity, sensitivity to change, and reliability of a short-scale to measure three basic dimensions of mood. *European Journal of Psychological Assessment*, *23*, 258–267.

Wright, J. H., Wright, A. S., Albano, A. M., Basco, M. R., Goldsmith, L. J., Raffield, T., et al. (2005). Computer-assisted cognitive therapy for depression: Maintaining efficacy while reducing therapist time. *The American Journal of Psychiatry*, *162*, 1158–1164.

Zelenski, J. M., & Larsen, R. J. (2000). The distribution of basic emotions in everyday life: A state and trait perspective from experience sampling data. *Journal of Research in Personality*, *34*, 178–197.

# Chapter 15
# Emotion Regulation and Mentalization in Somatoform Disorders

**Claudia Subic-Wrana**

## 15.1 Introduction

When in 1973 Sifneos coined the term "alexithymia," he referred to an impairment he thought to be characteristic of patients with psychosomatic disorders. When conducting clinical interviews with these patients, he had observed that they were severely hampered when it came to describing their feelings and he hypothesized that their diminished ability to be consciously aware of their emotions and to put them in words underpinned the onset and course of their psychosomatic disturbances. In particular, regarding patients with somatoform disorders, Sifneos' observation led him to conclude that their alexithymic characteristics led them to misinterpret bodily sensations relating to affective arousal as signs of bodily disturbance. Thus, alexithymic individuals do experience arousal often, but either do not attribute this to an affective state or, if they are aware of the presence of emotion, they do not know which emotion it is (Moormann, Bermond, & Albach, 2004). It can be hypothesized that this impairment in mentally representing affective arousal as different feeling states further hampers the ability of patients with somatoform disorders to regulate their emotions, which in turn may fuel the anxious awareness that they attach to the arousal-related bodily sensations as well as explain their urge to seek help within the medical system.

Mind reading or the ability to establish a theory of mind (ToM) is defined as the ability to infer mental states – such as feelings, thoughts, and intentions – in self and in others in order to predict their behavior. This ability is also called mentalization and it theoretically and empirically originates from the field of cognitive developmental psychology and was introduced into the clinical field by Fonagy and colleagues in their ground-breaking work "Affect Regulation, Mentalization, and the Development of the Self" (Fonagy, Gergely, Jurist, & Target, 2002).

C. Subic-Wrana (✉)
Clinic for Psychosomatic Medicine and Psychotherapy, University of Mainz,
Untere Zahlbacher Str. 8, 55131 Mainz, Germany
e-mail: subic-wrana@psychosomtik.klinik.uni-mainz.de

I. Nyklíček et al. (eds.), *Emotion Regulation and Well-Being*,
DOI 10.1007/978-1-4419-6953-8_15, © Springer Science+Business Media, LLC 2011

This work laid the theoretical foundation for the application of mentalization to clinical developmental psychology and underpinned it with a thorough review of the large body of empirical work on the construct conducted within developmental psychology and attachment research. In their clinical work, Fonagy and colleagues applied the concept to the understanding and treatment of borderline states and related personality disorders (Bateman & Fonagy, 2006), linking states of emotional hyperarousal to an impaired capacity to mentalize.

While patients with borderline personality disorders may be hampered in differentiating their feelings and may have severe difficulties enduring emotional ambivalence, they are at least conscious of their occasionally extremely intense feeling states, although deficits in mentalizing make it difficult for them to down-regulate this intense affective arousal on their own. A first indication that alexithymic persons who are not consciously aware of their affective arousal also suffer from deficits in mentalizing was provided by Hill et al. who observed (2004) that mentally able adults with Asperger's syndrome – an autistic spectrum disorder – scored high on alexithymia scales. Since there is evidence that adults and children with Asperger's syndrome are severely hampered in their mentalizing capacity (Baron-Cohen, 1995; Castelli et al., 2002) despite having highly developed cognitive abilities, Hill et al.'s observation links a diminished capacity to be aware of one's affective arousal with deficits in mind-reading abilities. There is currently little empirical knowledge as to whether Hill's finding in autistic patients can also be applied to patients with psychosomatic disorders; indeed the reception of the concept of mentalization and its impairments in the field of psychosomatic medicine has only just begun. Therefore, this chapter will focus on the relationship between high alexithymia or low emotional awareness and deficits in mentalizing with regard to somatoform disorders as a "classical" psychosomatic disorder. It will address whether the impaired ability of somatizing patients to be aware of and to express their feelings is related to an impaired ability to read others' minds; review first empirical data that suggest such an association; and discuss how the tendency of patients with somatoform disorders to misinterpret emotional arousal as physical symptoms hampers their implicit or intuitive understanding of social interaction.

## 15.2 Impaired Emotional Awareness and Representational Capacities in Psychosomatic Disorders as "Sunken Clinical Knowledge"

As early as 1948, Ruesch characterized somatizing patients from a psychoanalytic point of view as "infantile personalities" who not only fail to understand physical signs of affective arousal as emotional states rather than anxiety provoking bodily symptoms, but who are also hindered in making sense of social interaction. Ruesch explained the urgent need of these patients to have somebody to whom they can cling as being due to their severe difficulties in properly understanding what is going on inside them and in their relations to others. Ruesch's description links somatization with deficits in the ability to mentalize, that is, to represent self and others as feeling, thinking, and acting intentionally.

Krystal (1978) and Mitscherlich (1966) conceptualized the pathways that may lead to psychosomatic disturbances as reactions to an overwhelming experience of helplessness that lead to resomatization and desymbolization as desperate means of defense. Here, representational activities that have been acquired during development are deactivated, and thinking about extremely painful experiences and the conscious experience of the related feelings are replaced by the experience of an overall negative psychosomatic state, for example, by undifferentiated somatoform pain. Krystal (1997) also stated that children who are neglected or traumatized early in life may never mentally mature to a level at which they will be able to mentally represent affect and related fantasies or cognitions as symbols or words.

In the same line, McDougall (1980) conceptualized psychosomatic disturbances as being evoked by anxieties that are raised by instinctual needs and corresponding affects that cannot be symbolically represented due to the lack of an own psychic space allowing representational activities. She considers the typical psychosomatically disturbed patient to have been the child of an "addictive" mother who was eager to fulfill the physical needs of the child immediately at the same time as neglecting the child's psychic needs. In doing so, she thus functioned as a shield against external stimuli and inner impulses, instead of helping the child to make sense of or think about them.

All authors cited above have derived their theoretical conclusions from clinical work with psychosomatically disturbed patients, although they often do not explicitly differentiate between somatoform disorders and other psychosomatic states in the conclusions they draw. While arguing from somewhat different points of view, Krystal and Mitscherlich link psychosomatic symptoms to traumatization; while McDougall places greater emphasis on the characteristics of the typical caregiver–child relationship from which psychosomatic states may develop, they all point out that the general ability of these patients to represent mental contents is disturbed. In their view, patients with psychosomatic symptoms are not only impaired in representing affective arousal as conscious feeling states but are also generally impaired in thinking about themselves and others. The terminology used by these authors is based on different psychoanalytic theories; translated into modern terminology, however, they all indicate that the psychosomatically disturbed patients they treated were characterized by a more general impairment in mentalizing and not exclusively by an "alexithymic" impairment in representing affective arousal as conscious feeling states. Ruesch explicitly connects the impairments shown by somatizing patients in mentally representing their emotions with their difficulties to make sense of social interaction by inferring the thoughts, feelings, and intentions of others in order to predict their behavior.

## 15.3 Definitions and Explanations: Alexithymia, Emotional Awareness, and Mentalization

### *15.3.1 Alexithymia*

As mentioned above, Ruesch related psychosomatic conditions to "arrested development" (Ruesch, 1948, p. 134) which he saw to be caused by conditions such as a lack of consistent parenting or trauma that overwhelm the child's sense of mastery. He connected these experiences to deficits in social learning and to an "infantile" form of "self-expression" that manifests as somatization. Independently, Marty and de M'Uzan from the French Psychosomatic School described a specific cognitive style ("pensee operatoire") in individuals prone to psychosomatic disorders; a style characterized by a lack of fantasy and a preoccupation with the concrete details of external events (Marty & de M'Uzan, 1963). Not much later, Sifneos and Nemiah observed the marked difficulty of psychosomatic patients to verbally express their feelings. Sifneos termed this difficulty "alexithymia," a Greek term for "without words for emotion" (Sifneos, 1973). Nemiah, Freyberger, and Sifneos (1976) defined alexithymia as comprising (1) difficulties in identifying and describing feelings, (2) difficulties in distinguishing between feelings and bodily sensations of emotional arousal, (3) a deficient imagination, as evidenced by a lack of fantasies, and (4) an externally oriented cognitive style.

Several theories have been developed to explain how the difficulty of being consciously aware of feelings and of verbally expressing them is connected to the onset and duration of psychosomatic disorders. According to MacLean, the adaptive regulation of emotions requires the processing of emotional arousal (mediated by limbic regions) by the neocortex or "word brain," which symbolically encodes experience with language, allowing the experience to be organized and transformed. MacLean (1949) hypothesized that psychosomatic conditions result from impaired communication between the limbic system and the neocortex. Similarly, Sifneos and Nemiah proposed that dysregulated physiology with ensuing disease results from the failure to process emotion symbolically, via, for example, language or fantasy (Nemiah & Sifneos, 1970).

Taylor, Bagby, and Parker (1997) classified illnesses associated with alexithymia as "disorders of affect regulation." They regard medical, mental, and psychosomatic illnesses as disorders of psychobiological dysregulation and hypothesize a causal connection between deficient cognitive processing of emotions, dysregulation of the affective system, and dysregulation of behavioral and physiological systems (Taylor et al., 1997). With the development of the Toronto Alexithymia Scale (TAS; a self-report questionnaire), Taylor and his coworkers defined alexithymia as a personality trait and standardized its measurement. The first version of the TAS was developed based on a review of the literature and the selection of content areas thought to define the construct. The original version of the TAS comprised four factors: (1) difficulty in identifying and distinguishing between feelings and bodily sensations; (2) difficulty in describing feelings; (3) reduced daydreaming; and

(4) externally oriented thinking (Bagby et al., 1986). Since the daydreaming factor proved to be inconsistent with the other three factors of the scale, Taylor and colleagues made several revisions and finally presented the TAS-20 (a 20-item self-report scale) which yielded three factors: (1) difficulty in identifying feelings; (2) difficulty in describing feelings to others; and (3) externally oriented thinking (Bagby, Parker, et al., 1994; Bagby, Taylor, et al., 1994). Today, the TAS-20 is the most common measure in the field of alexithymia research. It has been translated into numerous languages, applied to participants with varying cultural backgrounds, and used to demonstrate that alexithymic features are common not only in individuals with psychosomatic disorders but also in patients with several physical and psychic diseases. Since the TAS-20 defines alexithymia as a personality trait, it has also frequently been applied in normal populations and healthy participants in order to investigate its relationship to other personality traits or to study impairments in emotion regulation in healthy individuals (for an overview, see Lane & Taitano, 2003). Critically, it has to be remarked that eliminating the daydreaming/fantasy factor from the TAS-20 has deprived the alexithymia construct – as it is defined by the TAS – from a core characteristic contained in the original definition by Nemiah et al. (1976); a characteristic that might be crucial for understanding the connection between alexithymic features and deficits in mentalization.

### *15.3.2 Emotional Awareness*

The definitions of alexithymia and the hypotheses surrounding its origin usually do not refer to an explicit theory on the normal development of affective processing. In contrast, Lane and Schwartz (1987) as well as Bucci (1997) have formulated testable theories on normal affective development that provide insight into the differences between normal cognitive–emotional development and its alexithymic impairments.

Lane and Schwartz (1987) proposed that the processing of emotion develops hierarchically through levels that involve cognitive mechanisms of increasing complexity and that organize affective experience. These levels structurally resemble Piaget's stages of normal cognitive development and are characterized by a progressive trend toward increasing differentiation and integration of an individual's schemata for processing information (Cowan & Piaget, 1978). In ascending order, the five "levels of emotional awareness" are (1) physical sensations, (2) action tendencies, (3) single emotions, (4) blends of emotion, and (5) blends of blends of emotional experience (the capacity to appreciate complexity in the experience of self and others). Emotional awareness is conceptualized as a separate domain of cognitive development that is consistent with the observation that highly intelligent individuals may sometimes lack sophistication in their ability to be aware of and describe their emotions (Lane & Schwartz, 1987). The model is hierarchical in the sense that each level adds to and modifies the function of previous levels, although each successive level does not eliminate the one before it.

Based on evidence from cognitive neuroscience, Bucci (1997) has proposed a "multiple code theory" of emotion in which emotions are nonverbally represented as sub-symbolic processes involving extero- and interoceptive sensations and as symbolic processes involving first imagery (nonverbal-symbolic, e.g. dreams) and later verbal symbols. Bucci states that alexithymia and a related tendency to somatize may occur when the "referential activity" that links the non-symbolic (e.g. visceral reaction to anxiety provoking sensual impressions) and symbolic channels (e.g. identification of the bodily sensation as anxiety) is disturbed. She points to the defense character of this disturbance when she hypothesizes that the referential activity is distorted because the so-called emotional schemes – typical reactions of the caregiver to the needs and affects of the child that have model character for the referential activity – are not mentally represented as memories if they are dominated by negative affects.

The models developed by Bucci (1997) and Lane and Schwartz (1987) differentiate implicit, sub-symbolic paths of affect regulation from explicit, pre-symbolic or symbolic modes of affect regulation. If affect is only regulated implicitly, conscious awareness of feelings does not occur, although affect might influence the mood states, the physical sensations, and the behavior of the individual.

The model developed by Lane and Schwartz can be empirically tested using the Levels of Emotional Awareness Scale (LEAS; Lane et al., 1990). This performance measure consists of 20 vignettes describing emotion provoking interactions between two persons. Participants are asked to write down how they would feel as the protagonist of each scene and how "the other" would feel. Answers are quantified using scoring rules derived from the levels of emotional awareness theory. Based on a sample of 294 inpatients undergoing psychotherapeutic treatment, the LEAS has been shown to demonstrate diagnosis-related sensitivity for differences in emotional awareness. Of six diagnostic subsamples, patients with somatoform disorders had the lowest LEAS scores at the onset of treatment and were the only group to achieve significantly higher LEAS scores at the end of treatment. By controlling for negative affect, it was further demonstrated that LEAS scores were not confounded by negative affect (Subic-Wrana et al., 2005).

### *15.3.3 Mentalization*

Mentalization or mentalizing is a relatively new term used to describe the origin and functioning of the representational activity that allows an individual to think about him/herself and others. In psychoanalytically informed theory, mentalization is a sophisticated developmental model describing the origin of affect regulation, symbolization, and a coherent sense of the self. The neurosciences adopted the term to describe the brain activity that is observed when participants are confronted with tasks that require them to infer others' mental states. Such experiments have accordingly primarily focused on a sub-aspect of mentalizing, such as testing whether a theory of mind (ToM) is used to explain the observed behavior of others.

Mentalization as a theoretical developmental model that explains how an individual develops the ability to think about him/herself and others as "having a mind" has been conceptualized and applied to psychopathology and psychotherapy by Fonagy and his coworkers (1996, 2002). They understand mentalizing as a mostly implicit, pre-conscious, or unconscious but also conscious process that allows one's own and others' actions to be interpreted as meaningful on the basis of intentional mental states such as desires, feelings, reason, and beliefs. Mentalizing also includes meta-cognitive skills, that is, being able to think about thinking. To mentalize in this sense means being open to the opaqueness of mental states and includes being aware that they can rapidly change, that they are not as stable as physical "things," and that the inference of one's own and others' mental states helps to understand social interaction at the same time as being highly prone to error. Important cornerstones in the development of mentalizing will be discussed in the next section.

Mentalization in a somewhat narrower sense has been and is a field of interest within modern cognitive developmental psychology. Here, experiments and empirical studies have been designed that help to address the question concerning the age at which a child is able to apply a ToM to others in order to predict their behavior. An important step in this direction is the ability to solve a false belief task. This ability has been shown to emerge in normally developing children at the age of 3–5 years. In such tasks, children are shown, often in the form of a puppet play performed by the experimenter, what someone else usually expects (e.g. the boy Peter expects the bottle he takes from the refrigerator to contain milk). In the next step of the experiment, the child who undergoes the false belief task observes a change in the facts upon which the usual belief rely (e.g. a second puppet enters the scene, drinks the milk from the bottle, fills it with water, and puts it back into the refrigerator). The crucial probe for the false belief task is subsequently made and it is tested whether the child is able to infer that someone who has not watched this change of the "usual" facts will still believe that the facts are "as usual" (e.g. the Peter-puppet appears again and opens the refrigerator in order to drink milk from the bottle). The child undergoing the experiment is asked what the Peter-puppet expects to find in the bottle. Children who are mature enough to form a ToM will answer that the Peter puppet expects milk and will, therefore, be disappointed to find water in the bottle. Children who have not yet reached this cognitive-developmental stage will answer that the Peter-puppet will expect to find water in the bottle and thus demonstrate that they tend to explain the behavior of others in a goal-directed way, that is, based on physical facts that they can observe in the outside world.

The distinction between a goal-directed and a theory-of-mind (ToM)-centered explanation of the behavior of others represents a crucial step in the achievement of mentalizing abilities; children who are able to state that Peter will be disappointed because he expected milk instead of water demonstrate that they have developed a qualitatively new approach in understanding the motives and reactions of others and are now able to refer inner states to them. In an important application of this cognitive-developmental concept of first-order mentalizing/goal-directedness and second-order mentalizing/ToM to the clinical field of autism research, Baron-Cohen (1995) demonstrated that cognitively able children with Asperger's syndrome – an autism-spectrum disorder – were not able to solve false belief tasks successfully, while normally developing children and children with Down syndrome were able to. Based on this experiment, Baron-Cohen not only provided strong support for the hypothesis that an impairment to read the mind of others is a core deficit in autism, but also demonstrated that the ability to infer the mental states of others (ToM) is (relatively) independent of general intelligence.

The principle behind false belief tasks has been explained in detail since they represent a straight-forward experimental method that distinguishes between first- (goal-directed) and second-order (ToM) mentalizing. When studying brain activity during mentalizing processes, applying tasks that require goal-directed and/or ToM activity in order to be successfully solved reveals which neuronal networks are involved when ToM activity, as a measurable aspect of the broad psychoanalytic developmental concept of mentalization, is investigated. In their overview, Frith and Frith (2006) conclude that most neuroimaging studies of ToM activity have shown involvement of the anterior paracingulate cortex, the temporal parietal junction, and the temporal poles.

## 15.4 Development of Mentalization: Social Feedback Theory, Psychic Equivalence, and Pretend Mode

A cornerstone of mentalization as a psychoanalytically informed theory of human development is the "social feedback theory" formulated by Gergely and Watson (1996). Here, it is proposed that the infant is born without knowledge of his/her own inner world or that of others and that the psychic structures that allow the child – and later the adolescent and adult – to think about his or her own feelings, thoughts, and intentions as well as those of others must be established through internalization of the child–caregiver relationship. If the caregiver is able to make sense of the utterances and sensorimotor reactions of the nursling, acts in a way that fulfills the basic needs of the child, and provides the child with symbolic understanding of this interaction (e.g. thinking about what is happening and communicating it to the child), then the child will gradually grow to understand its own needs and will find appropriate ways to respond to them.

Gergely and Watson specifically point out that the first psychic contents to be mentally represented are emotions. The only means with which the newborn can communicate with his/her caregivers are undifferentiated affects which roughly indicate that the child is in a good or bad state. Gergely and Watson reviewed evidence that the caregiver's mirroring of the child's display of these global affective states sensitizes the child to categorical differences among their own emotional states; "bad" becomes differentiated, for instance, into fear, anger, and pain, and "good" into happiness and interest. Mirroring includes utterances and actions of the caregiver; when soothing words of the caregiver in reaction to the child's crying in the dark are related to putting on the light, while other words are related to the changing of diapers that are wet with cold and biting urine, this provides the child with the cognitive means to represent fear and pain mentally as categorical different negative feelings. In addition, the difference between consciously guided mirroring of the child's affects by the caregiver and the caregiver's automatic facial display of his/her own affect elicited by the child is essential when it comes to the decoupling function that allows the child to distinguish between his/her own inner states and those of others.

Fonagy and colleagues (2002), who refer to the "social feedback" theory of Gergely and Watson, particularly stress that "marked" mirroring of the child's affective state is necessary in order to build the foundation for a sufficiently functioning mentalizing capacity. Compared to the caregiver's spontaneous emotional reaction to interactions with the child, the "marked" mirroring of the caregiver is often somewhat exaggerated or posed and thus signalizes, for instance, that the child is afraid (e.g. because a stranger has entered the room), but that there is no real danger (e.g. because he/she is someone familiar to the caregiver). "Marked" reactions to the child's affective states to a certain degree remove the emotion in question from direct social interplay – as construed by the often implicit facial or vocal expressions of affect – and signalize that this emotion can be looked at, thought about, and therefore mastered. Marked reactions of the caregiver are especially helpful when it comes to strong negative emotions, because they help the child think about and symbolize them as a first and important step to regulating them.

Fonagy and colleagues named the primary mode of psychic functioning that the child acquires when he/she is able to represent psychic contents mentally the mode of "psychic equivalence" (2002). In this mode, mental contents are connected with characteristics of the physical world. The differentiation between the psychic and the physical world is weak; emotions and related thoughts may elicit fear because, as of yet, no categorical difference has been established between doing something and thinking something. If a toddler in a state of rage wishes that his newborn sister would disappear, he may react to this wish with signs of intense fear and guilt, because he is aware neither that his thoughts will have no consequences in the physical world if they are not followed by actions, nor that his thoughts and feelings about his sister will quickly change if he starts to think about other aspects of his relationship to her. Perspective taking, an ability which is not under the deliberate command of a child who is thinking in the mode of psychic equivalence, becomes of interest when a child acquires the "pretend mode" (Fonagy et al., 2002). In this developmental stage (mostly starting at the age of between 2½ and 3 years), children deepen their understanding of the differences between play and reality. In the context of role plays and pretend situations, they test out and learn that pretending something and doing it for real are two very different things. The toddler who in the mode of psychic equivalence experienced fear in connection with his wish to send away his little sister can now pretend that she is left alone on a lonely island while he travels around with a big ship without experiencing guilt or fear. The pretend mode in which the child can handle emotions and related wishes in a "marked" way helps him/her to internalize the difference between characteristics of thoughts and characteristics of the physical world and is, therefore, extremely important for the ability to regulate one's emotions. Extensive use of this mode is associated with the danger of losing contact with one's physical existence (as in severe depersonalization) or with consequences of actions that are performed in a "pretend" state of mind.

Fonagy and colleagues (2002) state that differentiated mentalizing becomes possible when the two modes of psychic functioning – psychic equivalence and the pretend mode – can be integrated. In their developmental approach, mentalization is not a stable ability that can be applied in an unchangeable way once it has been acquired, but is rather a psychic capacity that might be subject to change under the pressure of the circumstances with which an individual has to cope. Physical illness as well as severe interpersonal conflicts may hamper an individual's capacity to mentalize his needs, intentions, and related emotions. Psychotherapy may help to reinstate hampered mentalizing capacity or to establish it in the case that it has not previously sufficiently developed.

## 15.5 Hypothesis About Emotional Awareness and Mentalization in Somatoform Disorders

Both the levels of emotional awareness theory (Lane & Schwartz, 1987) and the mentalization approach of Fonagy and colleagues (2002) posit that developing cognitive skills enables an individual to be aware of his or her emotions in order to regulate them by thinking about them. The scope of mentalization is wider than that of the levels of emotional awareness theory, offering a model of the emerging capacity to reflect upon self and others in all psychic content domains; at its core, however, mentalization provides a theory on how emotion regulation can be achieved. This is reflected in its emphasis upon affects as the first psychic contents to be mentally represented and in its implicit hypothesis that thinking about the self and others is needed to regulate the strong affects that are elicited when the wishes and intentions of an individual are not met in his/her social interaction with others. In the terminology of the mentalizing approach, patients with somatoform disorders function in the mode of psychic equivalence. Bodily sensations related to affective arousal cannot be mentalized (e.g. "the muscles in my back are aching, what has put me under so much tension?" or "my heart is beating so fast, could the quarrel with my boss have upset me more than I am aware of?") but are rather viewed as physical defects (e.g. "there is something wrong with my back or my heart and I have to go to the doctor"). In the levels of emotional awareness approach, somatizing patients are not able to transfer implicit signs of emotional arousal (e.g. a faster heartbeat) into an explicit mode of emotional processing (e.g. "my heart is beating so fast, I am upset") and, therefore, misinterpret them as signs of bodily malfunctions. The examples demonstrate that the levels of emotional awareness approach more closely consider the emotional contents with which the bodily sensation are associated, while the mentalizing approach also addresses the social interaction, represented either in thoughts or intentions or just experienced, which is related to the feeling indicated by the bodily sensation.

Having placed the two theoretical approaches in relation to one another, it might be hypothesized that patients with somatoform disorders are not only hampered in their conscious awareness of their feelings, but that they also are handicapped when it comes to using their emotions to understand themselves and others.

The mentalizing approach developed by Fonagy and colleagues stresses the importance of the caregiver–child relationship as the source from which the ability to represent the self and others as feeling, thinking, and acting intentionally emerges. If the primary attachment system is disturbed, development of mentalization becomes impaired. Failures in the attachment system and their consequences for the development of mentalizing capacity have been studied thoroughly in patients with borderline personality disorders. Here, empirical evidence shows that the majority of these patients have either an unresolved or an insecure attachment status (Fonagy et al., 1996), with a large proportion showing the former. In terms of attachment theory, an unresolved attachment status indicates that the individual has suffered from experiences of trauma that turn the primary source of security (the caregiver–child relationship) into a danger zone in which he/she has been exposed to abuse or neglect. In insecure attachment, the proximity-seeking child has repeatedly experienced that the caregiver does not function as a source of safety but either reacts in an ambivalent way or dismisses the signals of the child. Psychotherapeutic work with patients suffering from somatoform disorders often reveals adverse childhood experiences. Many patients report having been raised in a climate of emotional neglect and, in particular, patients with somatoform pain disorders have often suffered from severe physical abuse in their childhood. Therefore, a first hypothesis regarding impairments in the mentalizing capacity of patients with somatoform disorders connects these impairments with adverse childhood experiences that turned the caregiver–child relationship into a source of uncertainty and danger. If the later-to-be somatoform patient is unable to find safety and understanding for his/her needs and feelings, then (a) the child–caregiver relationship is not able to serve as a role model for trying to understand own needs and feelings and (b) relations to others are dismissed as a possible source of psychic or physical pain and thus do not become a primary source of learning when it comes to understanding self and others.

The first hypothesis that links impaired mentalizing capacity in patients with somatoform disorders with insecure or unresolved attachment has a more general quality, given the evidence that patients with severe psychosomatic or psychiatric disorders are generally characterized by a high load of childhood trauma (Widom et al., 2007). More specific hypotheses can be derived regarding failures in the process of mirroring and the marking of affects that might occur in the relationship between caregivers and children who, later in life, might tend to somatize. In order to make implicit processing of emotions explicit, the child needs to connect implicit markers of emotional arousal, such as physical sensations or action tendencies, with nonverbal and verbal symbols of feelings; according to the mentalization approach, this is achieved by the marked reactions of caregivers to children's emotion-related utterances. If these utterances go undetected by caregivers (e.g. in the case of emotional neglect, when caregivers fail to be empathetic to children's mood states) or if caregivers themselves are not able to mark these utterances because they themselves are not able to mentally represent the utterances as feelings (e.g. the "sickness" of a child facing a separation from the caregiver is not encoded and marked as being related to anxiety but is instead treated as illness), then these children will also fail to develop mental representations of bodily sensations as belonging to distinct feeling states. In the next section, first empirical support for these hypotheses will be presented.

## 15.6 Mentalization Deficits in Somatoform Patients: Empirical Indications and First Empirical Evidence

To date, no studies have been published which provide empirical support for the hypothesis that patients with somatoform disorders suffer from impairments in emotional awareness *and* in mentalizing capacity. Below, studies linking insecure attachment and childhood maltreatment with alexithymia will be reviewed. Finally, a study on mentalizing deficits in healthy alexithymic students and first, unpublished evidence of mentalizing deficits in somatoform patients will be discussed.

Taylor and Bagby (2004) suggest that studies on early stages of development and attachment research may become important areas of alexithymia research in the future. This is evidenced by investigations using self-report questionnaires in which strong relationships between insecure attachment and alexithymia measured using the TAS-20 have been reported for healthy individuals and for patients suffering from depression and anxiety disorders (Troisi et al., 2001; Wearden et al., 2005; Picardi et al., 2005). In a large community sample ($n$ = 620; Briere & Rickards, 2007), highly significant associations were found between emotional abuse (mostly by the mother) and self-reported ego-structural deficits that included deficits in affect regulation. In psychiatric patients, a moderate but significant relationship has been observed between a negative parenting style and both alexithymia and depression (Kooiman et al., 2004). In a self-report survey of 100 female students, alexithymia was found to moderate the relationship between physical and emotional abuse in childhood and ongoing self-injury (Paivio & McCulloch, 2004). In a further self-report survey of female students ($n$ = 500), it was shown that alexithymia correlated with emotional childhood abuse and the amount of self-perceived distress; when testing for statistical mediator models, alexithymia and self-perceived distress were found to best explain the association between childhood abuse and disturbed eating behavior (Hund & Espelage, 2006). Both of these studies are interesting since self-injury and disturbed eating behavior may be understood as indicators of difficulties in mentalizing negative emotions. In healthy police cadets, childhood trauma proved predictive of heightened physiological (skin conductance and eye blink magnitude) and negative emotional reactions to startling sounds (Pole et al., 2007). The authors conclude that childhood trauma may lead to long-lasting alterations in emotional and physiological reactivity to distress and that these alterations may be related to an alexithymic style of emotion processing.

A prospective study conducted by Lemche et al. (2004) demonstrated the relationship between a negative parenting style and disturbed emotion regulation due to an impaired mentalizing capacity. Here, the authors related the attachment status of 42 children at 12 months of age to mentalizing capacity at several time points thier between the ages of 12 and 36 months. They specifically tested the development of the ability to put emotions into words and to use verbal strategies for the regulation of affect. Insecurely attached children or children with disorganized attachment (display of chaotic patterns in relating to primary caregivers) showed severe developmental arrest in mentalizing compared to securely attached children. At the end of their third year of life, some of these children were not able to express emotions in words other than in a rudimentary manner. The authors conclude that alexithymia might be the result of impaired mentalizing that is formed by the attachment and parenting style of the parents.

In a functional Magnetic Resonance Imaging (fMRI) study, Moriguchi et al. (2006) studied the mentalizing capacity of healthy alexithymic individuals. They specifically investigated neuronal activity in high-alexithymic vs. low-alexithymic healthy students who were required to solve a ToM task that had previously been shown to distinguish between cognitively able adults with Asperger's autism and matched healthy controls with regard to their ToM capacity (2002). The task was developed by Frith and Happé and first used and published by Castelli, Happé, Frith, and Frith (2000) and consists of silent animations featuring a small red and a large blue triangle moving across a white background. In some of the animations, the movement of the triangles can be understood by using a goal-directed approach (e.g. the action of one triangle can be interpreted as being determined by the action of the second triangle, with, for example, one triangle chasing the other). In contrast, the interaction of the triangles in another set of the animations only makes sense if the onlooker refers to what the triangles might think, feel, or intend (e.g. one triangle wants to deceive the other). These latter animations are referred to as ToM animations. High-alexithymic individuals performed worse on this task than low-alexithymic individuals, inferring less thoughts, feelings, and intentions from the movement of the triangles in the ToM animations and, therefore, showing greater difficulty in understanding what was going on between the triangles. The high-alexithymic students also displayed less activity in the neuronal network shown to be related to ToM/mentalizing.

In a study conducted by the present authors, we administered the Frith–Happé animations task and the LEAS (Lane et al., 1990) to 30 patients with somatoform disorders and to 30 healthy controls, matched for age, sex, and educational level. As had been the case for high-alexithymic students, the somatoform patients performed significantly worse on the ToM task compared to healthy individuals, whereas patients and controls did not differ with respect to the goal-directed tasks. Patients also displayed a significantly lower level of emotional awareness on the LEAS (Subic-Wrana et al., 2010).

## 15.7 Conclusion

The clinical observation that patients with somatoform disorders not only fail to connect bodily signs of emotional arousal to feelings they are consciously aware of, but also have difficulties making sense of social interaction by inferring the feelings, thoughts, and intentions of self and others can be theoretically underpinned by the mentalization approach. This developmental model posits that the ability to mentally represent emotions, which is acquired in the child–caregiver relationship, constitutes the cornerstone for the regulation of emotional arousal by helping to understand the mental states of the self and others. While empirical support for this understanding of the cognitive–emotional impairments in patients suffering from somatoform disorders is sparse, first studies trying to link alexithymia with insecure attachment and decreased mentalizing capacity suggest that applying the mentalization concept to the theoretical understanding, empirical investigation, and psychotherapeutic treatment of somatoform disorders might prove worthwhile.

## References


Bagby, R. M., Parker, J. D., & Taylor, G. J. (1994) The twenty-item Toronto Alexithymia Scale – I. Item selection and cross-validation of the factor structure. *Journal of Psychosomatic Research, 38*, 23–32.

Bagby, R. M., Taylor, G. J., & Parker, J. D. (1994) The twenty-item Toronto Alexithymia Scale – II. Convergent, discriminant, and concurrent validity. *Journal of Psychosomatic Research, 38*, 33–40.

Bagby, R. M., Taylor, G. J., & Ryan, D. (1986) Toronto Alexithymia Scale: Relationship with personality and psychopathology measures. *Psychotherapy and Psychosomatics, 45*, 207–215.

Bateman, A., & Fonagy, P. (2006) *Mentalization-based treatment for borderline personality disorder. A practical guide*. New York: Oxford University Press.

Baron-Cohen, S. (1995) *Mindblindness*. Cambridge, MA: MIT Press.

Briere, J., & Rickards, S. (2007) Self-awareness, affect regulation, and relatedness: Differential sequels of childhood versus adult victimization experiences. *Journal of Nervous and Mental Disease, 195*, 497–503.

Bucci, W. (1997) Symptoms and symbols: A multiple code theory of somatization. *Psychoanalytic Inquiry, 12*, 151–172.

Castelli, F., Happé, F., Frith, U., & Frith, C. (2000) Movement and mind: A functional imaging study of perception and interpretation of complex intentional movement patterns. *NeuroImage, 12*, 314–325.

Castelli, F., Frith, C., Happé, F., & Frith, U. (2002) Autism: Asperger syndrome and brain mechanisms for the attribution of mental states to animated shapes. *Brain, 125*, 1839–1849.

Cowan, P. A., & Piaget, J. (1978) *With feeling: Cognitive, social, and emotional dimensions*. New York: Rinehart & Winston.

Frith, C. D., & Frith, U. (2006) The neural basis of mentalizing. *Neuron, 50*, 531–534,

Fonagy, P., Leigh, T., Steele, M., Steele, H., Kennedy, R., Mattoon, G., & Target, M. (1996) The relation of attachment status, psychiatric classification and response to psychotherapy. *Journal of Consulting and Clinical Psychology, 64*, 22–31.

Fonagy, P., Gergely, G., Jurist, E. L., & Target, M. (2002) *Affect regulation, mentalization and the development of the self*. New York: Other Press.

Gergely, G., & Watson, J. S. (1996) The social biofeedback theory of parental affect-mirroring. *International Journal of Psycho-Analysis, 77*, 1181–1121.

Hill, E., Berthoz, S., & Frith, U. (2004) Brief report: Cognitive processing of own emotions in individuals with autistic spectrum disorder and in their relatives. *Journal of Autism and Developmental Disorders, 34*, 229–235.

Hund, A. R., & Espelage, D. L. (2006) Childhood emotional abuse and disordered eating among undergraduate females: Mediating influence of alexithymia and distress. *Childhood Abuse and Neglect, 30*, 393–407.

Kooiman, C. G., van Rees Vellings, S., Spinhoven, P., Draijer, N., Trijsburg, R. W., & Rooijmans, H. G. (2004) Childhood adversities as risk factors for alexithymia and other aspects of affect dysregulation in adulthood. *Psychotherapy and Psychosomatics*, *73*, 107–116.

Krystal, H. (1978) Trauma and affects. *Psychoanalytic Study of the Child*, *33*, 81–116.

Krystal, H. (1997) Desomatization and the consequences of infantile psychic trauma. *Psychoanalytic Inquiry*, *12*, 12–150.

Lane, R. D., & Schwartz, G. E. (1987) Levels of emotional awareness: A cognitive-developmental theory and its application to psychopathology. *American Journal of Psychiatry*, *144*, 133–143.

Lane, R. D., Quinlan, D. M., Schwartz, G. E., Walker, P. A., & Zeilin, S. B. (1990) The Levels of Emotional Awareness Scale: A cognitive-developmental measure of emotion. *Journal of Personality Assessment*, *55*, 124–134.

Lane, R., & Taitano, K. (2003) Alexithymie. In R. H. Adler, J. M. Herrmann, K. Köhle, W. Langewitz, O. W. Schonechke, T. von Uexküll, & W. Wesiack (Eds.), *Psychosomatische Medizin* (pp. 279–294) Munich, Germany: Urban & Fischer.

Lemche, E., Klann-Delius, G., Koch, R., & Joraschky, P. (2004) Mentalizing language development in a longitudinal attachment sample: Implications for alexithymia. *Psychotherapy and Psychosomatics*, *73*, 366–374.

MacLean, P. D. (1949) Psychosomatic disease and the 'visceral brain': Recent developments bearing on the Papez theory of emotion. *Psychosomatic Medicine*, *11*, 338–353.

Marty, P., & de M'Uzan, M. (1963) La pensee operatoire. *Revue Francaise Psychoanalyse*, *27*(suppl.), 1345 ff.

McDougall, J. (1980) *Plea for a measure of abnormality*. New York: International University Press.

Mitscherlich, A. (1966) *Krankheit als Konflikt*. Frankfurt: Edition Suhrkamp.

Moormann, P. P., Bermond, B., & Albach, F. (2004) The Reality Escape Model: The intricate relation between alexithymia, dissociation, and anesthesia in victims of sexual abuse. In I. Nyklíček, L. Temoshok, & A. Vingerhoets (Eds.), *Emotional expression and health: Advances in theory, assessment, and clinical applications* (pp. 82–98). London: Brunner-Routledge.

Moriguchi, Y., Ohnishi, T., Lane, R. D., Maeda, M., Mori, T., Nemoto, K., Matsuda, H., & Komaki, G. (2006) Impaired self-awareness and theory of mind: An fMRI study of mentalizing in alexithymia. *NeuroImage*, 32, 1472–1482.

Nemiah, J. C., Freyberger, H., & Sifneos, P. E. (Eds.). (1976) *Alexithymia: A view of the psychosomatic process* (Vol. 3). London: Butterworths.

Nemiah, J. C, & Sifneos, P. E. (1970) Affect and fantasy in patients with psychosomatic disorder. In O.W. Hill (Ed.), *Modern trends in psychosomatic medicine* (Vol. 2, pp. 26–34). New York: Appleton-Century-Crofts.

Paivio, S. C., & McCulloch, C. R. (2004) Alexithymia as a mediator between childhood trauma and self-injurious behaviors. *Childhood Abuse and Neglect*, *28*, 339–345.

Picardi, A., Toni, A., & Caroppo, E. (2005) Stability of alexithymia and its relationships with the "big five" factors, temperament, character, and attachment style. *Psychotherapy and Psychosomatics*, *74*, 371–378.

Pole, N., Neylan, T. C., Otte, C., Metzler, T. J., Best, S. R., Henn-Haase, C., & Marmar, C. R. (2007) Associations between childhood trauma and emotion-modulated psychophysiological responses to startling sounds: A study of police cadets. *Journal of Abnormal Psychology*, *116*, 352–361.

Ruesch, J. (1948) The infantile personality. *Psychosomatic Medicine*, *10*, 134–144.

Sifneos, P. E. (1973) The prevalence of "alexithymic" characteristics in psychosomatic patients. *Psychotherapy and Psychosomatics*, *22*, 255–262.

Subic-Wrana, C., Bruder, S., Thomas, W., Lane, R. D., & Köhle, K. (2005) Emotional awareness deficits in inpatients of a psychosomatic ward: A comparison of two different measures of alexithymia. *Psychosomatic Medicine*, *67*, 483–489.

Subic-Wrana, C., Beutel, M. E., Knebel, A., & Lane, R. D. (2010) Theory of mind and emotional awareness deficits in patients with somatoform disorders. Psychosomatic Medicine, 72, 404–411

Taylor, G. J., Bagby, R. M., & Parker, J. D. A. (Eds.). (1997) *Disorders of affect regulation: Alexithymia in medical and psychiatric illness*. Cambridge: Cambridge University Press.
Taylor, G. J., & Bagby, R. M. (2004) New trends in alexithymia research. *Psychotherapy and Psychosomatics*, *73*, 68–77.
Troisi, D., D'Argenio, A., Peracchio, F., & Petti, P. (2001) Insecure attachment and alexithymia in young men with mood symptoms. *Journal of Nervous and Mental Disease*, *189*, 311–316.
Wearden, A. J., Lamberton, N., Crook, N., & Walsh, V. (2005) Adult attachment, alexithymia, and symptom reporting: An extension to the four category model of attachment. *Journal of Psychosomatic Research*, *58*, 279–288.
Widom, C. S., DuMont, K., & Czaja, S. J. (2007) A prospective investigation of major depression disorder and comorbidity in abused and neglected children grown up. *Archives of General Psychiatry*, *64*, 49–56.

# Chapter 16
# Emotion Perception and Health

**Mariska E. Kret, Charlotte B.A. Sinke, and Beatrice de Gelder**

## 16.1 Introduction

In everyday life, we are continuously confronted with other people. One of the most important sources of social information is facial expressions: humans are predominantly visual animals, and we spend a great deal of time looking at and analyzing faces. Moreover, many facial expressions are universally consistent. For this reason, emotion research has predominantly focused on faces. However, bodily expressions are just as well recognized, they can be seen from a distance and are, from an evolutionary perspective, much older. Body language, therefore, has a high communicative role, albeit we are less aware of it. Models on facial expression processing might also work for understanding bodily expressions. However, whereas faces illustrate the mental states of people, body postures in addition imply motion and show an action intention.

Almost everyone experiences depressive or anxious moments or even episodes. Depression and anxiety influence recognition and perception of emotional expressions. Research has shown that small diversities in personality type can already account for these differences.

We would like to put forward that brain responses to emotional expressions are driven not only by external cues but also by the personal state of mind and significance of the current social context. Individual differences such as personality type and psychopathology play an important role. The nature of emotion perception cannot be fully understood by focusing separately on social, cultural, contextual, individual, and interpersonal factors. The percept of an emotion is embodied, and its bodily grounded nature provides a foundation for social communication. "*What you see is what you get*" does not apply here. People neither "see" the same, nor do they attend to the same.

M.E. Kret (✉)
Department of Medical Psychology and Cognitive Neuroscience, Tilburg University,
P.O. Box 90153, 5000 LE Tilburg, Netherlands
e-mail: m.e.kret@uvt.nl

I. Nyklíček et al. (eds.), *Emotion Regulation and Well-Being*,
DOI 10.1007/978-1-4419-6953-8_16, © Springer Science+Business Media, LLC 2011

All the topics we just mentioned will be discussed in this chapter. They show us that recognizing emotional meaning from others is vital and that facial and bodily expressions are of crucial importance for normal communication. This is clearly impaired in disorders such as autism, schizophrenia, Huntington's disease, Parkinson's disease, depression, and anxiety. But before we discuss emotion perception in these disorders, we first provide an overview of the literature on emotional face and body processing in healthy people. Investigations of neurological differences in facial and bodily expression perception will enrich basic clinical research and can lead to the development of new observational and diagnostic tools.

## 16.2 Processing Faces and Bodies

### *16.2.1 Inversion Effect*

Social communication includes intuitively grasping signals of hostility and reacting with empathy to signals of distress. Humans are especially sensitive to the gestural signals and facial expressions made by other people, and use these signals as guides for their own behavior. Communicative ability also relies heavily on decoding messages provided by bodily signals. The neural network underlying body perception overlaps with areas involved in perceiving facial expressions (Peelen, Atkinson, Andersson, & Vuilleumier, 2007; van de Riet, Grèzes, & de Gelder, 2009). The major concept used to argue for the specificity of processing is configuration. Evidence shows that faces and bodies are not processed as a collection of features (such as objects): when presented upside down, recognition drops significantly and is relatively more impaired than for inverted objects (Reed, Stone, Bozava, & Tanaka, 2003). The face and body inversion effect can be seen back in the form of an increase of the N170,[1] an important electrophysiological component known to be involved in processing faces (Righart & de Gelder, 2007). Using magneto encephalography, this effect was visible already at 70–100 ms post-stimulus onset (Meeren, Hadjikhani, Ahlfors, Hamalainen, & de Gelder, 2008). For faces, it was observed in well-known face-selective areas: inferior occipital gyrus (including occipital face area) and fusiform gyrus (including fusiform face area), whereas for bodies, in the precuneus and posterior cingulate cortex. Hence, whereas face inversion modulates early activity in face-selective areas in the ventral stream, body inversion evokes activity in dorsal areas, suggesting different early cortical pathways for face and body perception.

[1]The N170 is a negative brain potential peaking at 170 ms after stimulus onset at the lateral occipito-temporal sites (including the fusiform and inferior occipital gyri). The N170 to inverted faces is larger and more delayed than to upright faces, but not inverted objects (Watanabe, Kakigi, & Puce, 2003). A similar effect has been observed for bodies (Stekelenburg & de Gelder, 2004).

### *16.2.2 Emotional Modulation of Face- and Body-Selective Areas*

Several studies have reported emotional modulation of the fusiform face area and the occipital face area (Vuilleumier, Armony, Driver, & Dolan, 2001). The effect of emotional information of bodily expressions on activation of body areas has not been studied often. The first functional magnetic resonance imaging (fMRI) study addressing this issue observed increased activation of the fusiform gyrus and the amygdala for fearful expressions (Hadjikhani & de Gelder, 2003). A follow-up experiment additionally showed the involvement of motor areas (de Gelder, Snyder, Greve, Gerard, & Hadjikhani, 2004). Moreover, when directly comparing emotional and neutral bodies with faces (van de Riet et al., 2009), emotional bodies activate motor-related structures such as the inferior frontal gyrus, caudate nucleus, and putamen.

Although our findings of emotional modulation of the fusiform body area have been replicated (for an overview see de Gelder et al., 2009), emotional modulation of the extra striate body area, specifically involved in processing bodies (Downing, Jiang, Shuman, & Kanwisher, 2001), remains still unclear. We observe emotional modulation of this area by using dynamic (Grèzes, Pichon, & de Gelder, 2007; Kret, Pichon, Grèzes, & de Gelder, in press; Pichon, de Gelder, & Grèzes, 2008) but not static body expressions (van de Riet et al., 2009).

## 16.3 Impaired Emotion Processing in the Clinical Population

Increased vigilance and enhanced autonomic activity are part of an adaptive response to threat. In various pathological conditions, the anxiety response is disproportionate to the stressor, because of either a misinterpretation of threat, or hyper- or hypo-responsiveness at any of a variety of points in the complex network of neural pathways that serve the stress response. Imaging techniques offer unique opportunities to explore the neurofunctional basis of personality differences and psychopathology, and show that perceiving emotions is greatly regulated by top down processes being different from person to person.

### *16.3.1 Autism*

Autism is a neurodevelopmental disorder characterized by impaired social interaction and communication, and restricted and repetitive behavior, the signs begin to appear before the age of three years (American Psychiatric Association, 2000). People with autism have social impairments and lack social intuition.

Autistic individuals look less at faces than controls and when they do so, perceptual processes and exploratory ocular movements focus much on irrelevant features (Senju & Johnson, 2009). Autistic people tend to look away from relevant parts of the face such as the eyes (Spezio, Adolphs, Hurley, & Piven, 2007). Also, in a naturalistic scene, autistic individuals spend less time viewing people in pictures (Riby & Hancock, 2008) or videos of social interactions (Riby & Hancock, 2009).

Having difficulties extracting social cues from others is something all individuals with different disorders of the autism spectrum have in common. Individuals with Asperger syndrome, an autism spectrum disorder where linguistic and cognitive development is relatively preserved, have deficits in the recognition of identity, gender, age, and expressions in faces (Celani, Battacchi, & Arcidiacono, 1999). Hubert et al. (2007) reported that autistic individuals performed much worse than controls in recognizing bodily emotions from point-light displays,[2] even though they performed as well as controls in recognizing simple actions and object manipulations.

One explanation for these deficits is a lack of interest in other people (Jemel, Mottron, & Dawson, 2006). Functional abnormalities have been found in the amygdala and mirror neuron system in response to neutral (Kleinhans et al., 2008) and emotional faces (Dapretto et al., 2006). Moreover, compromised functioning of regions in and around the superior temporal sulcus (STS) (Zilbovicius et al., 2006), as shown by reduced activation in this area in response to body (Freitag et al., 2008) and emotional face movements (Pelphrey, Morris, McCarthy, & Labar, 2007), and functional abnormalities of the fusiform cortex have been reported (Pierce, Muller, Ambrose, Allen, & Courchesne, 2001). Increased activation to fearful versus neutral body images in the fusiform gyrus and amygdala was absent in this group (Hadjikhani et al., 2009). Moreover, atypical functional connectivity was observed, including absence of change in connectivity strength when viewing fearful compared to neutral bodies between amygdala and STS, premotor cortex and inferior frontal gyrus. Autism spectrum disorders are thus characterized by shortcomings in socio-cognitive abilities in general, and emotion recognition in particular (Grèzes, Wicker, Berthoz, & de Gelder, 2009).

### 16.3.2 Schizophrenia

Schizophrenia is characterized by abnormalities in the perception or expression of reality. Distortions in perception most commonly manifest as auditory hallucinations, paranoia, and bizarre delusions, or disorganized speech and thinking with social or occupational dysfunction. Onset typically occurs in young adulthood, with 0.4–0.6% of the population being affected (Bhugra, 2005).

Social cognition has become a high priority area in schizophrenia research (Green & Leitman, 2008). Evidence suggests that schizophrenics may have problems integrating

[2] Biological motion refers to the unique visual phenomenon of a moving, animate object. Often, the stimuli used in biological motion experiments are comprised of just a few moving dots that reflect the motion of some key joints of the moving organism, which is known as a point-light display (see Atkinson, Dittrich, Gemmel, & Young, 2004).

visual features into perceptual wholes using configural information (Shin et al., 2008), such as difficulties in understanding facial expressions, which may influence socio-cognitive abilities (Mueser, Penn, Blanchard, & Bellack, 1997).

Some studies have investigated emotion perception in language; deficits have been reported in the categorization of emotional voices, and correlations between deficits in hearing and seeing emotions were found (de Gelder, Vroomen, Annen, Masthof, Hodiamont, 2003; de Gelder et al., 2005). In the healthy population, a vocal emotional expression influences categorization of a facial expression (de Gelder, Vroomen, & Teunisse, 1995) and vice versa (de Gelder & Vroomen, 2000). In schizophrenics, the multisensory integration of facial and vocal emotional information is impaired (de Jong, Hodiamont, Van der Stock, & de Gelder, 2009). Schizophrenia patients also show deficits in gender discrimination and emotion identification from body shapes and motion (Bigelow et al., 2006). Deficits in affect categorization of socially relevant stimuli go beyond facial features to include basic emotion recognition of human postures, complex social scenes, and body motion.

MRI studies have shown the fusiform gyri to be smaller in schizophrenia patients, where volume reduction is proportional to impairment at remembering face identities (Lee et al., 2002; Onitsuka et al., 2006). Functional imaging studies report that compared to controls, the extent of activation in fusiform gyrus, amygdala, parahippocampal gyrus, right superior frontal gyrus, and lentiform nucleus was significantly smaller in patients during facial emotion processing (for a meta-analysis, see Li, Chan, McAlonan, & Gong, 2009). Schizophrenia is associated with functionally important abnormalities in face processing in the domains of emotion recognition and complex social judgements (for a meta-analysis, see Marwick & Hall, 2008).

### *16.3.3 Neurodegenerative Genetic Movement Disorders*

Healthy people automatically mimic others' emotional expressions – as measured by electromyography (EMG) – with surprising speed and accuracy. When observing happy facial or bodily expressions, muscular activity over the zygomaticus major (cheek) region increases. When observing angry (or fearful) expressions, increased muscular activity over the corrugator supercilli (brow) region is observed (Tamietto & de Gelder, 2009). This emotional contagion has been defined as "the tendency to automatically mimic and synchronize expressions, vocalizations, postures, and movements with those of another and, consequently, to converge emotionally" (Hatfield, Cacioppo, & Rapson, 1993). Adopting the facial expressions of specific emotions (even via unobtrusive manipulations) affects emotional judgments and memories (Schnall & Laird, 2007). Manipulated body postures can affect behavior: slumped postures lead to more "helpless behaviors" (Riskind & Gotay, 1982). More evidence comes from a recent study by Harmon-Jones and Peterson (2009) in which participants heard insulting remarks about an essay they had written. Those who were sitting in a chair exhibited more left frontal cortex activity (which has been correlated with experiencing anger) than did those who were lying flat on their backs. These findings suggest that body postures may affect our emotions and the brain activity associated with them. If patients with a movement disorder cannot *produce* emotional facial expressions (so far, nothing has been reported about bodily expression deficits), it may well be that they also have a deficit in *perceiving* the emotion.[3]

#### 16.3.3.1 Huntington's Disease

Huntington's disease is a rare neurodegenerative genetic disorder that is the most common genetic cause of repetitive abnormal movements called chorea. The prevalence varies from one person per million in populations of Asian and African descent, to 70 per million in Western European populations. The earliest symptoms, appearing around the age of 40 years, are a lack of coordination and unsteady gait. As the disease advances, uncoordinated movements become more apparent, along with a decline in mental abilities and an increase in behavioral and psychiatric problems (Walker, 2007). The disease attacks primarily caudate nucleus and putamen, leading to an impairment in motor-(Vonsattel et al., 1985) and emotional tasks (Kampe, Frith, Dolan, & Frith, 2001).

Deficits in the perception of emotions have been widely reported, especially for disgust (Gray, Young, Barker, Curtis, & Gibson, 1997). Huntington's disease patients are impaired in recognizing instrumental and angry whole body postures and this deficit was correlated with measures of motor deficit (de Gelder, Van den Stock, de Diego Balaguer, & Bachoud-Levi, 2008). Research has clearly indicated that action recognition involves similar brain areas that are involved in performance of that same action by the observer (Rizzolatti & Craighero, 2004). The observed impairment in recognition of instrumental actions evokes the concept of motor resonance at the center of motor cognition abilities, which are implemented in the premotor cortex, parietal cortex, and STS. Degeneration of the motor areas in Huntington's disease, predominantly striatum and its connections to parietal and premotor cortex and STS, is consistent with the importance of action representation for intact recognition of whole body postures.

#### 16.3.3.2 Parkinson's Disease

Parkinson's disease is another degenerative disorder of the central nervous system that is characterized by muscle rigidity, tremor, a slowing of physical movement and, in extreme cases, a loss of physical movement (akinesia). The primary symptoms are

[3] People with autism also show less mimicking but this is not due to physical inabilities. Autistic people have less motor control (clumsiness) but this is not even close to the severe deficit apparent in Huntington's disease and has a different cause.

the result of decreased stimulation of the motor cortex by the basal ganglia, normally caused by a deficient dopamine system. Parkinson's disease is chronic and progressive. While many forms of the disease are "idiopathic," "secondary" cases may result from toxicity most notably caused by drugs, head trauma, or other medical disorders (Jankovic, 2008). Crude prevalence rate estimates range from 65.6/100,000 to 12,500/100,000 (for a meta-analysis, see von Campenhausen et al., 2005).

Parkinson's disease patients have a reduced ability in making spontaneous emotional expressions and have monotonous, flat, and poorly inflected speech. Jacobs, Shuren, Bowers, and Heilman (1995) demonstrated that these patients are impaired in imaging, perceiving, and expressing emotional faces. Dujardin and colleagues (2004) established that early in the course of Parkinson's disease, emotional facial processing is disturbed and untreated patients are significantly impaired in decoding these. It is generally argued that the loss of dopaminergic neurons, resulting in dysfunction of fronto-subcortical systems, not only leads to motor disturbances but also to emotional information processing deficits (Dujardin and colleagues 2004; Lawrence, Goerendt, & Brooks, 2007). Parkinson's disease patients report less arousal compared to controls while perceiving emotional pictures (Wieser et al., 2006). Suzuki, Hoshino, Shigemasu, and Kawamura (2006) showed that these patients were impaired at recognizing the facial expression of disgust. Sprengelmeyer et al. (2003) investigated the effect of dopamine medication and observed impaired recognition of emotional facial expressions. This deficit was more severe in non-medicated than in medicated patients. More specifically, the recognition of anger and fear was disrupted in medicated Parkinson's disease participants, and the recognition of fear, sadness, disgust, and anger was impaired in patients without medication. Dujardin et al. (2004) observed that Parkinson's disease participants without medication were less accurate than healthy participants in perceiving facial expressions of anger, sadness, and disgust. More recently, Lawrence et al. (2007) reported that the recognition of anger was impaired in Parkinson's disease patients who had been temporarily removed from dopamine replacement therapy.

Reduced dopaminergic-binding sites in the orbitofrontal cortex and amygdala (Ouchi et al., 1999), and abnormal clumps of degenerating neurons in the amygdala of Parkinson's disease patients (Mattila, Rinne, Helenius, & Röyttä, 1999) have been reported. In line with this, Tessitore et al. (2002) observed that in these patients, an emotional task was not associated with amygdala activation, but dopaminergic repletion was shown to restore this response. However, several studies failed to demonstrate any difference between patients and controls in facial emotion tasks (Adolphs, Schul, & Tranel, 1998).

The above-described patients cannot fully control their movements, and show impairments in recognizing emotional expressions. This leads us to wonder what would happen to emotion perception in people who are physically restricted to make movements.

Hennenlotter et al. (2009) studied women who had received botox injections for cosmetic reasons, thus rendering them unable to flex the corrugator muscle. For imitating angry expressions, activity in the left amygdala was lower in those who had received botox compared to those who had not. This suggests that pulling an angry expression modulates the amygdala, via the neural command to flex the face muscles and/or via feedback from the positioning of the facial muscles and movement of the skin.

These results suggest a close relationship between motor abilities and activation of the emotion circuit, but further studies are required.

### *16.3.4 Anxiety, Depression, and Personality Differences*

It has been estimated that 9.5% of adults in the USA have a depressive disorder and 18.1% an anxiety disorder. Anxiety disorders frequently co-occur with depression, substance abuse, or other anxiety disorders. Nearly three quarters of these patients will have their first episode by the age of 21.5 years (Kessler, Chiu, Demler, & Walters, 2005).

Elevated levels of trait anxiety are associated with an increased ability to accurately recognize fearful facial expressions (Surcinelli, Codispoti, Montebarocci, Rossi, & Baldaro, 2006). Patients with depression are impaired in recognizing facial expressions in general (Mikhailova, Vladimirova, Iznak, Tsusulkovskaya, & Sushko, 1996).

People differ in how they perceive emotions. For example, individuals with anxiety disorders show increased amygdala activity when confronted with threatening faces (Etkin & Wager, 2007). This pattern is also visible in the healthy population in individuals with high trait anxiety (Etkin et al., 2004). The role of the amygdala in depression is less clear. Whereas some studies report increased amygdala response for threatening versus neutral expressions related to depressive symptoms or negative affect (Canli et al., 2005; Peluso et al., 2009), others report decreased activity (de Gelder et al., 2008; Thomas et al., 2001) or no difference (Lee et al., 2004). Several studies report decreased cortico-limbic connectivity in depression in response to emotional stimuli, although antidepressant treatment can re-establish this connectivity (Anand, Li, Wang, Gardner, & Lowe, 2007). Decreased activation in the anterior cingulate cortex has also been reported in depression (Drevets, Savitz, & Trimble, 2008). Object deep brain stimulation of the subcallosal cingulate gyrus is currently being investigated for the treatment of major depressive disorder (Hamani et al., 2009).

People with Type D ("distressed") personality (21% of the general population) are more likely to experience feelings of depression and anxiety and tend to feel inhibited in social interaction. Consequently, Type D individuals have elevated levels of both negative affectivity and social inhibition. Hence, individuals with a Type D personality have the tendency to experience negative emotions across time and situations but inhibit the expression of emotions and behavior because of fear of rejection or disapproval which has proved to be unhealthy in the long term. (Denollet, 2005) de Gelder et al. (2008) observed a correlation between the negative affectivity subscale and amygdala de-activation for fear static facial and bodily expressions. Kret et al. (submitted) observed more differences by using dynamic stimuli. They confirmed a decreased activation pattern in brain areas important for emotion perception including the amygdala and insula in relation to negative affectivity and threat perception. Second, they showed that social inhibition may be marked by a sensitivity to over-mentalize and empathize when perceiving threat. Negative affectivity and social inhibition are differentially related to emotion-specific brain activation that may be relevant to both physical and mental health. The network of brain regions involved in emotion regulation may be relevant to the relationship between medical and psychological disorders. Therefore, their assessment should be considered in neuroimaging studies on emotion regulation and stress reactivity (Kret, Denollet, Grèzes & de Gelder, submitted).

## 16.4 Affective Gist of the Scene Influences Emotion Perception

### *16.4.1 Emotional Context*

Research on scene effects has a long tradition in object recognition. Repetitive co-occurrence of a given object in a scene makes our brain generate expectations (Biederman, Rabinowitz, Glass, & Stacy, 1974; Palmer & Rosenquist, 1975). A scene can facilitate object detection and recognition (Biederman, Mezzanotte, & Rabinowitz, 1982; Boyce & Pollatsek, 1992; Boyce, Pollatsek, & Rayner, 1989; Palmer & Rosenquist, 1975). Scenes can be processed and scene gist recognized rapidly (Bar et al., 2006).

Like recognizing objects is dependent on contextual cues, emotion perception does not proceed on information from one cue alone. Knowledge of the social situation, scenes (Aviezer et al., 2008), body postures (Meeren, van Heijnsbergen, & de Gelder, 2005), other emotional faces (Russel & Fehr, 1987), voices (de Gelder & Vroomen, 2000), or linguistic labels (Barrett, Lindquist, & Gendron, 2007) influences emotion perception and which emotion is seen in the structural configuration of the participant's facial muscles. Righart and de Gelder (2006, 2008) report that the presence of a fearful expression in a fearful context enhances the N170 amplitude. The effect was absent for the contexts-only condition, indicating that the increased amplitude resulted from the *combination* of a fearful face in a fearful context (Righart & de Gelder, 2006, 2008). That scenes are indeed important is also shown in fMRI studies where participants interpreted facial expressions differently and different brain areas were activated depending on the context (Kim et al., 2004; Mobbs et al., 2006).

As mentioned before, individuals differ in how many and which cues they use in emotion perception. A recent study examined context effects in Huntington patients while categorizing emotional faces (Aviezer et al., 2009). Disgust faces were embedded on images of people conveying sadness and anger as expressed by body language and additional paraphernalia. Additionally, sad and angry faces were embedded on context images conveying disgust. Despite the deficient explicit recognition of isolated disgust and anger faces, the perception of the emotions expressed by the faces was affected by context in Huntington patients in a similar manner as in controls. These findings suggest that despite their impaired explicit recognition of facial expressions, Huntington patients display relatively preserved processing of the same facial configurations when embedded in a context. The scenes used in this study were just simple objects. When dynamic complex naturalistic scenes including other people are used, other processes play a role. This will be discussed in the next paragraph.

### *16.4.2 Social Emotional Context and Observing Interactions*

Is our emotional reaction influenced when we watch a single individual fleeing from danger while bystanders are just passively staying where they are? Do we ignore the social scene to focus only on the emotion of the target figure or are we unwittingly influenced by the social scene, viewing individual action through the filter it provides us? Studies on crowd behavior (McDougall, 1920; Schachter & Singer, 1962) indicate that social scenes provide a context in which individual actions are better understood, prompting an adaptive reaction in the observer. Using point-light displays, Thornton and Vuong (2004) have shown that the perceived action of a walker depends upon actions of nearby "to-be-ignored" walkers. Another point-light study by Clarke, Bradshaw, Field, Hampson, and Rose (2005) demonstrated that the recognition of a person's *emotional* state depends upon another person's presence. A recent study by Kret and de Gelder (2010) reports that the social group in which we encounter a person influences how we perceive his body language. Images of emotional body postures were briefly presented as part of social scenes showing neutral or emotional group actions. These were better recognized when the actions in the scenes expressed an emotion congruent with the bodily expression of the target figure. These studies show the importance of a social (emotional) scene. Similar brain areas are involved when subjects experience disgust (Wicker et al., 2003) or pain (Jackson, Meltzoff, & Decety, 2005) as when they observe someone else experiencing these emotions. Such a process may contribute to observers' ability to perceive rapidly ambiguity between a person's body language and its social context. This incongruity may create a conflict in emotional contagion processes triggered by the target figure and help to explain the slower and less accurate reaction in the observer.

In most studies, observers see a face or body that is faced toward him- or herself. This way, an emotional expression has most impact on the observer since it asks for an immediate reaction. But what happens when a threat is not directed toward you? This question has been studied by Sinke, Sorger, Goebel, and de Gelder (2010). Video clips were used in which a male grabbed the handbag of a female which was done in either an aggressive or a teasing way, as if the two knew each other. The actors faced each other and did not attend to the observer. When you walk on the street, you may have your thoughts on an upcoming deadline instead of on the persons on the other side of the street. Will you then still be able to recognize a threat? To investigate this second question, three small dots, presented for 40 ms, were added to each movie. Participants in the first task categorized the situation (threatening or teasing). In the second task, they categorized the color of the dots. Results showed that the right amygdala was activated more during the threatening interactions independent of the task. This is in line with previous studies that the amygdala acts as a warning signal to react. Furthermore, during unattended threat, the amygdala seemed to pass this threat information through to body sensitive visual regions in fusiform gyrus, middle occipitotemporal gyrus, and STS. Furthermore, this heightened activation for unattended threat was paired with better behavioral performance on the dot task during threatening interactions, which shows more clearly that the amygdala response has a direct influence on people's actions. In conclusion, bodily expressions are easily recognized even though your attention is not explicitly on the situation and the threat is not directed toward you, which has high survival value, at least in the normal population.

### *16.4.3 Perceiving Social Contexts and Observing Interactions in Patients*

But how are social interactions recognized in patient groups such as those with autism and Williams syndrome? Autism is characterized by social withdrawal and lack of interest in socially relevant information, while Williams syndrome is a rare genetic disorder where patients show propulsion toward social stimuli and interactions. As far as we know, only behavioral studies have been performed using stimuli showing social interactions with these patients. One study tracked eye gaze of both children with autism and those with Williams syndrome looking at pictures of socially relevant scenes (Riby & Hancock, 2008). As found before, children in the former group spent less time looking at faces than normally developed children. On the contrary, children with Williams syndrome spent more time than controls looking at faces. These different visual preferences for important social information could mean that both groups interpret the social cues differently. Also, when using video clips instead of pictures, these same atypicalities in gaze remain (Riby & Hancock, 2009).

Pictures of emotional social scenes were used in a study comparing individuals with autism or schizophrenia with healthy controls (Sasson et al., 2007). Subjects categorized emotion depicted in the scene. Just as persons with autism, schizophrenics do not look as much as controls at faces. For the former group, it does not even make a difference whether those faces are blurred or not, while people with schizophrenia, like healthy controls, do orient faster to face regions when the faces contain information. They only show a delay in this orienting (Sasson et al., 2007). No differences in the emotion judgment task were found between groups or between emotions. We have preliminary data showing that on the one extreme, socially anxious individuals and on the other extreme, violent offenders are influenced by the social scene in a normal fashion. However, when the scene showed a fight, they got distracted by it more than the matched controls (Kret et al., in prep a/b).

The perception of interactions or complex social, emotional scenes is a yet unexplored field in psychological neuroscience. As far as we know, researches that have been done in this field are behavioral studies that focused on autism, Williams syndrome, and schizophrenia. It would be interesting to investigate this topic in more disorders and to investigate to what extent people with, for example, social phobia will be helped by additional social information in perceiving others' emotions.

### *16.4.4 Gender*

The presence of a clear context and other people helps us recognize others' emotions and this may work in the same manner or differently in healthy people and in patients. However, this is not the whole story; gender–emotion stereotypes have potential consequences for the way people evaluate male and female expressions.

A growing body of research consistently demonstrates that stereotypes about emotions are gender specific (Fischer, Rodriguez Mosquera, van Vianen, & Manstead, 2004). In particular, happiness, sadness, and fear are believed to be feminine, whereas anger would be masculine (Birnbaum, Nosanchuk, & Croll, 1980).

Earlier studies confirm the involvement of amygdala and fusiform gyrus in face and body perception (van de Riet et al., 2009; Meeren et al, 2008). A recent study by Kret, Pichon, Grèzes and de Gelder (submitted) revealed how this activity is modulated by gender. Participant's hemodynamic brain activity was recorded while observing videos showing facial or body expressions of fear, anger, or neutral signals by female and male actors. As indicated by recognition data obtained afterwards, male and female participants recognized all expressions equally well. Overall, a higher BOLD response in pre-supplementary motor area, extrastriate body area and superior temporal sulcus was found when participants observed male versus female actors expressing threat. But interestingly, in these regions, as well as in the fusiform face/body area, we observed an interaction between category, emotion and observer; more activation for male threatening versus neutral body stimuli in the male participants was observed. Threatening bodies and not faces triggered highest activity in the superior temporal sulcus, specifically in male observers. The amygdala was more active for facial than bodily expressions, independent of emotion, yet specifically for male observers watching female faces. This is consistent with findings that amygdala activity in male observers was increased for viewing female faces with relatively large pupils indicating an index of interest (Demos et al., 2008). Possibly, female faces provide more information to relevant males than male faces, whereas the distinction at the level of the face between male and female faces is less important for female observers. Other studies have reported that AMG is face but not emotion specific (van der Gaag et al., 2007). But the striking fact here is that the other areas that reflect sensitivity of the male observers are all emotion sensitive. This disjunction between amygdala face-gender and superior temporal sulcus, extrastriate body area, pre-supplementary motor area gender-emotion sensitivity indicates that the amygdala indeed plays a different role than being at the service of emotion encoding and fits with the notion that it encodes salience and modulates recognition and social judgment, hence the face-gender effect.

Common belief is that men express emotion because the situation warrants it, whereas females express emotions because they are just being emotional (Barrett & Bliss-Moreau, 2009). Our results believe this intuition. So, if we see an emotional male, something "real" must be going on and the observer has to decide whether to flight or fight, explaining the enhanced responses to male threatening body expressions in superior temporal sulcus, extrastriate body area and pre-supplementary motor area. While our results are similar to previous reports that show male observers to be more reactive to threatening signals than females (Aleman & Swart, 2008; Fine et al., 2009), previous studies used faces and did not take the gender of the actor into account. Whereas superior temporal sulcus and extrastriate body area showed a main effect of emotion, pre-supplementary motor area specifically showed increased activation for threatening versus neutral male actors as observed in male participants. It is well known that activity in the pre-supplementary motor area increases with action preparation to generate an escape response (Kwan et al., 2000) and it has been found responsive to threatening body expressions before (Grèzes et al., 2007). This is the first study that shows that males show a strong preparation to move or act as measured by the pre-supplementary motor area response when they are confronted with another males threatening body expression.

Not much research has been done on gender differences in emotion perception in patients. In a study to investigate differences in facial mimicry, males and females who scored extreme on the autism-spectrum quotient questionnaire were tested (Hermans, van Wingen, Bos, Putman, & van Honk, 2009). Autistic traits are continuously distributed across the population (Constantino & Todd, 2003) and the authors suspected that people who score high on these traits will show less mimicry. Electromyographic activity from the corrugator supercilii and zygomaticus major muscles was measured while participants watched pictures of angry and happy faces. Only the female high scorers showed reduced automatic mimicry to angry facial expressions, but the effect was caused by the high mimicry of female low scorers. Therefore, the authors reason that the male group had already reached a ceiling effect.

Vaskinn et al. (2007) examined gender effects when comparing emotion perception in participants with schizophrenia and bipolar disorder with that in healthy controls. In general, women from the schizophrenia and healthy group performed the emotion perception tasks better than men. No gender differences were found in the bipolar disorder group. There was no deficit in emotion processing in patients with bipolar disorder, while schizophrenics showed undamaged visual but impaired auditory perception.

It has recently been observed that men compared to women with Parkinson's disease and healthy control men display specific impairments in the recognition of fearful expressions (Clark, Neargarder, & Cronin-Golomb, 2008). A relationship between gender differences and anxiety traits has been found on prefrontal hemodynamic response to fearful facial stimuli (Marumo, Takizawa, Kawakubo,

Onitsuka, & Kasai, 2009). Specifically, greater right ventrolateral and premotor activation was found in females than males. Anxiety traits correlated with frontopolar activation in both groups.

Thus, gender differences also seem to exist in emotion perception in clinical groups, but this field is yet underexplored and needs more attention in the future. Further research should also take into account the gender of the actor, especially in clinical populations.

## 16.5 Conclusion

In this chapter, we gave a selective overview of emotional processing of facial and bodily expressions in relation to psychological and neurological disorders.

In healthy people, there are important similarities and differences in the neurofunctional basis of faces and bodies. Both are strong cues that grab our attention. But they can also be processed without attention, which shows their evolutionary significance. The scene in which we perceive emotions can facilitate our recognition and the presence of other people expressing the same emotion naturally helps us perceive another's emotion correctly.

The perception of emotions is not a pure bottom-up process. Several top-down processes, such as knowledge of the social situation and personality type, play a role. Emotion perception is disrupted in many different disorders. But already in healthy people, differences in emotion perception exist as a result of differences in person characteristics.

Different disorders such as autism, schizophrenia, and Parkinson's or Huntington's disease have taught us a lot about the close link between emotion and motor circuits in the brain. Since bodily expressions imply an action tendency in the expresser, as well as a reaction to this in the observer, they involve more brain areas than facial expressions. Still, not much research has been done on the recognition of bodily expressions in these disorders, which is definitely an issue for future research.

## References

Adolphs, R., Schul, R., & Tranel, D. (1998). Intact recognition of facial emotion in Parkinson's disease. *Neuropsychology*, *12*, 253–258.

Aleman, A. & Swart, M. (2008). Sex differences in neural activation to facial expressions denoting contempt and disgust. PLoS One 3, e3622.

American Psychiatric Association. (2000). Diagnostic criteria for 299.00 autistic disorder. *Diagnostic and statistical manual of mental disorders* (4th, text revision (DSM-IV-TR)). Stad: Uitgever.

Anand, A., Li, Y., Wang, Y., Gardner, K., & Lowe, M. J. (2007). Reciprocal effects of antidepressant treatment on activity and connectivity of the mood regulating circuit: an FMRI study. *Journal of Neuropsychiatry and Clinical Neurosciences*, *19*, 274–282.

Atkinson, A. P., Dittrich, W. H., Gemmel, A. J., & Young, A. W. (2004). Emotion perception from dynamic and static body expressions in point-light and full-light displays. *Perception*, 33, 717–746.

Aviezer, H., Bentin, S., Hassin, R. R., Meschino, W. S., Kennedy, J., Grewal, S., Moscovitch, M. (2009). Not on the face alone: perception of contextualized face expressions in Huntington's disease. *Brain*, *132*, 1633–1644.

Aviezer, H., Hassin, R., Ryan, J., Grady, G., Susskind, J., Anderson, A., Bentin, S. (2008). Angry, disgusted or afraid? Studies on the malleability of emotion perception. *Psychological Science*, *19*, 724–732.

Bar, M., Kassam, K. S., Ghuman, A. S., Boshyan, J., Schmid, A. M., Dale, A. M., Halgren, E. (2006). Top-down facilitation of visual recognition. *Proceedings of the National Academy of Sciences*, *103*, 449–454.

Barrett, L. F., & Bliss-Moreau, E. (2009). She's emotional. He's having a bad day: attributional explanations for emotion stereotypes. *Emotion*, *9*, 649–658.

Barrett, L. F., Lindquist, K. A., & Gendron, M. (2007). Language as context in the perception of emotion. *Trends in Cognitive Sciences*, *11*, 327–332.

Bhugra, D. (2005). The global prevalence of schizophrenia. *PLoS Medicine*, *2*, e151; quiz e175.

Biederman, I., Mezzanotte, R. J., & Rabinowitz, J. C. (1982). Scene perception: detecting and judging objects undergoing relational violations. *Cognitive Psychology*, *14*, 143–177.

Biederman, I., Rabinowitz, J. C., Glass, A. L., & Stacy, E. W. (1974). On the information extracted from a glance at a scene. *Journal of Experimental Psychology*, *103*, 597–600.

Bigelow, N. O., Paradiso, S., Adolphs, R., Moser, D. J., Arndt, S., & Heberlein, A. (2006). Perception of socially relevant stimuli in schizophrenia. *Schizophrenia Research*, *83*, 257–267.

Birnbaum, D., Nosanchuk, T., & Croll, W. (1980). Children's stereotypes about sex differences in emotionality. *Sex Roles*, *6*, 435–443.

Boyce, S. J., & Pollatsek, A. (1992). Identification of objects in scenes: The role of scene background in object naming. *Journal of Experimental Psychology: Human Memory and Cognition*, *18*, 531–543.

Boyce, S. J., Pollatsek, A., & Rayner, K. (1989). Effect of background information on object identification. *Journal of Experimental Psychology: Human Perception and Performance*, *15*, 556–566.

Canli, T., Cooney, R. E., Goldin, P., Shah, M., Sivers, H., Thomason, M. E., Gotlib, I. H. (2005). Amygdala reactivity to emotional faces predicts improvement in major depression. *Neuroreport*, *16*, 1267–70.

Celani, G., Battacchi, M. W., & Arcidiacono, L. (1999). The understanding of the emotional meaning of facial expressions in people with autism. *Journal of Autism and Developmental Disorders*, *29*, 57–66.

Clark, U. S., Neargarder, S., & Cronin-Golomb, A. (2008). Specific impairments in the recognition of emotional facial expressions in Parkinson's disease. *Neuropsychologia*, *46*, 2300–2309.

Clarke, T. J., Bradshaw, M. F., Field, D. T., Hampson, S. E., & Rose, D. (2005). The perception of emotion from body movement in point-light displays of interpersonal dialogue. *Perception*, *34*, 1171–1180.

Constantino, J. N., & Todd, R. D. (2003). Autistic traits in the general population: a twin study. *Archives of General Psychiatry*, *60*, 524–530.

Dapretto, M., Davies, M. S., Pfeifer, J. H., Scott, A. A., Sigman, M., Bookheimer, S. Y., Iacoboni, M. (2006). Understanding emotions in others: mirror neuron dysfunction in children with autism spectrum disorders. *Nature Neuroscience*, *9*, 28–30.

de Gelder, B., Snyder, J., Greve, D., Gerard, G., & Hadjikhani, N. (2004). Fear fosters flight: A mechanism for fear contagion when perceiving emotion expressed by a whole body. *Proceedings of the National Academy of Sciences*, *101*, 16701–16706.

de Gelder, B., Van den Stock, J., de Diego Balaguer, R., & Bachoud-Levi, A. C. (2008). Huntington's disease impairs recognition of angry and instrumental body language. *Neuropsychologia*, *46*, 369–373.

de Gelder, B., Van den Stock, J., Meeren, H. K. M., Sinke, C. B. A., Kret, M. E., & Tamietto, M. (2009). Standing up for the body. Recent progress in uncovering the networks involved in processing bodies and bodily expressions. *Biobehavioral Review, 33*, 3475–3484.

de Gelder, B., & Vroomen, J. (2000). Bimodal emotion perception: Integration across separate modalities, cross-modal perceptual grouping or perception of multimodal events? *Cognition and Emotion, 14*, 321–324.

de Gelder, B., Vroomen, J., Annen, L., Masthof, E., & Hodiamont, P. (2003). Audio-visual integration in schizophrenia. *Schizophrenia Research, 59*, 211–218.

de Gelder, B., Vroomen, J., de Jong, S. J., Masthoff, E. D., Trompenaars, F. J., & Hodiamont, P. (2005). Multisensory integration of emotional faces and voices in schizophrenics. *Schizophrenia Research, 72*, 195–203.

de Gelder, B., Vroomen, J., & Teunisse, J. P. (1995). Hearing smiles and seeing cries. The bimodal perception of emotion. *Bulletin of the Psychonomic Society, 29*, 309.

de Jong, J. J., Hodiamont, P. P., Van den Stock, J., & de Gelder, B. (2009). Audiovisual emotion recognition in schizophrenia: reduced integration of facial and vocal affect. *Schizophrenia Research, 107*, 286–293.

Demos, K. E., Kelley, W. M., Ryan, S. L., Davis, F. C., & Whalen, P. J. (2008). Human amygdala sensitivity to the pupil size of others. *Cerebal Cortex, 18*, 2729–2734.

Denollet, J. K. L. (2005). DS14: Standard assessment of negative affectivity, social inhibition, and Type D personality. *Psychosomatic Medicine, 67*, 89–97.

Downing, P. E., Jiang, Y., Shuman, M., & Kanwisher, N. (2001). A cortical area selective for visual processing of the human body. *Science, 293*, 2470–2473.

Drevets, W. C., Savitz, J., & Trimble, M. (2008). The subgenual anterior cingulate cortex in mood disorders. *CNS Spectrums, 13*, 663–681.

Dujardin, K., Blairy, S., Defebvre, L., Duhem, S., Noel, Y., Hess, U., et al. (2004). Deficits in decoding emotional facial expressions in Parkinson's disease. *Neuropsychologia, 42*, 239–250.

Etkin, A., Klemenhagen, K. C., Dudman, J. T., Rogan, M. T., Hen, R., Kandel, E. R., Hirsch, J. (2004). Individual differences in trait anxiety predict the response of the basolateral amygdala to unconsciously processed fearful faces. *Neuron, 44*, 1043–55.

Etkin, A., & Wager, T. D. (2007). Functional neuroimaging of anxiety: A meta-analysis of emotional processing in PTSD, social anxiety disorder, and specific phobia. *The American Journal of Psychiatry, 164*, 1476–1488.

Fine, J.G., Semrud-Clikeman, M., & Zhu, D.C. (2009). *Behavioral Brain Research, 201*, 137–146.

Fischer, A. H., Rodriguez Mosquera, P. M., van Vianen, A. E., & Manstead, A. S. (2004). Gender and culture differences in emotion. *Emotion, 4*, 87–94.

Freitag, C. M., Konrad, C., Haberlen, M., Kleser, C., von Gontard, A., Reith, W., & Krick, C. (2008). Perception of biological motion in autism spectrum disorders. *Neuropsychologia, 46*, 1480–1494.

Gray, J. M., Young, A. W., Barker, W. A., Curtis, A., & Gibson, D. (1997). Impaired recognition of disgust in Huntington's disease gene carriers. *Brain, 120*, 2029–2038.

Green, M. F., & Leitman, D. I. (2008). Social cognition in schizophrenia. *Schizophrenia Bulletin, 34*, 670–672.

Grèzes, J., Pichon, S., & de Gelder, B. (2007). Perceiving fear in dynamic body expressions. *NeuroImage, 35*, 959–967.

Grèzes, J., Wicker, B., Berthoz, S., & de Gelder, B. (2009). A failure to grasp the affective meaning of actions in autism spectrum disorder subjects. *Neuropsychologia, 47*, 1816–1825.

Hadjikhani, N., & de Gelder, B. (2003). Seeing fearful body expressions activates the fusiform cortex and amygdala. *Current Biology, 13*, 2201–2205.

Hadjikhani, N., Joseph, R. M., Manoach, D. S., Naik, P., Snyder, N., Dominick, K., & de Gelder, B. (2009). Body expressions of emotion do not trigger fear contagion in autism spectrum disorder. *Social, Cognitive and Affective Neuroscience, 4*, 70–78.

Hamani, C., Mayberg, H., Snyder, B., Giacobbe, P., Kennedy, S., & Lozano, A. M. (2009). Deep brain stimulation of the subcallosal cingulate gyrus for depression: anatomical location of active contacts in clinical responders and a suggested guideline for targeting. *Journal of Neurosurgery*, *111*, 1209–1215.

Harmon-Jones, E., & Peterson, C. K. (2009). Supine body position reduces neural response to anger evocation. *Psychological Science*, *20*, 1209–1210.

Hatfield, E., Cacioppo, J. T., & Rapson, R. L. (1993). Emotional contagion. *Current Directions in Psychological Science*, *2*, 96–99.

Hennenlotter, A., Dresel, C., Castrop, F., Baumann, A. O., Wohlschlager, A. M., & Haslinger, B. (2009). The link between facial feedback and neural activity within central circuitries of emotion – new insights from botulinum toxin-induced denervation of frown muscles. *Cerebral Cortex*, *19*, 537–542.

Hermans, E. J., van Wingen, G., Bos, P. A., Putman, P., & van Honk, J. (2009). Reduced spontaneous facial mimicry in women with autistic traits. *Biological Psychology*, *80*, 348–353.

Hubert, B., Wicker, B., Moore, D. G., Monfardini, E., Duverger, H., Da Fonseca, D., & Deruelle, C. (2007). Brief report: recognition of emotional and non-emotional biological motion in individuals with autistic spectrum disorders. *Journal of Autism and Developmental Disorders*, *37*, 1386–1392.

Jackson, P. L., Meltzoff, A. N., & Decety, J. (2005). How do we perceive the pain of others? A window into the neural processes involved in empathy. *NeuroImage*, *24*, 771–779.

Jacobs, D. H., Shuren, J., Bowers, D., & Heilman, K. M. (1995). Emotional facial imagery, perception, and expression in Parkinson's disease. *Neurology*, *45*, 1696–1702.

Jankovic, J. (2008). Parkinson's disease: Clinical features and diagnosis. *Journal of Neurology, Neurosurgery & Psychiatry*, *79*, 368–376.

Jemel, B., Mottron, L., & Dawson, M. (2006). Impaired face processing in autism: fact or artifact? *Journal of Autism and Developmental Disorders*, *36*, 91–106.

Kampe, K. K., Frith, C. D., Dolan, R. J., & Frith, U. (2001). Reward value of attractiveness and gaze. *Nature*, *413*, 589.

Kessler, R. C., Chiu, W. T., Demler, O., & Walters, E. E. (2005). Prevalence, severity, and comorbidity of twelve-month DSM-IV disorders in the National Comorbidity Survey Replication (NCS-R). *Archives of General Psychiatry*, *62*, 617–627.

Kim, H., Somerville, L. H., Johnstone, T., Polis, S., Alexander, A. L., Shin, L. M., & Whalen, J. (2004). Contextual modulation of amygdala responsivity to surprised faces. *Journal of Cognitive Neuroscience*, *16*, 1730–1745.

Kleinhans, N. M., Richards, T., Sterling, L., Stegbauer, K. C., Mahurin, R., Johnson, L. C., & Aylward, E. (2008). Abnormal functional connectivity in autism spectrum disorders during face processing. *Brain*, *131*, 1000–1012.

Kret, M. E., & de Gelder, B. (2010). Social context influences recognition of bodily expressions. *Experimental Brain Research*, *203*, 169–80.

Kret, M. E., Pichon, S., Grèzes, J., & de Gelder, B. (in press). Similarities and differences in perceiving threat from dynamic faces and bodies. An fMRI study. NeuroImage.

Kret, M. E., Stekelenburg, J., Roelofs, K., & de Gelder, B. The role of social anxiety in perceiving emotions (in prepration).

Kret, M. E., Denollet, J., Grezes, J., de Gelder, B. (under review). The role of negative affectivity and social inhibition in perceiving social threat: an fMRI study.

Kret M. E., Pichon S., Grèzes J., de Gelder B. (submitted). Men fear other men most: Gender specific brain activations in perceiving threat from dynamic faces and bodies. An fMRI study.

Kret, M. E., & de Gelder, B. (submitted). The perception of facial and bodily expressions of emotion in violent offenders.

Lawrence, A. D., Goerendt, I. K., & Brooks, D. J. (2007). Impaired recognition of facial expressions of anger in Parkinson's disease patients acutely withdrawn from dopamine replacement therapy. *Neuropsychologia*, *45*, 65–74.

Lee, C. U., Shenton, M. E., Salisbury, D. F., Kasai, K., Onitsuka, T., Dickey, C. C., McCarley, R. W. (2002). Fusiform gyrus volume reduction in first-episode schizophrenia: a magnetic resonance imaging study. *Archives of General Psychiatry, 59*, 775–781.

Lee, B. T., Seok, J. H., Lee, B. C., Cho, S. W., Yoon, B. J., Lee, K. U., Chae, J. H., Choi, I. G., Ham, B. J., Neural correlates of affective processing in response to sad and angry facial stimuli in patients with major depressive disorder. *Prog Neuropsychopharmacol Biol Psychiatry 32*, 778–85.

Li, H., Chan, R. C., McAlonan, G. M., & Gong, Q. Y. (2009). Facial emotion processing in schizophrenia: a meta-analysis of functional neuroimaging data. *Schizophrenia Bulletin*.

Marumo, K., Takizawa, R., Kawakubo, Y., Onitsuka, T., & Kasai, K. (2009). Gender difference in right lateral prefrontal hemodynamic response while viewing fearful faces: A multi-channel near-infrared spectroscopy study. *Neuroscience Research, 63*, 89–94.

Marwick, K., & Hall, J. (2008). Social cognition in schizophrenia: A review of face processing. *British Medical Bulletin, 88*, 43–58.

Mattila, P. M., Rinne, J. O., Helenius, H., & Röyttä, M. (1999). Neuritic degeneration in the hippocampus and amygdala in Parkinson's disease relation to Alzheimer pathology. *Acta Neuropathologica, 98*, 157–164.

McDougall, W. (1920). *The group mind*. New York: G.P. Putnam's Sons.

Meeren, H. K., Hadjikhani, N., Ahlfors, S. P., Hamalainen, M. S., & de Gelder, B. (2008). Early category-specific cortical activation revealed by visual stimulus inversion. *PLoS One, 3*, e3503.

Meeren, H. K., van Heijnsbergen, C. C., & de Gelder, B. (2005). Rapid perceptual integration of facial expression and emotional body language. *Proceedings of the National Academy of Sciences of the United States of America, 102*, 16518–16523.

Mikhailova, E. S., Vladimirova, T. V., Iznak, A. F., Tsusulkovskaya, E. J., & Sushko, N. V. (1996). Abnormal recognition of facial expression of emotions in depressed patients with major depression disorder and schizotypal personality disorder. *Biological Psychiatry, 40*, 697–705.

Mobbs, D., Weiskopf, N., Lau, H. C., Featherstone, E., Dolan, R. J., & Frith, C. D. (2006). The Kuleshov effect: The influence of contextual framing on emotional attributions. *Social Cognitive and Affective Neuroscience, 1*, 95–106.

Mueser, K. T., Penn, D. L., Blanchard, J. J., & Bellack, A. S. (1997). Affect recognition in schizophrenia: a synthesis of findings across three studies. *Psychiatry, 60*, 301–308.

Onitsuka, T., Niznikiewicz, M. A., Spencer, K. M., Frumin, M., Kuroki, N., Lucia, L. C., Shenton, M. E., & McCarley, R. W. (2006). Functional and structural deficits in brain regions subserving face perception in schizophrenia. *The American Journal of Psychiatry, 163*, 455–462.

Ouchi, Y., Yoshikawa, E., Okada, H., Futatsubashi, M., Sekine, Y., Iyo, M., & Sakomoto, N. (1999). Alterations in binding site density of dopamine transporter in the striatum, orbitofrontal cortex, and amygdala in early Parkinson's disease: compartment analysis for beta-CFT binding with positron emission tomography. *Annals of Neurology, 45*, 601–610.

Palmer, L. A., & Rosenquist, A. C. (1975). Single-unit studies in the cat. *Neurosciences Research Program Bulletin, 13*, 214–220.

Peelen M. V., Atkinson, A. P., Andersson, F., & Vuilleumier, P. (2007). Emotional modulation of body-selective visual areas. *Social Cognitive and Affective Neuroscience*, 2, 274–83.

Pelphrey, K. A., Morris, J. P., McCarthy, G., & Labar, K. S. (2007). Perception of dynamic changes in facial affect and identity in autism. *Social Cognitive and Affective Neuroscience, 2*, 140–149.

Peluso, M. A., Glahn, D. C., Matsuo, K., Monkul, E. S., Najt, P., Zamarripa, F., Li, J., Lancaster, J. K., Fox, P. T., Gao, J. H., & Soares, J. C. (2009). Amygdala hyperactivation in untreated depressed individuals. *Psychiatry Research, 173*, 158–161.

Pichon, S., de Gelder, B., & Grèzes, J. (2008). Emotional modulation of visual and motor areas by still and dynamic body expressions of anger. *Social Neuroscience, 3*, 199–212.

Pierce, K., Muller, R. A., Ambrose, J., Allen, G., & Courchesne, E. (2001). Face processing occurs outside the fusiform "face area" in autism: evidence from functional MRI. *Brain, 124*, 2059–2073.

Reed, C. L., Stone, V. E., Bozova, S., & Tanaka, J. (2003). The body-inversion effect. *Psychological Science, 14*, 302–308.

Riby, D., & Hancock, P. J. (2009). Looking at movies and cartoons: Eye-tracking evidence from Williams syndrome and autism. *Journal of Intellectual Disabilities*, *53*, 169–181.

Riby, D. M., & Hancock, P. J. (2008). Viewing it differently: Social scene perception in Williams syndrome and autism. *Neuropsychologia*, *46*, 2855–2860.

Righart, R., & de Gelder, B. (2006). Context influences early perceptual analysis of faces – An electrophysiological study. *Cerebral Cortex*, *16*, 1249–1257.

Righart, R., & de Gelder, B. (2007). Impaired face and body perception in developmental prosopagnosia. *Proceedings of the National Academy of Sciences*, *104*, 17234–17238.

Righart, R., & de Gelder, B. (2008). Rapid influence of emotional scenes on encoding of facial expressions: An ERP study. *Social Cognitive and Affective Neuroscience*, *3*, 270–278.

Riskind, J. H., & Gotay, C. C. (1982). Physical posture: Could it have regulatory or feedback effects on motivation and emotion? *Motivation and Emotion*, *6*, 273–298.

Rizzolatti, G., & Craighero, L. (2004). The mirror-neuron system. *Annual Review of Neuroscience*, *27*, 169–192.

Russel, J. A., & Fehr, B. (1987). Relativity in the perception of emotion in facial expressions. *Journal of Experimental Psychology*, *116*, 233–237.

Sasson, N., Tsuchiya, N., Hurley, R., Couture, S. M., Penn, D. L., Adolphs, R., & Piven, J. (2007). Orienting to social stimuli differentiates social cognitive impairment in autism and schizophrenia. *Neuropsychologia*, *45*, 2580–2588.

Schachter, S., & Singer, J. E. (1962). Cognitive, social, and physiological determinants of emotional state. *Psychological Review*, *69*, 379–399.

Schnall, S., & Laird, J. D. (2007). Facing fear: Expression of fear facilitates processing of emotional information. *Social Behavior and Personality*, *35*, 513–524.

Senju, A., & Johnson, M. H. (2009). Atypical eye contact in autism: Models, mechanisms and development. *Neuroscience and Biobehavioral Reviews*, *33*, 1204–1214.

Shin, Y. W., Na, M. H., Ha, T. H., Kang, D. H., Yoo, S. Y., & Kwon, J. S. (2008). Dysfunction in configural face processing in patients with schizophrenia. *Schizophrenia Bulletin*, *34*, 538–543.

Sinke, C. B. A., Sorger, B., Goebel, R., & de Gelder, B. (2010). Tease or threat? Judging social interactions from bodily expressions. *NeuroImage*, *49*, 1717–1727.

Spezio, M. L., Adolphs, R., Hurley, R. S., & Piven, J. (2007). Analysis of face gaze in autism using "Bubbles." *Neuropsychologia*, *45*, 144–151.

Sprengelmeyer, R., Young, A. W., Mahn, K., Schroeder, U., Woitalla, D., Buttner, T., & Przuntek, H. (2003). Facial expression recognition in people with medicated and unmedicated Parkinson's disease. *Neuropsychologia*, *41*, 1047–1057.

Stekelenburg, J. J., & de Gelder, B. (2004). The neural correlates of perceiving human bodies: an ERP study on the body-inversion effect. *Neuroreport*, *15*, 777–780.

Surcinelli, P., Codispoti, M., Montebarocci, O., Rossi, N., & Baldaro, B. (2006). Facial emotion recognition in trait anxiety. *Journal of Anxiety Disorders*, *20*, 110–117.

Suzuki, A., Hoshino, T., Shigemasu, K., & Kawamura, M. (2006). Disgust-specific impairment of facial expression recognition in Parkinson's disease. *Brain*, *129*(Pt 3), 707–717.

Tamietto, M., & de Gelder, B. (2009). Emotional contagion for unseen bodily expressions: Evidence from facial EMG. *Proceedings of the FG 2008 meeting*, Amsterdam.

Tessitore, A., Hariri, A. R., Fera, F., Smith, W. G., Chase, T. N., Hyde, T. M., & Mattay, V. S. (2002). Dopamine modulates the response of the human amygdala: A study in Parkinson's disease. *Journal of Neuroscience*, *22*, 9099–9103.

Thomas, K. M., Drevets, W. C., Whalen, P. J., Eccard, C. H., Dahl, R. E., Ryan, N. D., & Casey, B. J. (2001). Amygdala response to facial expressions in children and adults. *Biological Psychiatry*, *49*, 309–316.

Thornton, I. M., & Vuong, Q. C. (2004). Incidental processing of biological motion. *Current Biology*, *14*, 1084–1089.

van de Riet, W. A. C., Grèzes, J., & de Gelder, B. (2009). Specific and common brain regions involved in the perception of faces and bodies and the representation of their emotional expressions. *Social Neuroscience*, *4*, 101–120.

van der Gaag, C., Minderaa, R.B., & Keysers, C. (2007). Facial expressions: What the mirror neuron system can and cannot tell us. *Social Cognitive and Affective Neuroscience*, *2*, 93–103.

Vaskinn, A., Sundet, K., Friis, S., Simonsen, C., Birkenaes, A. B., Engh, J. A., & Andreassen, O. A. (2007). The effect of gender on emotion perception in schizophrenia and bipolar disorder. *Acta Psychiatrica Scandinavica*, *116*, 263–270.

von Campenhausen, S., Bornschein, B., Wick, R., Botzel, K., Sampaio, C., Poewe, W., & Dodel, R. (2005). Prevalence and incidence of Parkinson's disease in Europe. *European Neuropsychopharmacology*, *15*, 473–490.

Vonsattel, J. P., Myers, R. H., Stevens, T. J., Ferrante, R. J., Bird, E. D., & Richardson, E. P., Jr. (1985). Neuropathological classification of Huntington's disease. *Journal of Neuropathology & Experimental Neurology*, *44*, 559–577.

Vuilleumier, P., Armony, J. L., Driver, J., & Dolan, R. J. (2001). Effects of attention and emotion on face processing in the human brain: An event-related fMRI study. *Neuron*, *30*, 829–841.

Walker, F. O. (2007). Huntington's disease. *The Lancet*, *369*, 218–228.

Watanabe, S., Kakigi, R., & Puce, A. (2003). The spatiotemporal dynamics of the face inversion effect: a magneto- and electro-encephalographic study. *Neuroscience*, *116*, 879–895.

Wicker, B., Keysers, C., Plailly, J., Royet, J. P., Gallese, V., & Rizzolatti, G. (2003). Both of us disgusted in My insula: the common neural basis of seeing and feeling disgust. *Neuron*, *40*, 655–664.

Wieser, M. J., Muhlberger, A., Alpers, G. W., Macht, M., Ellgring, H., & Pauli, P. (2006). Emotion processing in Parkinson's disease: dissociation between early neuronal processing and explicit ratings. *Clinical Neurophysiology*, *117*, 94–102.

Zilbovicius, M., Meresse, I., Chabane, N., Brunelle, F., Samson, Y., & Boddaert, N. (2006). Autism, the superior temporal sulcus and social perception. *Trends in Neurosciences*, *29*, 359–366.

# Chapter 17
# Emotional Eating

**Michael Macht and Gwenda Simons**

## 17.1 Introduction

Hannah, a 29-year-old obese woman, reported to her psychologist that she had up to five episodes of binge eating per week. During binging, she would lose control and devour large amounts of food and, on average, consume 6,000 kcal in one episode (i.e., 3 times the recommended daily energy intake). These episodes of binge eating were typically preceded by intense emotional stress: Late at night, she would get flashbacks of sexual abuse during her childhood. Eating was her way to cope with these distressing flashbacks.

Since long time, psychotherapists assert, in line with the above example, that overweight persons might eat in order to cope with states of anxiety, depressive moods, anger, and other negative emotions (Kaplan & Kaplan, 1957). Some of these patients are aware of the difference between "real hunger" and emotion-driven desire to eat: "It is my mouth that wants it; I know that I have had enough" (Bruch 1973, p. 127). They feel that negative emotions exert a greater influence on their eating than hunger and satiety. According to Hilde Bruch, the influential expert on eating disorders, such a habitual pattern of eating to cope with negative emotions can ultimately lead to obesity. This appears to be a popular lay notion as well, as indicated, for example, by the German colloquialism "Kummerspeck" (literally: grief bacon) which is used to indicate the weight people gain from emotion-related overeating. Scientists refer to the phenomenon of eating in order to cope with emotions as "emotional eating."

Emotional eating theory (e.g., Bruch, 1973; Slochower, 1983) makes two core assumptions: First, negative emotions increase the motivation to eat (sometimes experienced as intense craving) and subsequently induce eating. Second, eating

M. Macht (✉)
Institute of Psychotherapy and Medical Psychology, University of Würzburg, Klinikstr. 3, 97070, Würzburg, Germany
e-mail: macht@psychologie.uni-wuerzburg.de

G. Simons
Department of Experimental Psychology, University of Oxford, England, UK, South Parks Road, Oxford OX1 3UD, UK
gwenda.simons@psy.ox.ac.uk

I. Nyklíček et al. (eds.), *Emotion Regulation and Well-Being*,
DOI 10.1007/978-1-4419-6953-8_17, © Springer Science+Business Media, LLC 2011

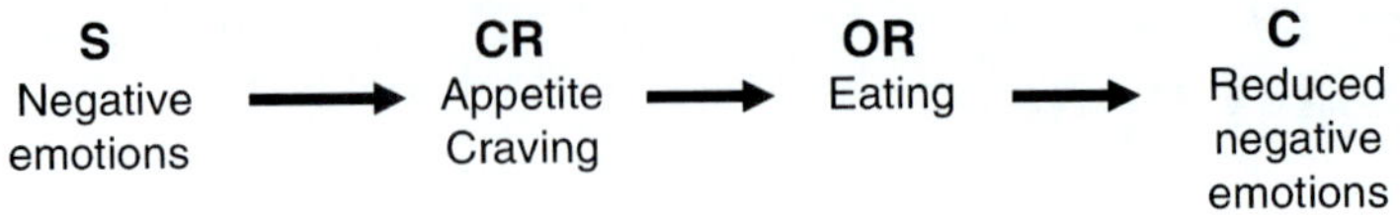


**Fig. 17.1** Principle of emotional eating: *S* stimulus; *CR* conditioned response; *OR* operant response; *C* consequence

reduces the intensity of negative emotions. These assumptions can also be expressed in terms of learning theory (Booth, 1994): the experience of a negative emotion elicits classically conditioned responses (e.g., craving) that are followed by an operant eating response that is reinforced by reduced intensity of the negative emotion. Figure 17.1 illustrates this chain of events.

In this chapter, we will explore the existing evidence from both healthy and clinical samples supporting the theory of emotional eating. We will discuss the possible causes of emotional eating as well as the physiological and psychological mechanisms that are likely to be involved (i.e., why does emotional eating work as an emotion regulation strategy?), before discussing some of its therapeutical implications.

## 17.2 Eating as an Emotion Regulation Strategy

Eating small or large amounts of food is just one of the many possible regulation strategies humans might apply in order to deal with our emotions and moods. Emotion regulation refers to both automatic and controlled processes and might affect the initiation of emotions/feeling states, their maintenance, and their intensity and duration (Gross & Thompson, 2007). In automatic emotion regulation, levels of emotions are registered without awareness and they are also adjusted at a non-conscious level (Parkinson & Totterdell, 1999). The term "controlled emotion regulation," in contrast, refers to the strategies that people deliberately and intentionally apply. These strategies influence their emotions and moods, and they "are implemented or terminated as a function of consciously monitored changes in affect" (p. 278).

Eating certain foods may act as a pleasant distractor and as such be used to regulate (elevate) negative emotions or moods (Tice & Bratslavsky, 2000). Participants in Parkinson's and Totterdell's study (1999) qualified comfort eating as a controlled (i.e., deliberate) affect-regulation strategy similar to other distraction-oriented behavioral strategies such as "doing enjoyable things" or "tidying up".

Although overall emotional eating seems to fit the profile of a controlled emotion regulation strategy, there are also instances where it appears to be a more or less automatic process. This is especially the case when emotional eating episodes have become habitual or indeed compulsive. In fact, most researchers will acknowledge that many instances of emotion (affect) regulation are likely to involve combinations of both type of processes (Parkinson, Totterdell, Briner, & Reynolds, 1996) or fall on a continuum from controlled to automatic emotion regulation (Gross, 1998).

## 17.3 Evidence for Emotional Eating

From the literature on emotion regulation in general, one may conclude that eating to regulate mood and emotions is probably commonplace and certainly not restricted to clinical populations. Indeed, numerous studies have shown that negative emotions stimulate food consumption (for a review, see Canetti, Bachar, & Berry, 2002 or Macht, 2008). These findings seem to support the first assumption of the emotional eating theory, which states that negative emotions increase the motivation to eat. However, it should be noted that at least some of the findings may be explained by emotional disinhibition of restrained eating rather than by a tendency to eat emotionally (Macht, 2008). In other words, people who increase food intake in response to emotions may do so not only because their emotions induce emotional eating, but also because they disrupt restrained eating patterns.

There is (separate) evidence supporting the second assumption of emotional eating theory (i.e., eating reduces the intensity of negative emotions). For example, Pines and Gal (1977) offered students sandwiches during an examination. Compared to a control group that received no food, students who ate sandwich reported a reduction in their levels of anxiety. Similar findings were reported by Agras and Telch (1998), Herman and Polivy (1975), and Slochower and Kaplan (1980).

In conclusion, there is evidence in support of each of the emotional eating assumptions. However, emotional eating theory additionally proposes a mutual relationship: Negative emotions elicit eating, which in turn reduces their intensity. To our knowledge, the full chain of events, as shown in Figure 17.1, has so far not been demonstrated in a well-controlled experimental study. In the laboratory, it is difficult to induce negative emotions that are comparable in intensity and duration to the emotional experiences that are thought to be the cause of emotional eating in real life. It is even more difficult to offer eating as a strategy to cope with these induced emotions without disclosing the specific goals of the study and hence potentially influencing the findings. If they feel observed, emotional eaters may hesitate to exhibit their usual eating response. In fact, at least for binge eaters, emotional eating tends to occur mainly when they are alone and feel unobserved. It is, therefore, not surprising that most of our knowledge of emotional eating is based on clinical observations and questionnaire studies in both clinical and normal populations.

There are a number of questionnaires which measure emotional eating. For example, Jackson and Hawkins (1980) developed the Mood Eating Scale to study the relationship between mood and eating. Table 17.1 gives some examples of items from this scale. Participants were requested to indicate on five-point scales to which extent they agreed with these statements. Similar measures have been developed by Van Strien, Bergers, and Defares (1986), Stunkard & Messick (1985), Macht (1999), and others. Findings from studies using these questionnaires suggest that a substantial part of the general population eat, at least occasionally, in order to cope with negative emotions. For example, in a survey conducted in Finland, 30% of women and 25% of men reported to eat in order to cope with

**Table 17.1** Example items from the mood eating scale (Jackson & Hawkins, 1980)

| |
|---|
| Eating can make me feel somewhat relieved when I am overwhelmed with things to do |
| I find myself eating more than usual during periods of great stress (e.g., breaking up with a lover, final exam week, starting college or a new job, getting married) |
| I seem to eat more than usual when I feel things are out of control |
| I snack a lot while studying for an exam |

stress (Laitinen, Ek, & Sovio, 2002). Slightly smaller percentages were found in a representative survey in Germany (Pudel & Westenhöfer, 1993). Thus, on the basis of questionnaire and survey data, it can be concluded that emotional eating is a common phenomenon.

However, data from surveys and questionnaire studies can be criticized for various methodological reasons. For example, Allison and Heshka (1993) suggested that overweight or obese persons may report more emotional eating because they are complying with social demands and expectations. Their exposure to psychological theories on obesity treatment (and treatment concepts) might produce inflated self-reports of emotional eating among these obese persons, simply because they learn from the popular literature or their therapists that emotional eating may be the cause of their obesity. A similar phenomenon has been described in relation to obtaining knowledge about the premenstrual stress syndrome. Watching a 10-min videotape describing this syndrome resulted in increased reports of premenstrual symptoms in a sample of Mexican women (Marván & Esobedo, 1999).

Another potential problem is that the questionnaires ask respondents to provide ratings of their eating patterns, retrospectively, over relatively long periods of time. Retrieval of this type of information from memory can be subject to a whole set of recall biases, which might violate the validity of self-reports (Barrett & Barrett, 2001). Field studies using experience-sampling methodology (ESM; Csikszentmihalyi & Larson, 1987) may partly solve some of these methodological problems (Macht, Haupt & Salewsky, 2004). In studies using ESM, participants typically report on their behavior or experiences during their normal everyday life, either when a pre-defined event occurs or in response to random or regularly timed signals (Wheeler & Reis, 1991).

In one such study, we assessed emotions in everyday life and examined the subjective motivation to eat associated with these emotional states (Macht & Simons, 2000). Participants rated their momentary emotional state and motivation to eat 5 times a day for a period of six consecutive days. A cluster analysis of the resulting 634 emotion profiles revealed three types of emotional states that were labeled "Anger-dominance," "Tension/Fear," and "Relaxation/Joy." A fourth cluster showing low levels of emotions was labeled "Unemotional state." During negative emotions, participants reported an increased tendency to cope with these emotions through eating compared to both positive and unemotional states.

A second ESM study examined changes in eating patterns in response to a real-life stressor (Macht, Haupt & Ellgring, 2005). Students awaiting an examination and control participants (no examination) were assessed 3–4 weeks before the examination (non-stress baseline) and again 3–4 days before the examination. They were given a pager, which beeped 10 times a day, on two successive days at random intervals. Upon each signal, they rated their emotional state and motivations to eat. If they had eaten since the last signal, they reported the perceived function of their actual eating behavior. Compared to control subjects, students awaiting an examination reported higher emotional stress and an increased tendency to eat in order to distract themselves from stress. The results from both these ESM studies thus support the existence of emotional eating in a non-clinical population under real-life conditions.

Nevertheless, results from clinical studies suggest that emotional eating plays a more important role for people with eating disorders than it does for healthy people. Using a stimulus response questionnaire (developed by Macht, 1999), patients with a variety of eating disorders reported an increased tendency to regulate negative emotions such as anger by eating compared to healthy controls (cf. Fig. 17.2; similar patterns of results were found for other negative emotions such as sadness and boredom). This was especially the case for the clinical conditions characterized by binge eating (bulimia nervosa and binge-eating disorder). In contrast, anorexics did not report higher levels of emotional eating than healthy controls (Weiland & Macht, et al., 2006).

Based on the findings of these and other studies, it appears that we can distinguish several degrees or levels of emotional eating ranging from occasional snacking to improve mood to binge-eating episodes in such clinical conditions as bulimia nervosa and binge-eating disorder.

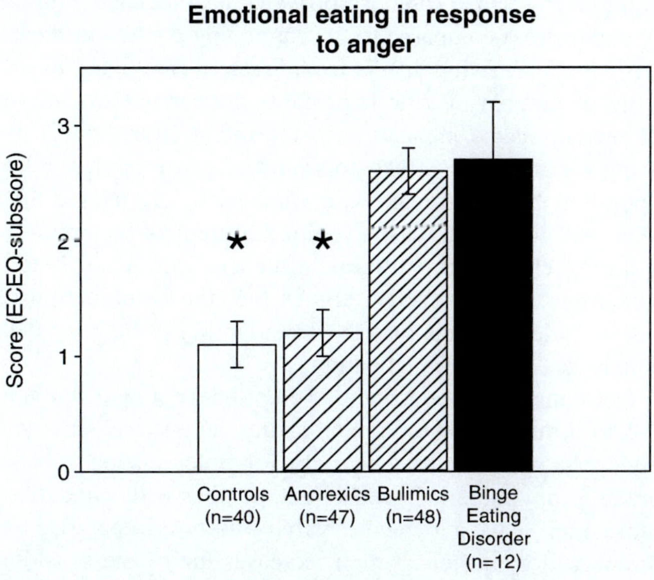


**Fig. 17.2** Emotional eating in response to anger in patients with eating disorders and in healthy controls (based on a conference presentation by Weiland & Macht (2006))

## 17.4 Etiology of Emotional Eating

As we have shown, there is evidence supporting the occurrence of emotional eating in both normal and clinical populations. However, there is very little data explaining the causes of emotional eating. According to psychodynamic theory, emotional eating originates from early feeding experiences. Early in childhood, food intake is intimately related to socio-affective stimuli such as the mother's attention and warmth. Harlow's classical experiments with monkeys showed that the separation of feeding and social interaction in early life is detrimental. Infant monkeys that were reared with access to plenty of food but without contact to their mothers showed fundamental behavioral deficits later in life. For example, they were unable to care for their own offspring (Harlow, 1958).

Referring to the possible origin of dysfunctional eating patterns in humans, Bruch (1973) stressed that "the important aspect is whether the response to the child's need was appropriate, or was superimposed according to what the mother felt he needed, often mistakenly" (p. 51). Children who are consistently fed when they are emotionally aroused and not necessarily when they are hungry could end up eating to cope with stress later in life. With this learning history, such adults may misuse eating to "solve" emotional and interpersonal problems. Although the psychodynamic explanation of the causes of emotional eating appears plausible, there is currently no empirical evidence that supports this hypothesis and many issues remain as yet unanswered.

It is, however, evident that stress responses in infants are a function of their caregiver's behaviors. For example, the caretaking context in hunter-gatherers societies such as the !Kung San, a tribe in Botswana, is associated with drastically less infant crying and distress compared to the caretaking context in Western industrial countries. Kung San caregiving differs from Western caregiving in several aspects, such as the higher amount of time the infants are carried around and the higher frequency of feeding at the instigation of the infant (Barr, 1990). Possibly, such early caretaking variables also affect stress and emotion regulation later in life.

It is also possible that emotional eating can be acquired later in life, even during adulthood. There is no logical reason to limit etiological factors to mother–infant interactions during childhood. Cultural influences may contribute to emotional eating. For example, Thayer (2001) argues that the combination of the rise of stress in modern society and the increased availability of highly palatable, energy-dense foods may lead to emotional eating.

A further factor that might contribute to emotional eating is our genetic makeup. Genes may exert influences on emotional eating via taste sensitivity. Research has found genetic variation in taste sensitivity for bitter tasting substances such as propylthiouracil. Propylthiouracil tasters (i.e., persons with a hereditary capacity to taste propylthiouracil) have a greater density of fungiform papillae on their tongue than propylthiouracil nontasters, which increases their taste sensitivity (Miller & Reedy, 1990). Preliminary data from our own laboratory suggest that this taste sensitivity is not restricted to bitter substances alone and that propylthiouracil tasters show more pronounced hedonistic reactions to sugar and appear to display more pronounced food-induced mood improvements than propylthiouracil nontasters. Speculatively, heightened taste responsivity may predispose a person to acquire the habit of emotional eating, whereas intense emotional stress and deficits in emotion regulation skills may contribute to a further development of pathological forms of emotional binge eating. Further research is needed to evaluate each of the above etiological hypotheses.

## 17.5 Mechanisms of Emotional Eating

Let us now turn to some of the possible mechanisms involved in emotional eating. One of the obvious reasons for emotional eating is that food, beyond its basic function to calm hunger, appears to have the capacity to alleviate emotional stress. It is less obvious which mechanisms mediate these effects. We suggest that emotional eating may involve both *physiological* and *psychological* mechanisms.

### *17.5.1 Physiological Mechanisms*

Nutrients affect energy metabolism, neurotransmitter systems, and hormone levels – and each of these changes may alter emotional state. Changes in neurological systems are thus a natural consequence of food intake.

#### 17.5.1.1 Serotonin Increase

The intake of meals very rich in carbohydrates but very poor in proteins (e.g., potatoes, rice, and many sweet foods) raises the tryptophan levels in the blood (relatively to other large neutral amino acids), which in turn leads to increased activity of the serotonergic brain systems. Serotonin is an important neurotransmitter that is related not only to hunger, pain, and sleep, but also to mood. This is why some antidepressants, such as fluoxetine, act by increasing the availability of serotonin in the brain, leading to an improved mood. Thus, eating carbohydrate-rich meals may similarly result in a reduction in depressive moods (Wurtman, 1982).

Some support for this hypothesis comes from an experiment conducted by Markus, Panhuysen, and Tuiten (1998). Participants consumed meals which were either carbohydrate rich and protein poor, or carbohydrate poor and protein rich for both breakfast and lunch. In the afternoon, they were asked to solve some difficult math problems while they were exposed to constant noise (a task designed to induce stress). The participants who consumed carbohydrate-rich meals displayed elevated levels of tryptophan in their blood as well as reduced stress reactions in comparison to the participants who consumed meals low in carbohydrates. However, this effect was limited to the participants scoring high on a questionnaire measuring stress-proneness. Thus, the serotonin hypotheses may have only limited validity, and carbohydrates may only decrease tension in susceptible people. Moreover, the effect of carbohydrates on serotonin levels in the brain was prevented when as little as 5% of the caloric intake was protein (Benton & Donohoe, 1999). Finally, few diets in real life "will regularly increase the availability of tryptophan, although occasionally a particular meal might stimulate the mechanism" (Benton, 2002, p. 300). To summarize, the serotonin hypothesis appears to play a minor role, at least in emotional eating. There are, however, other ways in which nutrients might have an effect on the neurochemical systems related to mood and emotions.

#### 17.5.1.2 Endocrine Effects

In a series of animal studies, Dallman, Pecoraro, et al. (2003) induced stress in rats by confining them in small clear-plastic cages for 3 h a day, for five consecutive days. After each daily stress induction, one group of rats was fed a standard diet and the other group, a diet enriched with lard and sugar. Animals that were offered the enriched food ate more than those on the standard diet and their weight increased rapidly. The rats on the sugar and fat diet further had lower levels of cortisol, an indication that the energy-dense food reduced physiological stress by influencing on the hypothalamic–pituitary–adrenal axis.

Since sweet, fatty foods seem to depress the endocrine stress response, as indicated by the reduced levels of cortisol, it can be speculated that people consume these foods in an effort to improve their emotional state. Indeed, comfort food typically has a high energy density (Wansink, Cheney, & Chan, 2003). Research demonstrating a positive relationship between the intake of sweet, fatty foods and emotional eating in humans was conducted by Oliver, Wardle, et al. (2000). Using the Dutch Eating Behavior Questionnaire (DEBQ; Van Strien et al., 1986), healthy participants were categorized as either emotional or non-emotional eaters. Participants in both groups were confronted with either a stress-inducing task (i.e., to prepare a 4-min speech they would have to give after lunch and which supposedly would be videotaped and evaluated) or relaxation while listening to a reading of an emotionally neutral text. After the experimental task, the participants were served a buffet lunch that included sweet, salty, and bland tasting foods that were either high or low in fat. Whereas the non-stressed, emotional, and non-emotional eaters displayed very similar eating patterns in the stress group, the emotional eaters ingested much more energy-dense (i.e., sweet and fatty) food than the non-emotional eaters. There was, however, no difference in the total amount of food consumed, suggesting that stress affects the quality of food choice but not the quantity. It remains unclear, however, whether the meal that participants consumed in this experiment had the capacity to exert similar endocrine effects as those observed in Dallman's animal studies. It is possible that endocrine effects only arise after a number of meals (i.e., during chronically increased intake of energy-dense food).

#### 17.5.1.3 Energy Increase

A single meal may also affect mood simply as a result of the energy it provides. Field studies have shown that the consumption of sweet snacks such as a bar of chocolate results in increased energy levels and reduced tiredness, specifically during the 30–60 min directly after consumption (Thayer, 1987; Macht & Dettmer, 2006). Laboratory studies have further shown that the manipulation of blood glucose levels causes participants' moods to change from a normal to a tense-tired state and back again to normal (Gold, MacLeod, Deary, & Frier, 1995). Thayer (2001) has argued that the consumption of sweet snacks increases feelings of energy and decreases feelings of tension, and thus helps to cope with negative mood states, in particular, with "tense tiredness," a feeling often experienced in modern society.

Taken together, these results are a clear indication that emotional eating is likely to be mediated by various physiological mechanisms. There is, however, one major problem with this explanation: nutrient-dependent emotional changes need time. They can only occur after food is digested, its components are absorbed into the bloodstream and transported to the brain. For an emotional eater, it would obviously be more effective if mood improvement immediately follows the consumption of food. Delayed effects may be useful for coping with chronic stress, but not for responding to negative emotions arising from unpredictable stimuli as they often occur in daily life. We need to look at other mechanisms to explain the more immediate effects of food intake that will gratify an emotional eater.

### *17.5.2 Psychological Mechanisms: A Hedonistic Hypothesis*

Based on observations of his son, Charles Darwin wrote: "It may be presumed that infants feel pleasure whilst sucking and the expression of their swimming eyes shows that this is the case" (Darwin, 1877, p. 288). One hundred years later, Steiner's systematic observations of newborns' facial reactions revealed that a sweet taste elicits emotionally positive responses (Steiner, 1977). The babies made sucking movements, licked their lips, and relaxed their faces, looking satisfied. In contrast, when the babies were given a bitter substance, they reacted with disgust, scrunching their eyebrows together and sticking out their tongues. Similar taste-elicited facial responses have been found in a number of primate species and are, therefore, considered to be universal. Even human adults react to sweet and bitter tastes with facial expressions similar to those displayed by primates and human infants. For example, adults display lip sucking actions more often while tasting a sweet chocolate drink compared to that while tasting either water or a bitter substance (Greimel, Macht, Krumhuber, & Ellgring, 2006).

Interestingly, sweet solutions have been found to calm stress responses in human infants rapidly. After an inoculation, infants were given either a sucrose solution or a pacifier. The magnitude of the calming by sucrose was striking. It reduced stress responses much more effectively than the pacifier (Smith, Fillion, & Blass, 1990).

In a recent research, we examined whether such calming effects from the consumption of sweet foods can also be observed in human adults (Macht & Müller, 2007). After a baseline rating of their emotional state, participants were shown a sad film clip in order to induce a negative mood state. After the emotion induction, the participants rated their emotional state again (manipulation check). Subsequently, the participants were given either a piece of chocolate to eat or 20 mL of water to drink after which they rated their emotional state for the final time. Results showed that compared to water, chocolate improved the experimentally induced negative emotional state. In a second experiment, using a similar set-up, the participants received either a piece of highly palatable or a piece of less palatable chocolate (determined in a pre-test). We found that chocolate improved mood only if it tasted well. Thus, palatability may be the crucial factor for food-induced improvement of mood. In fact, in our studies, emotional eaters showed more pronounced mood changes after eating chocolate than non-emotional eaters. These results support the assumption of a hedonistic mechanism in emotional eating.

*A Three-stage Model: Physiological and psychological mechanisms combined*

The above discussion suggests that emotional eating can be mediated by two types of mechanisms. In the first type, the nutrients may play a crucial role: Energy-dense foods lead to changes in metabolism, brain neurotransmitters, and neuroendocrine systems, which in turn exert influences on affect. In the second type, palatability is the key factor: Enjoyable foods elicit pleasant sensations that improve emotional state. In principle, both types of mechanisms may be involved in emotional eating. Indeed, energy-dense foods such as chocolate do not only supply the body with large amounts of carbohydrates and fat, but are also highly palatable.

However, different mechanisms may be activated by different eating patterns. As the research we have presented in this chapter suggests, there are at least three levels or degrees of emotional eating (varying from eating small amounts to binging on extreme amounts of food) that are likely to be associated with different mechanisms. This link between degree and mechanisms of emotional eating is shown in Fig. 17.3. On the first level, only the hedonic mechanism is involved. Small amounts of food or sweet snacks are consumed occasionally to cheer oneself up. Indeed, as little as 5 g of chocolate is enough to cause a slight improvement of a negative mood (Macht & Müller, 2007). At the second level, where emotional eaters habitually consume a whole meal to regulate their mood, physiological mechanisms

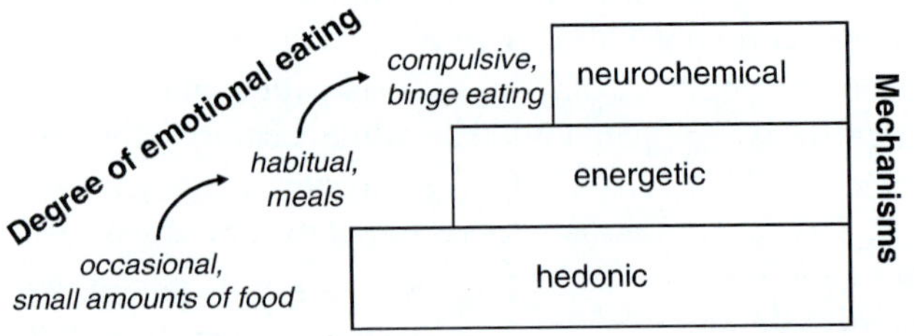


**Fig. 17.3** A three-stage model proposing a link between degree and mechanisms of emotional eating

become involved in addition to the hedonic mechanism. Energy levels increase, and tension and tiredness are reduced (Thayer, 1987; Macht & Dettmer, 2006). Finally, at the third level, emotional binge eating, which involves the compulsive consumption of chronically large amounts of energy-dense food, leads to additional neurochemical or neuroendocrine effects.

## 17.6 Therapeutical Implications

Although occasional consumption of a chocolate bar might be considered an effective way to regulate our mood with no negative consequences to our well-being other than perhaps the slight tightening of the waistband, emotional binge-eating and the associated obesity have severe consequences for our health and general well-being. For these obese patients, dieting alone is not enough and a restriction of food intake might even have the reverse effect (Polivy, 1996). Breaking of their diet might lead to further distress, which in turn induces a binge-eating episode. So it is foremost important to deal with the causes of their emotional eating and break the pattern. If we understand emotional binge eating as a maladaptive strategy to cope with negative emotions, improvement of emotion regulation skills is crucial for the treatment of binge eating. Research has shown that a training that is focused on improving emotion knowledge, self-monitoring of emotions, and providing patients with alternative emotion regulation strategies reduced pathological eating patterns in patients diagnosed with a binge-eating disorder (Telch, Agras & Linehan, 2000). Similarly, Hannah was able to abstain from binge eating as soon as she had learned to cope with emotional stress using alternative strategies.

Furthermore, because patients with eating disorders find it difficult or even impossible to enjoy eating and thereby loose an important source of well-being, it will also be beneficial to promote the ability to enjoy eating (i.e., eating for pleasure or hedonistic eating) in addition to adaptive emotion regulation skills. Both hedonistic and emotional eating seem to rely on the same principle: They serve to change an emotional state. The hedonistic eater eats to increase emotional well being; the emotional eater eats to reduce negative emotions. However, on closer inspection, there are a number of notable differences between the two types of eaters. In contrast to a hedonistic eater, an emotional binge eater does not care much about the selection or even the preparation of foods. The eater feels stressed, tense, and physically unwell; and eats quickly, losing control, without time to focus on the salient characteristics of the food and environment. And above all, while for the hedonistic eaters good company at the dinner table increases their feelings of well-being, the emotional binge eaters prefer to eat alone. Re-learning to enjoy eating can be an important part of therapy. But what is hedonistic eating exactly?

Hedonistic eating (or eating for pleasure) is characterized by pleasant sensations, and feelings such as joy, calmness, relaxation, and physical well-being. Features of the physical environment (comfortable setting, nice ambiance, etc.) and social activities (sharing a meal with others) are deliberately utilized to amplify

**Table 17.2** Core features of hedonistic eating

| |
|---|
| The foods selected for a pleasurable meal and its salient characteristics are specific to the individual |
| Environmental features and social activities increase the pleasure derived from eating |
| The person feels moderately hungry, calm, relaxed, physically well, and free of time pressure |
| Hedonistic eating is slow and focuses on the salient characteristics of foods |
| Positive sensations, emotions such as joy, and pleasant bodily sensations are elicited |

*Note*: Summarized from Macht, Meininger & Roth (2005)

these positive affective reactions. People who enjoy eating have the explicit intention to enjoy their meal and often engage in anticipatory activities before the meal. In a series of semi-structured interviews exploring the pleasures of eating, respondents mentioned anticipatory activities such as thinking about which foods to buy, preparing the food, reading the menu in a restaurant, thinking of the pleasure the eating of the meal is going to bring, drinking a glass of wine, and putting on nice clothes (Macht, Meininger, & Roth, 2005). Table 17.2 includes the core features of hedonistic eating derived from these interviews. These might be used as a kind of guideline to help patients reinstate non-pathological eating as an emotion regulation strategy with the aim to increase feelings of pleasure and well-being.

## 17.7 Concluding Remarks

In summary, we argue that eating in order to change negative moods and emotions is a fairly common phenomenon. However, individuals differ considerably in the quantities of food they consume in order to improve their mood, ranging from occasional snacking on small amounts of food to consuming large quantities during binge-eating episodes. The causes of these differences between individuals remain as yet unknown. There is further no clear evidence on the origin of emotional eating, although there are some promising leads. Theories point to the learning of links between emotion and eating in early childhood, but cultural influences, such as the abundance of food in certain societies and an omnipresence of stress and certain biological factors (e.g., taste sensitivity), may also play a role. The exact causes of emotional eating will only be discovered when methodological approaches to the study of emotional eating are improved. Innovative study designs that go beyond questionnaire studies are urgently needed to achieve this objective.

Whereas the causes of emotional eating remain unclear, we know a little more regarding the underlying mechanisms. During ingestion, food can elicit strong hedonic responses that improve emotional state. After ingestion, nutrients may change neurochemical and endocrine systems that are linked with mood and stress. Both these psychological (hedonic) and physiological (neurochemical) mechanisms may play a role at the same time. We propose, however, that their instigation depends on the degree of emotional eating. Whereas hedonic responses may occur in most instances of emotional eating, in order for neurochemical and neuroendocrine effects to come into play, a certain amount of food is needed as well as the repeated consumption of emotionally elicited meals. In pathological forms of emotional eating, the physiological pathways may override hedonic effects.

On the whole, although an old concept, emotional eating is not well-understood. It has gained attention from clinicians and now from the wider research community, but the phenomenon has not yet been studied extensively and many aspects remain unclear. More research is needed for a better understanding of this, often maladaptive, emotion regulation strategy. If this research takes into account possible relationships of emotional eating to obesity and addiction, its findings might help deal with the current obesity epidemic.

## References

Agras, W. S., & Telch, C. F. (1998). The effects of caloric deprivation and negative affect on binge eating in obese binge-eating disordered women. *Behavior Therapy*, *29*, 491–503.

Allison, D. B., & Heshka, S. (1993). Emotion and eating in obesity? A critical analysis. *International Journal of Eating Disorders*, *13*, 289–295.

Barrett, L. F., & Barrett, D. J. (2001). An introduction to computerized experience sampling in psychology. *Social Science Computer Review*, *19*, 175–185.

Barr, R. G. (1990). The early crying paradox: a modest proposal. *Human Nature*, *1*, 355–389.

Benton, D. (2002). Carbohydrate ingestion, blood glucose and mood. *Neuroscience and Biobehavioral Reviews*, *26*, 293–308.

Benton, E., & Donohoe, R. T. (1999). The effects of nutrients on mood. *Public Health Nutrition*, *2*, 403–409.

Booth, D. A. (1994). *Psychology of nutrition*. London: Taylor & Francis.

Bruch, H. (1973). *Eating disorders. Obesity and anorexia nervosa*. Riverside: Behavior Science Book Service.

Canetti, L., Bacher, E., & Berry, E. M. (2002). Food and emotion. *Behavioural Processes*, *60*, 157–164.

Cszikszentmihalyi, M. & Larson, R. 1987. Validity and reliability of the experience-sampling method. *Journal of Nervous and Mental Diseases*, *175*, 526–536.

Dallman, M. F., N. Pecoraro, et al. (2003). Chronic stress and obesity: a new view of "comfort food". *Proceedings of the National Academy of Sciences*, *100*, 11696–11701.

Darwin, C. (1877). A biographical sketch of an infant. *Mind*, *2*, 285–294.

Gold, A. E., MacLeod, K. M., Deary, I. J., & Frier, B. M. (1995). Changes in mood during acute hypoglycemia in healthy subjects. *Journal of Personality and Social Psychology*, *68*, 498–504.

Greimel, E., Macht, M., Krumhuber, E., & Ellgring, H. (2006). Facial and affective reactions to tastes and their modulation by sadness and joy. *Physiology and Behavior*, *89*, 261–269.

Gross, J. J. (1998). The emerging field of emotion regulation: an integrative review. *Review of General Psychology*, *2*, 271–299.

Gross, J. J., & Thompson, R. A. (2007). Emotion regulation: conceptual foundations. In J. J. Gross (Ed.), *Handbook of Emotion Regulation* (pp. 3–24). New York: Guilford Press.

Harlow, H. F. (1958). The nature of love. *American Psychologist*, 13, 673–685.

Herman, C. P., & Polivy, J. (1975). Anxiety, restraint and eating behavior. *Journal of Abnormal Psychology*, *84*, 662–672.

Jackson, L. J., & Hawkins, R. C. (1980). *Stress Related Overeating Among College Students: development of a Mood Eating Scale.* Paper presented at the 26th Annual Convention of the Southwestern Psychological Association.

Kaplan, H. I., & Kaplan, H. S. (1957). The psychosomatic concept of obesity. *Journal of Nervous and Mental Disease, 125*, 181–201.

Laitinen, J., Ek, E., & Sovio, U. (2002). Stress-related eating and drinking behavior and body mass index and predictors of this behavior. *Preventive Medicine, 34*, 29–39.

Macht, M. (1999). Characteristics of eating in anger, fear, sadness, and joy. *Appetite, 33*, 129–139.

Macht, M. (2008). How emotions affect eating: a five-way model. *Appetite, 50*, 1–11.

Macht, M., & Dettmer, D. (2006). Everyday mood and emotions after eating a chocolate bar or an apple. *Appetite, 46*, 332–336.

Macht, M., Haupt, C., & Ellgring, H. (2005). The perceived function of eating is changed during examination stress: a field study. *Eating Behaviors, 6*, 109–112.

Macht, M., Haupt, C., & Salewsky, A. (2004) Emotions and eating in everyday life: application of the experience-sampling method. *Ecology of Food and Nutrition, 43*, 327–337.

Macht, M., Meininger, J., & Roth, J. (2005). The pleasures of eating: a qualitative analysis. *Journal of Happiness Studies, 6*, 137–160.

Macht, M., & Müller, J. (2007). Increased negative emotional responses in PROP supertasters. *Physiology and Behavior, 90*, 466–472.

Macht, M., & Simons, G. (2000). Emotions and eating in everyday life. *Appetite, 35*, 65–71.

Markus, C. R., Panhuysen, G., & Tuiten, A. (1998). Does carbohydrate-rich, protein-poor food prevent a deterioration of mood and cognitive performance of stress-prone subjects when subjected to a stressful task? *Appetite, 31*, 49–65.

Marván, M. L., & Esobedo, C. (1999). Premenstrual symptomatology: role of prior knowledge about premenstrual syndrome. *Psychosomatic Medicine, 61*, 163–167.

Miller, I. J. & Reedy, F. E. (1990). Variations in human taste bud density and taste intensity perception. *Physiology and Behavior, 47*, 1213–1219.

Oliver, G., J. Wardle, et al. (2000). Stress and food choice: a laboratory study. *Psychosomatic Medicine, 62*, 853–865.

Parkinson, B., & Totterdell, P. (1999). Classifying affect-regulation strategies. *Cognition and Emotion, 13*, 277–303.

Parkinson, B., Totterdell, P., Briner, R. B., & Reynolds, S. (1996). *Changing moods: The psychology of mood and mood regulation*. Harlow: Longman.

Pines, C. J., & Gal, R. (1977). The effect of food on test anxiety. *Journal of Applied Social Psychology, 49*, 774–780.

Polivy, J. (1996). Psychological consequences of food restriction. *Journal of the American Dietetic Association, 96*, 589–592.

Pudel, V., & Westenhöfer, J. (1993) *Ernährungspsychologie*. [Nutrition Psychology] Göttingen: Hogrefe.

Slochower, J. (1983). *Excessive eating: the role of emotions and environment*. New York: Human Sciences Press.

Slochower, J., & Kaplan, S. P. (1980). Anxiety, perceived control, and eating in obese and normal weight individuals. *Appetite*, 1, 75–79.

Smith, B. A., Fillion, T. J., & Blass, E. M. (1990). Orally mediated sources of calming in 1- to 3-day-old human infants. *Developmental Psychology, 26*, 731–737.

Steiner, J. E. (1977). Facial expressions of the neonate infant indicating the hedonics of food-related chemical stimuli. In J. M. Weiffenbach (Ed.), *Taste and Development*. Bethesda: U.S. Department of Health, Education, and Welfare.

Stunkard, A. J., & Messick, S. (1985). The three-factor eating questionnaire to measure dietary restraint, disinhibition, and hunger. *Journal of Psychosomatic Research, 29*, 71–83.

Telch, C. F., Agras, W. S., & Linehan, M. M. (2000). Group dialectical behavior therapy for binge-eating disorder: a preliminary, uncontrolled trial. *Behavior Therapy, 31*, 569–582.

Thayer, R. E. (1987). Energy, tiredness, and tension effects of a sugar snack versus moderate exercise. *Journal of Personality and Social Psychology*, *52*, 119–125.

Thayer, R. E. (2001). *Calm energy – how people regulate mood with food and exercise*. Oxford: Oxford University Press.

Tice, D. M., & Bratslavsky, E. (2000). Giving in to feel good: the place of emotion regulation in the context of general self-control. *Psychological Inquiry*, *11*, 149–159.

Van Strien, T., Frijters, J. E. R., Bergers, G. P. A., & Defares, P. B. (1986). The Dutch Eating Behavior Questionnaire (DEBQ) for assessment of restrained, emotional and external eating behavior. *International Journal of Eating Behavior*, *5*, 295–315.

Wansink, B., Cheney, M. M., & Chan, N. (2003). Exploring comfort food preferences across age and gender. *Physiology and Behavior*, *79*, 739–747.

Weiland, R., & Macht, M. (2006) Emotionsbedingtes Essverhalten bei Bulimia nervosa, Anorexia nervosa und Binge-Eating-Störung [Emotion driven eating behavior in Bulimia nervosa, Anorexia nervosa and Binge-eating disorder][abstract]. In F. Lösel, D. Bender (Eds.) 45. *Kongress der Deutschen Gesellschaft für Psychologie* (S. 387). Lengerich: Pabst.

Wheeler, L., & Reis, H. T. (1991). Self-recording of everyday life events: origins, types, and uses. *Journal of Personality*, *59*, 339–354.

Wurtman, R. J. (1982). Nutrients that modify brain function. *Scientific American*, *246*, 50–59.

# Chapter 18
# Expressive Writing in Patients Diagnosed with Cancer

**Arden Corter and Keith J. Petrie**

## 18.1 Introduction

Cancer is a leading cause of death in most countries. Recent estimates suggest that by 2020, 15–20 million people will be diagnosed with cancer annually. Along with these global increases in cancer incidence, data also shows that in developed countries, mortality associated with cancer is decreasing due to the improvements in treatment and the benefits from screening programs (Donovan, Carter & Byrne, 2006). On average, half of people diagnosed with cancer will survive for more than 5 years, but this varies greatly by cancer site and sex.

Unfortunately, improvements in prognosis and increasing survival rates do not necessarily lead to decreases in psychological distress for cancer patients. Symptoms of depression are common in cancer patients, with between 5 and 50% of patients reporting signs of depression, and at least half of these patients meeting the criteria for clinical depression (Deimling, Kahana, Bowman & Schaefer, 2002; Stommel, Kurtz, Given & Given, 2004). Depression can detrimentally affect patients' quality of life, and there is also some evidence that it may have a negative impact on prognosis (Andersen, Kiecolt-Glaser & Glaser, 1994).

The diagnosis of cancer impacts on psychological and emotional well-being as individuals may experience a loss in their sense of control and self-efficacy (Zabora, Brintzenhosfeszoc, Curbow, Hooker & Piantadosi, 2001). Fears of death and worries about reoccurrence often dominate patients concerns. Cancer also affects physical functioning and appearance. The effects of the disease as well as the treatment can be devastating in their own right (Salsman, Segerstrom, Brechting, Carlson & Anrykowski, 2009).

Marital relationships can also be negatively affected by the diagnosis of cancer. Cancer in a partner can bring up ambivalent feelings in a spouse of fear and aversion to the cancer, at the same time as the awareness of the need to provide support to their loved one (Wortman & Dunkel-Schetter, 1979). This process can

K.J. Petrie (✉)
Department of Psychological Medicine, Faculty of Medical and Health Sciences,
University of Auckland, Private Bag 92019, New Zealand
e-mail: kj.petrie@auckland.ac.nz

I. Nyklíček et al. (eds.), *Emotion Regulation and Well-Being*,
DOI 10.1007/978-1-4419-6953-8_18, © Springer Science+Business Media, LLC 2011

result in intimacy difficulties and many patients also report problems with sexual functioning, as treatment and surgery for cancer can affect body self-esteem and reduce sexual desire (Andersen, Anderson & deProusse, 1989).

## 18.2 Difficulties in Sharing Emotions

While the diagnosis and treatment of cancer often brings with it a rise in emotional distress, many patients find the expression of negative emotions difficult. For some patients, there may be no real or perceived social support network with whom emotions may be shared. In other instances, such as discussing fears of death with family members, emotional disclosure may be perceived as inappropriate or difficult because of the distress it may cause for intimate others. Disclosure may also lead to a sense of being misunderstood, if the target of disclosure is unsupportive (Rodriguez & Kelly, 2006).

Some cancer patients may face issues of social rejection, isolation, and stigmatization, which in turn lead to feelings of loneliness and isolation (Ussher, Kirsten, Butow and Sandoval, 2006). Writing on a cancer blog Web site (http://cancerforums.net) a woman discusses her difficulty in discussing her thoughts and feelings about her breast cancer with others:

> *There were so many months of tests after that [diagnosis]: 5 MRIs, biopsies, injections, prognoses and predictions but it is the scar that summarizes the aloneness and betrayal of those months. I learned, for example, that no one wants to tell you the truth about the "C" word. Partners, family, friends and most doctors lapse quickly into words to placate, to hush one from speaking the awful truth that we are mortal; it is almost as if they are saying, with considerable desperation: "please, please, can't we talk about something else?" No one wants to really believe that someday we all will die, even themselves. I didn't want to believe it either but I did want to talk about it.*

As this quote demonstrates, cancer patients may find it difficult to speak about their cancer and associated feelings, even when they would like to talk about their illness. Recently, Henderson et al. (2002) studied the extent to which cancer patients talk about their illness, the targets of their disclosure, as well as variables that may constrain emotional disclosure. They found that between 20 and 30% of the 270 women with breast cancer in their sample reported little or no disease disclosure to social or health-related networks, including family, friends, and health professionals. Women held back from disclosing for a variety of reasons, including a desire for secrecy, difficulty in discussing their illness, or a lack of supportive contacts to talk to. One approach that is receiving increasing attention for its potential application to help patients cope with the experience of cancer is expressive writing (EW).

## 18.3 Expressive Writing

Over the last 20 years, hundreds of studies have examined the effects of EW on health and well-being. Generally, findings suggest that individuals assigned to write over 3–5 consecutive days about traumatic events experience positive psychological and physical health changes. Studies have reported that EW leads to benefits, such as fewer medical center visits, decreases in work-related absenteeism, enhanced immune responses, improvements in mood, as well as decreases in symptoms associated with chronic illness (for a review see Frattaroli, 2006).

The original study into EW was motivated by a theory of inhibition (Pennebaker & Beall, 1986). The basic premise was that, if holding back strong emotions leads to ill health, then by expressing negative emotions and feelings of personal upheaval, individuals could experience health benefits. Early studies of the effects of EW were conducted primarily with healthy participants. However, encouraged by positive results and excited by the potential clinical utility of EW, researchers turned their attention to assessing its efficacy in populations of patients with illnesses, such as fibromyalgia, HIV infection, chronic pain, and breast cancer. The results of broadened exploration into the psychophysiological and social effects of emotional disclosure are mixed, with some studies finding beneficial effects, others showing equivocal results and a few even finding detrimental effects of EW.

The most recent meta-analysis found a significant and positive average effect of EW ($r = 0.075$) (Frattaroli, 2006). This effect size compares with widely used medical treatments, such as taking aspirin to prevent death from a second heart attack, and to more time intensive and costly treatments, such as psychotherapy. The meta-analysis also found that EW was more effective for populations with physical health problems or with a history of trauma. Completing EW at home had a greater impact on psychological outcomes than participation in a controlled setting, and providing participants with greater privacy during writing was also associated with greater psychological benefit. Frattaroli also found that individuals who reported higher stress and lower optimism were more likely to benefit from EW. The review identified that beneficial effects of EW were most often found when assessed up to 1 month following writing, after which positive changes began to wear off.

In recent years, a number of studies have explored the effects of EW in various populations of cancer patients. Since 2002, approximately 20 studies have been published examining the effectiveness of EW for improving psychological outcomes of patients with different types of cancer.

## 18.4 Expressive Writing in Cancer Populations

The majority of studies assessing the effects of EW for cancer patients have been conducted with women with breast cancer. These are reviewed along with some research in prostate cancer populations, populations of mixed cancer patients, and those undergoing palliative care.

### *18.4.1 Breast Cancer*

A number of studies have been conducted to look at EW in patients diagnosed with breast cancer. In an early study, Walker et al. examined the benefits of EW for women whose cancer was at an early stage. The outcomes for an attention control group, where women spoke with a researcher about their events and plans on the final day of radiation treatment, were compared to the effects of two EW groups. In one, women participated in one 30-min EW session on the last day of treatment, and in the other, women wrote over three sessions during the last week of treatment. The study showed no benefits of EW over 28 weeks on measures of mood or intrusiveness of cancer-related thoughts, but the effects of EW on physical health were not assessed (Walker, Nail & Croyle, 1999).

A further study with breast cancer patients compared the effects of writing about deep thoughts and feelings (EW) to a benefit finding writing condition, and a control condition in which women wrote about the facts of their early stage breast cancer (Stanton et al., 2002). All groups wrote on four 20-min occasions in their preferred location and completed the writing within 5 months of their treatments for cancer. Results showed that at the 3 month follow-up both the EW and benefit finding groups showed significant reductions in symptoms and medical appointments for cancer-related morbidities compared to the control group. Interpreting the reductions in medical center visits, the authors suggest that emotional expression may have helped women to clarify and pursue their goals, to make more efficient use of scheduled appointments, or to address other concerns that may have contributed to help seeking behavior. A follow-up study using the data from this research made a more formal assessment of the mechanisms for the effects of writing. This study found that the use of negative emotion and cognitive processing words were associated with heart rate habituation within the writing session, which mediated the effects of writing on symptoms (Low, Stanton & Danoff-Burg, 2006).

Another study examined the effectiveness of EW as a stress management intervention for women undergoing the treatment for breast cancer (de Moor et al., 2008). The EW intervention was delivered in between surgery and beginning chemotherapy and women were assigned either to write for four sessions on their thoughts and feelings about their cancer and upcoming surgery or were given a neutral writing task. Four 20-min writing sessions were completed at participants' homes over a period of a week, approximately 3 weeks before scheduled surgery. Analyses revealed no effect of the intervention on distress but found the EW group to report greater use of sleeping medication following writing.

A recent study explores the effects of writing on women with breast cancer perceptions of emotional support, as well as effects on mood, quality of life, and health care utilization (Gellaitry, Peters, Bloomfield & Horne, 2010). The scores of EW participants on these measures were compared to those of a standard care control group at 1, 3, and 6 months assessments. Analyses showed a significant and positive effect of EW on women's perceptions of social support, which was negatively correlated with depression-dejection and anger-hostility scores and positively correlated with social and family well-being at 6 months postintervention. No other effects of the intervention were noted.

### 18.4.2 Prostate Cancer

Only two EW studies have been conducted with prostate cancer patients. The first of these was a pilot study delivering EW to individuals attending outpatient care for prostate cancer. Writing about their cancer, patients completed their writing at home and were tested at baseline, 3 and 6 months follow-up on physiological outcomes (e.g., PSA levels, t-cell proliferation), physical outcomes (e.g., symptoms), and psychological outcomes (e.g., quality of life, mood). Comparing results to no disclosure controls, this study found that EW participants showed improvements in pain and a trend toward lower health care utilization and reduced use of medications. There were no effects on psychological or physiological markers of patient well-being. However, the sample sizes were small so this study may have lacked power to detect effects.

In the second study, Solano et al. (2007) had patients who were about to undergo prostate surgery write for three consecutive days about their experience of being in the hospital. The study showed that intervention group patients who were at lower surgical risk had a reduced length of stay in hospital following the operation, lower symptom scores, and better medical evaluations as compared to a control group. However, intervention group patients at higher surgical risk showed a trend for a worse postoperative course on these outcome measures (Solano, Donati, Pecci, Persichetti & Colaci, 2003).

### 18.4.3 Other Cancer Populations

Where EW studies have been conducted in cancer treatment centers or clinics, the patient populations have often included diverse samples. For example, a recent study examined the feasibility and effectiveness of having patients engage in a structured EW exercise while waiting for an appointment at a cancer chemotherapy clinic (Morgan et al., 2008). Adult leukemia and lymphoma patients were approached in the waiting room and asked to complete a 20-min EW exercise along with baseline, post-writing and 3-week follow-up assessments. Results showed that participants generally enjoyed the writing and experienced changes in their thoughts and feelings about their cancer immediately after the writing. These benefits persisted at follow-up and were associated with reports of improved physical quality of life.

Another recent study examined whether writing about the impact of cancer would benefit cancer patients' experience of pain (Cepeda et al., 2008). The sample included a wide range of patients with different types of cancer at various stages of disease, but all had an above average pain intensity rating. The study found no differences in pain or well-being between the EW group and a control or usual care group. However, the results showed that participants who wrote more emotionally about their cancer experience showed a clinically meaningful pain reduction compared to those who used fewer emotion words in their writing.

### *18.4.4 Palliative Care*

An early pilot study examined the effects of EW for patients with metastatic renal cell carcinoma. Although there were no differences between an EW and a neutral writing group on the measures of mood or symptoms distress, the EW group reported less sleep disturbance and better sleep quality and duration (de Moor, Sterner, Hall, Warneke, Glani, Amato & Cohen, 2002).

Subsequently, Lacetti (2007) assigned women to write about their thoughts and feelings about having metastatic cancer and facing death. Results showed that women who used more positive words in their writing reported improved emotional well-being, but the significance of the findings are difficult to interpret without a control group. However, the authors report that participants viewed EW positively, and many intended to use it again.

One other study examined the feasibility of EW as an intervention for patients receiving palliative cancer care (Bruera, Willey, Cohen & Palmer, 2008). Participants were assigned to either an EW or neutral writing group and writing sessions were conducted with the help of prompts from a research nurse who telephoned participants 2 times per week for 2 weeks. As the study progressed, the researchers found that despite initial interest in participation, there was considerable attrition due to illness, hospitalization, and other factors. Additionally, review of the writing assignments suggested that participants did not write as expected in the EW group – most detailed the chronological events of their cancer rather than their personal thoughts and emotions. Based on the difficulties completing the study, the authors recommended that future EW research with palliative patients address issues such as: identification of appropriate times for receiving nursing phone calls; better patient education regarding study expectations; more flexible timing for EW sessions, including time between medical appointments; the possibility of using a secure internet Web site for logging it to post-writings; follow-up prompts to improve patient adherence; and processes to manage distress that may arise from the act of EW.

## 18.5 Methodological Issues

There are a number of methodological issues to consider in delivering and assessing the effectiveness of EW interventions within cancer populations. A number of these are common to other groups (Frattaroli, 2006).

The first issue is whether EW is useful for all types of cancer. Cancer is a diverse illness and the various subtypes affect a particular range of patients. To date, EW has only been tried in a relatively small number of different types of cancer, albeit many of the more common cancer diagnoses, such as breast and prostate. However, it is difficult to draw firm conclusions about the applicability of the intervention to other cancer types because these may differ markedly in the demographics of the population affected. Furthermore, the differing nature of the disease process, treatment demands, and prognosis may create marked differences between cancer types. The fact that many of the studies reviewed in this chapter reported that individual differences moderated the effects of EW does suggest that EW is unlikely to provide the same level of benefit across different cancer diagnoses (e.g., Low et al., 2006).

Another important issue is when and how the EW is conducted. From our review, we see that EW has been applied as an intervention at various points along the cancer continuum. Without more formal analysis, it is difficult to determine where writing should be placed to produce the best benefit. However, research suggests if done too closely to a traumatic experience, such as high-risk surgery, EW may actually engender more distress than it alleviates. In contrast, there is some evidence that when patients leave supportive medical care EW may help provide patients greater perceived social support (Gellaitry, et al., 2010). Given these findings, greater attention to the effectiveness of EW along different points of the cancer continuum is warranted. More work is also needed on how the EW context influences outcomes of cancer patients. Studies often vary the number of sessions and setting for writing from Pennebaker's original method although there is evidence that this may influence outcome (Corter & Petrie, 2008).

It is likely that the severity and stage of the cancer can also impact upon the benefits patients draw from EW, but there is a lack of data in this area. The physical demands of the illness and treatment vary enormously over the course of the disease of many cancers, and it is likely that the effects of writing vary accordingly. Many studies in the EW area have grouped patients facing different stages of the same cancer into the same trial and little effort has been made to systematically evaluate the impact of this variable on outcomes. This is clearly an area that needs attention in further studies of EW in patients with cancer.

## 18.6 Summary and Future Research

The diagnosis of cancer forces considerable adjustments on patients. Patients need to cope with the effects of the illness and treatment as well as integrate changes the illness brings to their personal goals and relationships. It is not surprising that the illness brings with it the potential for major emotional upheaval. The fact that more people are surviving the disease or living with the illness for many years means there is a need to develop effective psychological interventions that can alleviate the distress and help with the challenges to self-identity that cancer brings.

Compounding the emotional adjustments required in the face of a diagnosis of cancer, research shows that many patients have difficulty sharing their feelings about the illness with intimate others. The emotional writing paradigm developed by Pennebaker and colleagues offers to fill a potential need in this area by allowing patients to express their deepest thoughts and feelings through structured writing exercises that have been shown in other groups to be reasonably successful in improving psychological and health outcomes.

Does writing work in cancer patients? Looking at the data overall, it seems that writing is well accepted by patients and many seem to gain some personal benefit from EW. Most people seem willing to take part in EW research and based on findings from a few studies that have assessed patients' perceptions of the writing, the majority find it beneficial (e.g., Gellaitry, et al., 2010; Rosenberg et al., 2002). The data from studies conducted in breast and prostate cancer patients show some reduction in physical symptom reporting, lower need for medical care, and increases in perceived social support. The few studies that have been done in other cancer types and in palliative care are generally supportive of these findings with improvements in self-reported physical symptomatology, sleep and quality of life. No strong benefits have been shown for emotional distress or improved survival. There is some hint in the literature that the emotionality of writing may have an important influencing on outcome, and this should be measured in future research.

It is clear that the type of cancer, when the writing is conducted, and a number of individual difference variables will potentially influence the effectiveness of EW in patients with cancer. The patient's age, their educational level, and personality traits, such as optimism can act to influence coping with chronic illness (Carver and Antoni, 2004; Felton et al., 1984). Factors related to the disease itself in terms of its stage, physical characteristics, and symptomatology are also likely to influence the benefits from writing. More systematic study is needed on the effects of these variables on writing outcomes.

There are a large number of unanswered questions in the EW and cancer area. However, one interesting recent development is the fact that the internet has given researchers unprecedented access to the writings of patients with cancer. The development of Web-based patient support networks, such as www.sharedexperience.org, as well as patient online support groups, chat rooms, and newsgroups have provided greater access to look at the way patients are writing and what they are writing about. There is a growing realization that patient Web groups and blogs may provide important information that can help us understand the way people are talking and thinking about illnesses and treatments. We know that cancer support groups are much more frequent than other illnesses even after adjusting for prevalence of condition (Davison, Pennebaker & Dickerson, 2000). The use of this Web material and even writing interventions conducted over the Web are likely to increase rapidly in the future, and this is likely to lead to a greater understanding of the value of EW in helping patients with cancer diagnoses.

## References

Andersen, B. L., Anderson, B., & deProusse, C. (1989). Controlled prospective longitudinal study of women with cancer: I. Sexual functioning outcomes. *Journal of Consulting and Clinical Psychology*, *57*, 683–691.

Andersen, B. L., Kiecolt-Glaser, J., Glaser, R. (1994). A biobehavioral model of cancer stress and disease outcome. *American Psychologist*, *49*, 389–404.

Bruera, E., Willey, J., Cohen, M., & Palmer, L. J. (2008). Expressive writing in patients receiving palliative care: A feasibility study. *Journal of Palliative Medicine,11*, 15–19.

Carver, C. S, & Antoni, M. H. (2004). Finding benefit in breast cancer during the year after diagnosis predicts better adjustment 5 to 8 years after diagnosis. *Health Psychology, 23*, 595–598.

Cepeda, M. S., Chapman, C. R., Miranda, N., Sanchez, R., Rodriguez, C. H., Restrepo, A. E., Ferrer, L. M., Linares, R. A., & Carr, D. B. (2008). Emotional disclosure through patient narrative may improve pain and well-being: Results of a randomized controlled trial in patients with cancer pain. *Journal of Pain and Symptom Management, 35*, 623–631.

Corter, A. L., & Petrie, K. J. (2008). Expressive writing in context: The effects of a confessional setting and delivery of instructions affect participant experience and language in writing. *British Journal of Health Psychology, 13*, 27–30.

Davison, K. P., Pennebaker, J. W., & Dickerson, S. S. (2000). Who talks? The social psychology of illness support groups. *American Psychologist, 55*, 205–217.

Deimling, G. T., Kahana, B., Bowman, K. F., & Schaefer, M. L. (2002). Cancer survivorship and psychological distress in later life. *Psychooncology, 11*, 479–494.

de Moor, C., Sterner, J., Hall, M., Warneke, C., Gilani, Z., Amato, R. & Cohen L. (2002). A pilot study of the effects of expressive writing on psychological and behavioral adjustment in patients enrolled in a phase II trial of vaccine therapy for metastatic renal cell carcinoma. *Health Psychology, 21*, 615–619.

de Moor, J.S., Moye, L., Low, M. D., Rivera, E., Singletary, S. E., Fouladi, R. T., & Cohen, L. (2008). Expressive writing as presurgical stress management intervention for breast cancer patients. *Journal Social Intervention in Oncology, 6*, 59–66.

Donovan, R., Carter, O., & Byrne, M. (2006) People's perceptions of cancer survivability: implications for oncologists, *Lancet Oncology, 7*, 668–675

Felton, B. J., Revenson, T. A., & Hinrichsen, G. A. (1984). Stress and coping in the explanation of psychological adjustment among chronically ill adults. *Social Science and Medicine, 18*, 889–898.

Frattaroli, J. (2006). Experimental disclosure and its moderators: A meta analysis. *Psychological Bulletin, 132*, 823–865.

Gellaitry, G., Peters, K., Bloomfield, D., & Horne, R. (2010). Narrowing the gap: The effects of an expressive writing intervention on perceptions of actual and ideal emotional support in women who have completed treatment for early stage breast cancer. *Psycho-oncology, 19*, 77–84.

Henderson, B. N., Davison, K. P, Pennebaker, J. W., Gatchel, R. J., & Baum, A. (2002). Disease disclosure patterns among breast cancer patients. *Psychology and Health, 17*, 51–62.

Laccetti, M. (2007). Expressive writing in women with advanced breast cancer. *Oncology Nursing Forum, 34*, 1019–1024.

Low, C. A., Stanton, A. L., & Danoff-Burg, S. (2006). Expressive disclosure and benefit finding among breast cancer patients: Mechanisms for positive health effects. *Health Psychology, 25*, 181–189.

Morgan, N. P., Graves, K. D., Poggi, E. A., & Cheson, B. D. (2008). Implementing an expressive writing study in a cancer clinic. *The Oncologist, 13*, 196–204.

Pennebaker, J. W., & Beall, S. (1986). Confronting a traumatic event: Towards an understanding of inhibition and disease. *Journal of Abnormal Psychology, 95*, 274–281.

Rodriguez, R. R., & Kelly, A. E. (2006). Health effects of disclosing secrets to imagined accepting versus nonaccepting confidants. *Journal of Social and Clinical Psychology, 25*, 1023–1047.

Rosenberg, H. J., Rosenber, S. D., Ernstoff, M. S., Wolford, G. L., Ambur, R. J., Elshamy, M. R., Bauer-Wu, S. M., Ahles, T. A.. & Pennebaker, J. W. (2002). Expressive disclosure and health outcomes in a prostate cancer population. *International Journal of Psychiatry in Medicine, 32*, 37–53.

Salsman, J. M., Segerstrom, S. C., Brechting, E. H., Carlson, C. R., & Anrykowski, M. A. (2009). Postraumatic growth and PTSD symptomatology among colorectal cancer survivors: A 3-month longitudinal examination of cognitive processing. *Psycho-oncology, 18*, 30–41.

Solano, L., Donati, V., Pecci, F., Persichetti, S., & Colaci, A. (2003). Postoperative course after papilloma resection: Effects of written disclosure of the experience in subjects with different alexithymia levels. *Psychosomatic Medicine*, *65*, 477–484.

Solano, L., Pepe, L., Donati, V., Persichetti, S., Laudani, G., & Colaci, A. (2007). Differential health effects of written processing of the experience of a surgical operation in high- and low-risk conditions. *Journal of Clinical Psychology*, *63*, 357–369.

Stanton, A.L., Danoff-Burg, S., Sworowski, L. A., et al. (2002). Randomized, controlled trial of written emotional expression and benefit finding in breast cancer patients. *Journal of Clinical Oncology*, *20*, 4160–4168.

Stommel, M., Kurtz, M. E., Given, C. W., & Given, B. A. (2004). A longitudinal analysis of the course of depressive symptomatology in geriatric patients with cancer of the breast, colon, lung, or prostate. *Health Psychology*, *23*, 564–573.

Ussher, J., Kirsten, L., Butow, P., & Sandoval, M. (2006). What do cancer support groups provide which other supportive relationships do not? The experience of peer support groups for people with cancer. *Social Science and Medicine*, *62*, 2565–2576.

Walker, B. L., Nail, L. M., & Croyle, R. T. (1999). Does emotional expression make a difference in reactions to breast cancer? *Oncology Nursing Forum*, *26*, 1025–1032.

Wortman, C. B., & Dunkel-Shetter, C. (1979). Interpersonal relationships and cancer: A theoretical analysis. *Journal of Social Issues*, *35*, 120–155.

Zabora, J., BrintzenhofeSzoc K., Curbow, B., Hooker, C., & Piantadosi, S. (2001). The prevalence of psychological distress by cancer site. *Psychooncology*, *10*, 19–28.

# Chapter 19
# Secrets and Subjective Well-Being: A Clinical Oxymoron

**Andreas Wismeijer**

## 19.1 Introduction

In 1998, in Hilvarenbeek in the Netherlands, two criminals were assassinated in broad daylight as a result of a failed drug deal. Two young innocent bystanders who witnessed the liquidation were murdered as well. The murder remained unsolved for 5 years, until one of the murderers committed suicide, and confessed everything in his diary. In his diary he wrote that the weight of the secret had become too heavy, that he was obsessively ruminating over the murder, and that he no longer could live with the secret. Literally he wrote: "These two pairs of eyes keep haunting me. I hope I will get rest now."

The extreme example above illustrates how heavy a burden a secret can become. Yet, also small secrets have the ability to intrigue us. Secrets exercise a certain attraction and excitement by the mere fact that they are not accessible, and people go at great lengths in their attempts to reveal them. For centuries people have been fascinated by secrecy but it was not until the introduction of Pennebaker's inhibition theory (1989), which links the nondisclosure of distressing information with the increased risk of somatic disease, that behavioral scientists embraced the topic. Although still not a mainstream topic, Pennebaker's model proved to have a significant heuristic value, by causing an avalanche of empirical and conceptual studies trying to link nondisclosure with the development of pathophysiological processes.

However, these studies largely ignored the essence and the phenomenological aspects of secrets. The lack of theory-guided empirical research has backfired in the way that we now dispose of empirical results that are difficult to understand and sometimes even conflicting. For example, secrecy prevalence rates range from 32% to an astonishing 99% (Frijns & Finkenauer, 2009; Vangelisti, 1994) and secrets seem to affect somatic processes, yet not all secrets and not in everybody (van Heck

A. Wismeijer (✉)
Department of Developmental, Clinical, and Cross-Cultural Psychology, Tilburg University, P.O. Box 90153, 5000 LE Tilburg, Netherlands
e-mail: a.a.j.wismeijer@uvt.nl

I. Nyklíček et al. (eds.), *Emotion Regulation and Well-Being*,
DOI 10.1007/978-1-4419-6953-8_19, © Springer Science+Business Media, LLC 2011

& Vingerhoets, 2004). Finally, secrecy has repeatedly been shown to be either positively or negatively related to subjective well-being (SWB), depending on the kind of manifestation of secrecy one has focused on. These confusing results might be caused by the lack of a clear conception of what secrets are and thus which are the major distinctive features that determine the effects for the well-being of the individual. In short, a heterogeneous pool of secrets has been studied in different populations with different operationalizations and research methodologies, without a clear idea of how these differences may affect the findings (Wismeijer, 2008; Wismeijer & Vingerhoets, 2010).

## 19.2 What Is Secrecy?

Anything that exists, either in the real physical world or in imagination, can become a secret, whether they are facts, feelings, observations, obsessions or objects, as long as they are consciously hidden for others. This can be an obvious theme as adultery or having checked the email account of one's spouse, but can also refer to smoking or seeing a psychiatrist. In general, secrecy can be defined as a conscious and effortful process of social selective information exchange that requires cognitive resources and that can be experienced as an emotional burden. This definition integrates a large diversity of definitions of secrets that have arisen over the years and that all focused on a particular aspect (Frijns, 2004; Hillix, Harari, & Mohr, 1979; Margolis, 1974; Lane & Wegner, 1995). For example, according to Frijns (2004), secrecy is a *conscious* process that is intentional and deliberate because secret keeping requires the monitoring and screening of the (social) environment to prevent disclosing information: the secret-keeper has to determine what information to share, with whom and when. It is also *effortful* since it forces the individual to engage in strategic behavior to ensure that the secret remains a secret for those "not in the know." Cognitive resources such as suppressing secret-related thoughts are deployed to avoid unwanted or inappropriate disclosure. Inventive recovery tactics must be employed to do swift repair work in those instances when a slip of the tongue occurs (Lane & Wegner, 1995; Wegner, 1994; Wegner & Gold, 1995). Bouman (2003) conceived an alternative definition of secrecy where he sees secrecy as safety behavior that is functionally equivalent to avoidance and neutralizing behaviors, i.e., as behavior that is positively reinforced by the nonoccurrence of undesirable consequences. This view is particularly interesting as it suggests that once you keep something secret, it becomes increasingly harder to share the secret and confront the possible consequences, much like phobics who become ever more afraid of being confronted with the object of their fear.

Most laypersons assume that secrets stay secret during a lifetime, and even are taken into the grave. Indeed, to some extent there is evidence that a large barrier exists to share secrets of an intimate or compromising nature and that secrets are kept secret for prolonged periods of time. For example, several studies estimate that between 46 and 65% of long-term psychotherapy clients deliberately left things undisclosed in therapy (Hill, Thompson, Cogar, & Denman, 1993). However, secrets are generally not so exclusive and exceptional as one may think as Vrij, Nunkoosing, Paterson, Oosterwegel, & Soukara (2002) found that in a sample of college students the average duration of a secret is not more than 29 months (although with a standard deviation of 41 months). In addition, approximately 66% of secrets are shared with at least one person (Hillix et al., 1979). These results challenge the common belief that secrets are hardly disclosed and contain information that is exclusively known by and accessible for the secret-keeper.

## 19.3 Why We Keep Secrets: Protection

There are several good reasons to keep something secret, such as to increase one's status, to surprise somebody, or to have a strategic advantage such as in the case of army secrets. However, protection is one of the most important reason for secrecy (Norton, Feldman, & Tafoya, 1974). This protection may concern oneself, another, or a relationship (Afifi & Guerrero, 2000). The main reason for secrecy is to shield oneself against social disapproval (e.g., Wegner & Lane, 1995), embarrassment, and shame (e.g., Hill et al., 1993; Kelly, 1998). That is, one withholds information that is morally condemned by others and that may lead to social rejection or punishment (Warren & Laslett, 1977). By doing so, secrets provide a socio-protective function by reducing or preventing negative feedback, social disapproval, and stigmatization from others (Bok, 1989; Kelly, 2002; Kelly & McKillop, 1996; Larson & Chastain, 1990; Wegner & Gold, 1995; Wegner & Lane, 1995). This is corroborated by preliminary results of our data from over 400 Dutch senior citizens (aged 65 years and older) (Roeling, Wismeijer, Waringa, & Van Assen, 2010). In that study we asked the respondents to think of their most important secret and indicate for each reason in a list of 23 different reasons how much that reason was applicable to their secret. Examples are "because I worry how others will react," "to protect some body else," and "because it gives me a sense of control and power." This list was composed based on the scientific literature on why people keep secrets, as well as on interviews with secret-keepers. Factor analysis showed that the reasons for secrecy could be summarized into four factors: (1) self-protection, (2) protection of significant others, (3) status considerations, and (4) strategic use of secrecy. Self-protection and protection of significant others had significantly higher scores than the other two factors, suggesting that protection is indeed the most salient reason to keep secrets.

In this light it is interesting to mention research on social pain theory. Social pain theory suggests that social behavior and reactions to social exclusion in particular are regulated by a general threat-defense system that prepares the organism for potentially harmful situations (Herman & Panksepp, 1978; MacDonald & Leary, 2005; Panksepp, 1998). The interesting hypothesis is that these harmful situations are not limited to physical situations, but can also be social in nature. This pairing of physical and social threats may have developed because being separated from important social entities posed an enormous pressure on the survival of our ancestors with the result that "evolution has equated exclusion with extinction, meaning rejection may be treated as a mortal danger at the motivational level" (MacDonald & Leary, 2005, p. 214). Therefore, social pain theory regards the affective component of physical pain and social distress as managed by the same physiological system, since both kinds of pain share the same function of promoting adaptive approach or avoidance behavior in response to threats in order to protect the physical and social integrity.

Extending Bouman's (2003) notion of secrecy as safety behavior that is functionally equivalent to avoidance, secrecy can thus be seen as a strategy to increase the defensive distance between the organism and the social threat that might lead to exclusion. Secrecy helps to reduce or control the risk of being ostracized and socially excluded. Since not only physical threats but also social threats may have evolved to be perceived as life threatening, it is tentative to regard secrecy as a mechanism that taps on archaic motivational structures that are evolutionary linked to survival. This may explain the strong tendency people have to remain silent about topics they fear may lead to disapproval from others.

The protective function of secrets also explains why secrets do not always have to be associated with negative physical consequences. A study by Cole, Kemeny, and Taylor (1997) suggests that in certain cases, secrecy may even protect against negative health effects. They found that rejection-sensitive gay men who concealed their homosexuality, compared to rejection-sensitive gay men who reported being mainly or completely out of the closet, did not experience a significant decrease in objective health status while those out of the closet did. That is, the (anticipated) physical pain that is warded off by concealing something potentially ostracizing may buffer the potential detrimental effects of secrecy and result in a net benefit for well-being.

## 19.4 Consequences of Secrecy

Notwithstanding the above, the relation between secrecy and well-being has long been thought to be a detrimental one (Ellenberger, 1965). Both psychologists and laypersons believe that keeping secrets negatively affects bodily and cognitive processes, which may eventually lead to physical and mental illness (Farber & Hall, 2002, Finkenauer & Rimé, 1998; Kelly & Achter, 1995; Kelly & Yip, 2006; Lane & Wegner, 1995; Pennebaker, 1989). Indeed, a large body of empirical studies suggests that secrecy demands a high price for the individual in terms of negative intra- and interpersonal consequences (e.g., Frijns & Finkenauer, 2009; Lane & Wegner, 1995, Larson & Chastain, 1990, for a review see Smyth, 1998). Negative interpersonal consequences of secrecy for example become evident when secrets are being kept in a close relationship. While at first secrets increase the individual's attractiveness (Kelly & McKillop, 1996; Olson, Barefoot, & Strickland, 1976; Wegner, Lane, & Dimitri, 1994), in later and more intimate stages of the relationship the secret-keeper's partner may feel left out, and become increasingly distressed by this perceived lack of confidence (Finkenauer, 1998).

In addition, the negative intrapersonal consequences can manifest themselves in a host of negative mental and physical consequences such as rumination, obsession with the secret (Lane & Wegner, 1995), depression (Cramer, 1999; Larson & Chastain, 1990), and increased risk of somatic disease due to compromised immunocompetence (Christensen et al., 1996; Esterling, Antoni, Kumar, & Schneiderman, 1990; Petrie, Booth, & Pennebaker, 1995). Indeed there is evidence showing that secrecy is negatively associated with SWB and health (SWB; see Kelly & Yip, 2006, for an overview). For example, Cole, Kemeny, Taylor, Visscher, and Fahey (1996) demonstrated that seropositive gay men who concealed their homosexual status to a higher degree than other seropositive gay men experienced a more rapid disease progression over a 9-year period. In particular, they developed a critically low EDT lymphocyte level at an earlier stage, were earlier diagnosed with AIDS, and died earlier. Cole, Kemeny, Taylor, and Visscher (1996) found in another, 5-year longitudinal, study that concealing one's homosexual identity is related to a higher incidence of infectious diseases. Further, Finkenauer and Rimé (1998) found that respondents who could recall an emotionally demanding event they keep secret for others reported a lower SWB that those without such secrets. Finally, a host of correlational studies have shown that a stable disposition to conceal personal information is associated with or predicts lower physical and psychological well-being.

Three models are frequently cited as candidates to explain this debilitating influence of secrecy on SWB. The first model is the inhibition model by Pennebaker (1989) that focuses on the physical consequences of the nondisclosure of traumatic events. In this model, sharing life events is considered as naturally occurring behavior (cf. Wetzer, 2007; Zech, Bradley, & Lang, 2002). Inhibition of this natural tendency may be regarded as a minor stressor, which nevertheless places a burden on the person's physiology, which may manifest itself by an elevated blood pressure (Christensen & Smith, 1993), a compromised immunocompetence (Christensen et al., 1996; Esterling et al., 1990; Petrie et al., 1995), and increased skin conductance levels (Pennebaker, Hughes, & O´Heeron, 1987). An interesting finding in this respect is that HIV seropositive (HIV+) gay men who concealed their homosexuality showed a significantly lower immune function when they had an extensive social network they left unused, compared to those HIV+ gay men who also concealed their homosexuality but that did not have an extensive social network to rely on (Ullrich, Lutgendorf, Stapleton, & Horowitz, 2004). This may suggest that not speaking up when the opportunity is there may be more detrimental than not speaking up per se. Because of the presumed chronic and long-term nature of many secrets, the inhibition to share one's life events is thought to have a cumulative effect, capable of inducing pathophysiological processes eventually resulting in somatic symptoms (Pennebaker, 1989). Although this model has been of great heuristic importance, it has several important shortcomings that limit its use in explaining how secrets are related to SWB. Although probably being the most often cited model, it is currently not anymore regarded as a promising explicative model.

The preoccupation model of secrecy proposed by Lane & Wegner (1995) is a more promising alternative. In contrast to Pennebaker´s inhibition model that has its emphasis on the possible physical consequences, this model focuses mainly on the psychological sequelae of secrecy. It postulates that secrecy initiates intentional thought suppression to prevent a slip-of-the-tongue or actions that might reveal the secret. However, in his well-known white-bear paradigm studies, Wegner (1992, 1994) demonstrated that intentional thought suppression led to the paradoxical consequence of an increase rather than a decrease in intrusive thoughts about the suppressed information or secret. Since these thoughts in their turn also have to be suppressed, a vicious circle of ruminative thoughts is initiated that might lead to an obsessive preoccupation with the hidden information that can eventually result in psychopathology (Lane & Wegner, 1995). Results of a correlational study by Cramer (1999) point in this direction, in which positive correlations between secrecy and depression of .36 and .40 were found.

A third promising model to explain how secrecy may affect well-being is proposed by Brosschot and Thayer (2004). In their model, perseverative thinking (similar to rumination on the secret) leaves the individual in a continuous state of psychophysiological "action preparation" by continuously reactivating cognitive schemata related to the initial stressor that asks for appraisal. That is, perseverative thinking may continuously activate cognitive networks that, above a certain threshold, can trigger a feedforward process in which increasingly more cues of the relevant event are perceived. As a consequence, "perseverative thinking might convert the immediate psychological and physiological concomitants of life events and daily stressors into prolonged physiological activation, which in turn is necessary for the development of a chronic pathogenic state" (Brosschot & Thayer, 1998, p. 329). Although the study of perseverative thinking is still in its infancy, the concept tentatively might be the missing link between psychological factors and the chronic pathogenic state thought to be causally related to the development of physical complaints (Brosschot & Thayer, 2004). To the degree that this concept of perseverative thinking indeed equals rumination on a secret as proposed by Lane and Wegner (1995), it may explain how secrecy may be related to physical complaints: the excessive rumination on the secret that accompanies secrecy may cause continuous reactivation of cognitive schemata related to the secret, with prolonged physiological activation and the development of physical complains as a possible result. This fusion of the models of Lane and Wegner (1995) and Brosschot and Thayer (2004) may be helpful to understand the mechanism behind Pennebaker's (1989) claim that secrets exert a continuous and cumulative influence on well-being. In conclusion, it thus seems that the individual secret-keeper may pay a considerable price to obtain the advantages secrecy provides. This is evidenced by the extensive body of research that linked secrecy to a host of dependent SWB measures, from which we just reviewed only a fraction.

However, the picture is less clear-cut than it seems. Doubts have been raised about several assumptions made by the theories on secrecy and secrecy-related health effects. For example, the longevity of secrets may not be as high as Pennebaker (1989) and Lane and Wegner (1995) assume (Hillix et al., 1979; Vrij et al., 2002). In addition, empirical findings could not always be replicated or contradicted each other (Van Heck & Vingerhoets, 2004). What might cause this confusing state of affairs? The answer may lie in the fact that the literature regards all secrets as qualitatively equal: simply information that one conceals from others (Frijns, 2004). As we will show next, this assumption is arguable at best.

## 19.5 Secrets as Process or Trait

Kelly (1998, 2002) and Kelly and Yip (2006) make a compelling case that the results of previous studies on the relation between secrecy and SWB may be less reliable than supposed. They argue that it is essential to distinguish having a secret (secrecy as an act) and being a secretive person (secrecy as trait). Or, more precisely, keeping a major secret (KMS) and self-concealment (SC; Larson & Chastain, 1990). Although Kelly and Kelly and Yip did not explicitly define what makes a secret a major secret, it is safe to say that "major" refers to the perception of the individual that the secret is important or emotionally demanding, as opposed to trivial and neutral secrets. SC refers to a personality trait that is characterized by concealing negatively valenced personal information, independent of environmental circumstances (Larson & Chastain, 1990). The difference between KMS and SC is that one may occasionally keep secrets due to situational forces without necessarily being a secretive person. Hence, knowing that someone who scores high on KMS is not sufficiently informative without additional information about why one is keeping the secret. The difference between KMS and SC is of importance for understanding the relation between secrecy and SWB as both instances refer to different characteristics of the individual, and as we will see, are quite differentially related to SWB.

## 19.6 Self-Concealment and Subjective Well-Being

SC (Larson & Chastain, 1990) refers to the personality characteristic to conceal information from others, as opposed to seeing secrecy as a function of mainly situational determinants. The concept of SC is derived from the trait component of inhibition as studied by Pennebaker (1989) and is defined as the "predisposition to actively conceal from others personal information that one perceives as distressing or negative" (Larson & Chastain, 1990, p. 440). Self-concealed personal information is a subset of private personal information, consciously accessible to the individual and actively kept from the awareness of others. It is negative in valence, and if disclosed at all, usually only confided to a small number of persons because of its highly intimate content (Larson & Chastain, 1990). Since its introduction, the concept of SC has been commonly applied, predominantly in clinical psychological studies on anxiety and depressive symptoms.

Several studies have shown that SC is positively associated with various measures of psychological distress such as anxiety (e.g., Pennebaker, Colder, & Sharp, 1990; Ritz & Dahme, 1996), depression (e.g., Kelly & Achter, 1995), maladjustment (e.g., Kawamura & Frost, 2004), overall psychological distress (e.g., Cramer, 1999), loneliness and low self-esteem (Cramer & Lake, 1998), and physical complaints, even after controlling for traumatic events and self-disclosure (Larson & Chastain, 1990; Pennebaker et al., 1990). Further, recently Wismeijer, Van Assen, Sijtsma, and Vingerhoets (2009) found SC to be negatively related with self-reported life satisfaction, psychological well-being, health status, and positively with fatigue. Also, we showed that SC is positively associated with neuroticism (Wismeijer & Van Assen, 2008). In addition, SC is associated with a host of other maladaptive processes such as reluctance to seek social support, and experiencing lower satisfaction with received social support (Cepeda-Benito & Short, 1998; Kelly & Achter, 1995; Wallace & Constantine, 2005). The associations between SC and SWB are regularly in the range of medium to large, also in longitudinal studies (Wismeijer, Van Assen, Sijtsma, & Vingerhoets, 2010a, b). This demonstrates that SC is an important negative determinant of SWB, which is consistent with the literature (Kelly & Achter, 1995; Larson & Chastain, 1990; Pennebaker et al., 1990; Wallace & Constantine, 2005; Wismeijer & Van Assen, 2008; Wismeijer et al., 2009; Yukawa, Tokuda, & Sato, 2007).

## 19.7 KMS and Well-Being

In a study among therapy outpatients, Kelly (1998) did not find a significant correlation between KMS and a measure of SWB (the Global Severity Index of the Brief Symptom Inventory (BSI; Derogatis, 1993)), but she did find a negative correlation between SC and SWB. When controlling for SC and social desirability, however, KMS was positively associated with SWB. Even when baseline SWB was accounted for, KMS had a positive relation with SWB measured later in time, and SC had a negative relation with SWB. In a more recent study using undergraduates, Kelly & Yip (2006) found similar results. Again, they did not find a correlation between KMS and SWB, while SC correlated negatively with SWB. However, when SC was accounted for, KMS had a positive relation with SWB measured 9 weeks later, whereas SC had a negative relation with SWB measured 9 weeks later.

Using a prospective, 5-year longitudinal design, we found that SC was negatively associated with SWB during each assessment, and this relation also was found after having controlled for KMS (Wismeijer, Van Assen, Sijtsma, & Vingerhoets, 2010a, b). KMS was negatively related to SWB, but after controlling for SC this relation turned positive. KMS mediated the relation between SC and SWB. The mediation was inconsistent in that the effect of SC on SWB increased after controlling for the effect of KMS. Finally, we also found that, over a 5-year period, almost half of the relations between SC, KMS, and SWB remained significant predictors of SWB after controlling for SWB at the previous wave. Our results were obtained using a different measure for KMS, three different measures of SWB, a larger and different sample (representative of the Dutch general population), a considerably longer time span, and a different method of analysis that controls for measurement error. The corroboration of the findings of Kelly (1998) and Kelly & Yip (2006), notwithstanding these differences in methodology, hints at a reliable and robust phenomenon. Finally, in a recent study among over 300 HIV+ outpatients we found that KMS was negatively associated with SWB (Maas, Wismeijer, Aquarius, & Van Assen, 2010). However, after controlling for SC, this relationship either disappeared or turned positive. Furthermore, it was found that cognitive preoccupation was a significant mediator: cognitive preoccupation not only decreased the direct negative effect of SC on SWB, but also increased the positive effects of KMS on SWB.

How can we reconcile these results showing a positive relation between secrecy and SWB with the literature that historically negatively linked secrecy to SWB? The answer lies in the distinction between secrecy as a trait or as a process. The overall effect of secrecy on SWB is negative because it consists of an indirect positive effect of SC that is mediated by KMS, and a larger negative direct effect of SC. Hence, the negative associations between secrecy and SWB and between KMS and SWB, without controlling for SC, is misleading, and shows the danger of considering secrecy as a unidimensional concept. As Kelly and Yip (2006) suggested, past studies that found secrecy to be negatively associated with SWB may have found quite different results if they would have controlled for SC.

## 19.8 Explanatory Models

It becomes clear that SC and KMS indeed are two quite different manifestations of secrecy, not only conceptually but in particular in terms of predicting SWB. Understanding the mechanism by which each manifestation affects SWB and how they divert one from the other allows us to better disentangle SC and KMS.

### *19.8.1 Why Is SC Negatively Related with SWB?*

Several explanations for the debilitating effect of SC on SWB are reported in the literature. First, the lack of social support that self-concealers experience is a recurrent theme in the self-concealment literature (Cepeda-Benito & Short, 1998; Kelly & Achter, 1995; Wallace & Constantine, 2005). Social support has repeatedly been shown to promote SWB by influencing emotions, cognitions, and behaviors (Cohen, Gottlieb, & Underwood, 2000; Gallagher & Vella-Brodrick, 2008) by, for example, providing feedback about one's problems or mood states. The perceived and actual level of social support of self-concealers is lower compared with low self-concealers. The explanation for this is straightforward: consistently not sharing private information with others makes these others unsure of one's willingness to bond and hence reluctant to invest in a friendship that would provide the social support. Further, not communicating one's internal states and thoughts simply makes others unaware of the need for support. Although several studies exist that controlling for social support does not eliminate the relation between SC and SWB (Kelly, 2002), lack of social support appears to be a viable mechanism by which SC may negatively affect SWB.

An alternative explanation, related to the social support notion, is that SC induces the use of an inward directed coping strategy rather than an outward directed coping strategy such as asking a confidant advice on one's own mood state. Cepeda-Benito and Short (1998) found SC to be negatively associated with attitudes toward counseling and the tendency to seek counseling. Further, Kelly and Achter (1995) found that self-concealers have negative attitudes toward counseling when it was emphasized that the client had to disclose personal information during counseling. This negative attitude of self-concealers toward counseling may in part be mediated by other correlates of SC such as social anxiety, a strong preference to be alone, and perfectionism (Cramer & Lake, 1998; DiBartolo, Li, & Frost, 2008; Gesell, 1999).

Finally, in our own work we found that SC is associated with maladaptive mood regulation, characterized by scrutinizing one's negative moods without being able to label these and adequately act upon them (Wismeijer et al., 2009). Using the Mood Awareness Scale from Swinkels and Giuliano (1995) we found that SC is positively associated with mood monitoring and negatively associated with mood labeling. Mood monitoring refers to the stable tendency to scrutinize and focus on one's moods, and implies a great involvement in the mood state itself, to the point of the individual wallowing in it. Mood labeling, in contrast, refers to completeness in understanding one's moods and being able to adequately label or categorize them. Hence, the scrutiny of mood states associated with mood monitoring should not be confounded with an increased *understanding* of one's mood state; it simply means that the individual is more aware of being in a specific mood. More precisely, whereas mood monitoring is associated with persistent vigilance for affect and affect changes that may lead to premature and inadequate mood regulation, mood labeling is associated with accuracy in recognizing one's mood states, which may facilitate choosing appropriate mood regulation strategies (Van-Leeson, Totterdell, & Parkinson, 2006). Mood monitoring and mood labeling partly mediate the relation between SC and various measures of SWB; from 28 to 51% of the total relation between SC and SWB was mediated by mood monitoring and mood labeling together (Wismeijer et al., 2009). This suggests that SC predicts double trouble: negatively valenced mood states receive increased and continuous levels of attention, but a better understanding of the nature and cause of these mood states is not attained. The result may be a limited deployment of adequate emotion regulatory processes (Cepeda-Benito & Short, 1998), and a longer duration of the negative mood state (Nolen-Hoeksema, 2000).

One could argue that third variables, most notably higher order personality traits such as neuroticism and extraversion that are reported as the most important predictors of SWB (Vittersø, 2001), may explain the relation between SC and SWB. However, we reported empirical evidence that neuroticism (but not extraversion) only mediated a small part of the relation between SC and SWB, and that SC remained a significant predictor with a modest decrease of the regression coefficient (Wismeijer & Van Assen, 2008). Although this result does not exclude the existence of other third variables, it shows that the two major determinants of SWB did not explain the relation between SC and SWB. Summarizing, SC is a trait that includes a host of problematic internal behaviors (low self-esteem, social anxiety, high mood monitoring, low mood labeling) and external behaviors (lack of seeking counseling, lack of social support, preference for solitude), all adding up to the consistent finding that SC negatively predicts SWB.

### *19.8.2 Why Is KMS Positively Related with SWB?*

Several specific examples exist of the beneficial qualities of KMS. For example, keeping secrets is an important aspect of constructing healthy ego boundaries (Margolis, 1974). Further, in romantic relationships keeping some aspects of oneself secret enhances one's attractiveness in the short run (Olson et al., 1976; Wegner et al., 1994). However, related to SWB the strongest arguments why KMS may positively predict SWB are probably derived from the self-presentational view (Kelly, 2000; Schlenker & Weigold, 1992). This view suggests that hiding one's unfavorable aspects from others, especially from close and significant others (Leary & Kowalski, 1990), may help one feeling better about oneself (Kelly, 2000), as it aids in creating a desirable identity image. Kelly pointed out that keeping secrets may facilitate the construction of more desirable identity images, thus allowing the secret-keeper to see him/herself in a favorable light. The result may be an improved SWB.

An alternative but overlapping explanation is the socioprotective function of secrets. Keeping certain secrets may reduce or even prevent negative feedback, social disapproval, and stigmatization from others (Bok, 1989; Kelly, 2002; Kelly & McKillop, 1996; Larson & Chastain, 1990; Wegner & Gold, 1995; Wegner & Lane, 1995). This is particularly salient for high rejection-sensitive subjects who experience significant anticipated distress for the negative reactions of others following disclosure. Indeed, Cole et al. (1997) found that KMS functions as a buffer against negative health effects. They demonstrated that rejection-sensitive gay men who concealed their homosexuality did not experience a significant decrease in objective health status, while rejection-sensitive gay men who reported being out of the closet did. This shows that KMS is particularly beneficial by warding off negative feedback from others when one is sensitive to negative evaluation. Social pain theory that was discussed earlier makes a compelling case that everyone of us is evolutionarily bound to experience some degree of social evaluation anxiety. Hence, although KMS may be most beneficial for high rejection-sensitive individuals, the socio-protective function benefits us all.

## 19.9 General Discussion

Limited empirical scientific work has been done to understand one of the most basic mechanisms that we all use in our social interactions: secrecy. How can so little be known about a mechanism so important and omnipresent in daily social interactions? The laymen's view that secrets are detrimental for health, in combination with the myriad negative associations of secrecy with SWB, may have been so powerful that is has directly shined us in the eyes for decades. The potential positive aspects of secrecy have therefore largely been ignored, making secrecy a clinical oxymoron. Secrecy is so much under our skin that we failed to acknowledge the importance of secrecy in basic scientific and applied clinical research. In the last two decades though, research on secrecy has been steadily increasing and works are published in important journals such as *Psychological Bulletin* (Kelly & McKillop, 1996) and *Journal of Personality and Social Psychology* (Wegner et al., 1994). Important research findings such as those by Kelly (1998) and Kelly & Yip (2006) show that secrecy is a multifaceted phenomenon that must be treated as such. It has now been sufficiently shown that secrecy research must explicitly control for the difference between secrecy as a trait and as a process by measuring both.

Future research should hence put more efforts in adequately mapping the various components of secrecy. Although it is obvious that not all secrets are alike in their detrimental potential, hardly any theoretical or empirical effort has been done to come to a systematic classification of secrets that may be helpful in future research to unravel the specific qualities of secrets that render them toxic. This gap in our knowledge complicates a true understanding of the psychological and physical consequences of secrecy. We call for longitudinal studies in which respondents, in a nonthreatening and completely anonymous fashion, are asked to share their secrets and in which both self-reported and objective measures of physical and mental well-being are applied. In this way it can be determined which individual secrets seem to have a detrimental potential and which not.

In addition, more research is needed on how to operationalize KMS. Given the importance of KMS for SWB, it is surprising that no literature exists on what elements should constitute KMS. Simply keeping a secret does not make one keep a major secret. Does "major" mean that the secret must be experienced as emotionally negative? Or does the term refer to the extent of negative reactions from others one expects, and must major be defined in terms of anticipated social cost? Makes this hiding a desired pregnancy until the 12-week threshold not count as a major secret? Hence, I strongly call for basic research that focuses on constructing a taxonomy of the core aspects of secrecy. Interesting work done by Davidoff (1996) on how people conceptualize the severity of a disease may help us to obtain insight into what is meant by the seriousness of secrets. By applying a combination of the medical model of disease (incorporating etiology, anatomy, and pathophysiology) and the patient's personal experience of illness, this author identified four separate aspects that relate to disease severity: (1) distress (as caused by pain, anxiety, etc.), (2) disability (functional interference), (3) seriousness (threat to life), and (4) urgency (immediate need for medical intervention). One can partially adopt this framework to determine the seriousness of a secret by having the individual rate his or her secret on the (anticipated) amount of emotional distress it may cause, the degree in which having the secret interferes with performing daily duties (for example by avoiding certain individuals or situations, by excessive rumination that interferes with concentration, etc.) and to the extent in which the secret is threatening to oneself or others. The latter aspect may not necessarily have to refer to life-threatening issues, and can also incorporate psychosocial threats such as ego threats or threats to one's need to belong. Further research should determine if these factors contribute to successfully predicting the pathophysiological potential of a secret.

To this end, we have recently developed a self-report inventory, termed the Tilburg Secrecy Scale (TSS), that consists of 25 items measuring five separate dimensions of secrecy, including separate scales for KMS and SC (Wismeijer, Sijtsma, Van Assen, & Vingerhoets, 2008; Wismeijer, Van Assen, Sijtsma, & Vingerhoets, 2010a, b). This inventory further also measures one's preoccupation due to keeping the secret, the apprehension about disclosure, and a measure of the social distance between oneself and a possible confidant (e.g., one's partner or an acquaintance). The scale can be used for research purposes and clinical purposes and is suited for investigating questions such as: (1) Do major secrets exist without apprehension about disclosure? (2) Is cognitive preoccupation with a secret a stronger predictor of SWB than KMS or SC? (3) Can one be apprehensive about disclosure while at the same time not being cognitively preoccupied by the secret?

Finally, the literature has mainly focused on the negative effects of secrecy. Indeed, there is compelling evidence that having certain kinds of secrets is associated with reduced mental and physical well-being. However, it is important not to regard all secrets alike since some are likely to be more harmful than others. Currently, it remains unclear what makes a secret beneficial or harmful for well-being. An evolutionary psychological paradigm might be fruitful to guide this research. The work of MacDonald and Leary (2005), discussed earlier in this chapter, on social pain is one example of how evolutionary insights might lead us to a better understanding of secrets and how these may affect (patho-)physiological processes.

## 19.10 Conclusion

Secrecy is a clinically relevant phenomenon that can be studied from very different perspectives by several disciplines including psychology, sociology, anthropology, and medicine. Virtually anything has the potential to become a secret, from the most traumatic experience to the most trivial event: it depends on how the individual judges the perception of the information by others. Most secrets concern negatively valenced personal information that the secret-keeper conceals from others in order to protect him/her for the social consequences of revealing the secret. The relation between secrecy and SWB has long been thought to be negative, but recently it was found that one must distinguish secrecy as a trait from secrecy as a process. They appear to be mutually inversely related with SWB. The suggestion that some aspects of secrecy may be negatively related with SWB and others positively makes secrecy a topic that merits further scientific inquiry.

## References

Afifi, W. A., & Guerrero, L. K. (2000). Motivations underlying topic avoidance in close relationships. In S. Petronio (Ed.), *Balancing the secrets of private disclosures* (pp. 165–180). Mahwah: Erlbaum.

Bok, S. (1989). *Secrets: On the ethics of concealment and revelation*. New York: Vintage Books.

Bouman, T. K. (2003). Intra- and interpersonal consequences of experimentally induced concealment. *Behavior Research and Therapy 41*, 959–968.

Brosschot, J. F., & Thayer, J. F. (1998). Anger inhibition, cardiovascular recovery, and vagal function: a model of the link between hostility and cardiovascular disease. *Annals of Behavioral Medicine, 20*, 326–332.

Brosschot, J. F., & Thayer, J. F. (2004). Worry, perseverative thinking and health. In I. Nyklíček, L. Temoshok, & A. Vingerhoets (Eds.), *Emotional expression and health: Advances in theory, assessment and clinical applications* (pp. 99–114). New York: Brunner-Routledge.

Cepeda-Benito, A., & Short, P. (1998). Self-concealment, avoidance of psychological services, and perceived likelihood of seeking professional help. *Journal of Counseling Psychology, 45*, 58–64.

Christensen, A. J., Edwards, D. L., Wiebe, J. S., Benotsch, E. G., McKelvey, L., Andrews, M., & Lubaroff, D. M. (1996). Effect of verbal self-disclosure on natural killer cell activity: Moderating influence of cynical hostility. *Psychosomatic Medicine, 58*, 150–155.

Christensen, A. J., & Smith, T. W. (1993). Cynical hostility and cardiovascular reactivity during self-disclosure. *Psychosomatic Medicine, 55*, 193–202.

Cohen, S., Gottlieb, B., & Underwood, L. (2000). Social relationships and health. In L. Underwood, S. Cohen, & B. Gottlieb (Eds.), *Social support measurement and interventions: A handbook for health and social scientists*. New York: Oxford University Press.

Cole, S. W., Kemeny, M. E., & Taylor, S. E. (1997). Social identity and physical health: Accelerated HIV progression in rejection-sensitive gay men. *Journal of Personality and Social Psychology, 72*, 320–335.

Cole, S. W., Kemeny, M. E., Taylor, S. E., & Visscher, B. R. (1996). Elevated physical health risk among gay men who conceal their homosexual identity. *Health Psychology, 15*, 243–251.

Cole, S. W., Kemeny, M. E., Taylor, S. E., Visscher, B. R., & Fahey, J. L. (1996). Accelerated course of human immunodeficiency virus infection in gay men who conceal their homosexuality. *Psychosomatic Medicine, 58*, 219–231.

Cramer, K. M. (1999). Psychological antecedents to help-seeking behavior: A reanalysis using path modeling structures. *Journal of Counseling Psychology, 46*, 381–387.

Cramer, K. M., & Lake, R. P. (1998). The Preference for Solitude Scale: Psychometric properties and factor structure. *Personality and Individual Differences, 24*, 193–199.

Davidoff, F. (1996). Severity. The missing link between disease and illness. In F. Davidoff (Ed.), *Who has seen a blood sugar? Reflections on medical education* (pp. 146–151). Philadelphia: American College of Physicians.

Derogatis, L. R. (1993). *Brief Symptom Inventory (BSI): Administration, scoring, and procedures manual* (3rd ed.). Minneapolis: Nation Computer Systems.

DiBartolo, P. M., Li, C. Y., & Frost, R. O. (2008). How do the dimensions of perfectionism relate to mental health? *Cognitive Therapy and Research, 32*, 401–417.

Ellenberger, H. F. (1965). The pathogenic secret and its therapeutics. *Journal of the History of the Behavioral Sciences, 2*, 29–42.

Esterling, B. A., Antoni, M. H., Kumar, M., & Schneiderman, N. (1990). Emotional repression, stress disclosure responses, and Epstein-Barr viral capsid antigen titers. *Psychosomatic Medicine, 52*, 397–410.

Farber, B. A., & Hall, D. (2002). Disclosure to therapists: What is and is not discussed in psychotherapy. *Journal of Clinical Psychology*, 58, 359–370.

Finkenauer, C. (1998). *Secrets: Types, determinants, functions, and consequences.* Unpublished doctoral dissertation. Belgium: University of Louvain at Louvain-la-Neuve, Louvain-la-Neuve.

Finkenauer, C., & Rimé, B. (1998). Socially shared emotional experiences vs. emotional experiences kept secret: Differential characteristics and consequences. *Journal of Social and Clinical Psychology, 17*, 295–318.

Frijns, T. (2004). *Keeping secrets: Quantity, quality and consequences.* Unpublished doctoral dissertation. Amsterdam: Vrije Universiteit Amsterdam.

Frijns, T., & Finkenauer, C. (2009). Longitudinal associations between keeping a secret and psychosocial adjustment in adolescence. *International Journal of Behavioral Development, 33*, 145–154.

Gallagher, E. N., & Vella-Brodrick, D. A. (2008). Social support and emotional intelligence as predictors of subjective well-being. *Personality and Individual Differences, 44*, 1551–1561.

Gesell, S. B. (1999). The roles of personality and cognitive processing in secret keeping (anxiety). *Dissertation Abstracts International: Section B: The Sciences and Engineering, 60* (6-B), 2971.

Herman, B. H., & Panksepp, J. (1978). Effects of morphine and naloxone on separation distress and approach attachment: Evidence for opiate mediation of social affect. *Pharmacology, Biochemistry, and Behavior, 9*, 213–220.

Hill, C. E., Thompson, B. J., Cogar, M. C., & Denman, D. W. (1993). Beneath the surface of long-term therapy: Therapist and client report of their own and each other's convert processes. *Journal of Counseling Psychology, 40*, 278–287.

Hillix, W. A., Harari, H., & Mohr, D. A. (1979). Secrets. *Psychology Today, 13*, 71–76.

Kawamura, K. Y., & Frost, R. O. (2004). Self-concealment as a mediator in the relationship between perfectionism and psychological distress. *Cognitive Therapy and Research, 28*, 183–191.

Kelly, A. E. (1998). Client´s secret keeping in outpatient therapy. *Journal of Counseling Psychology, 45*, 50–57.

Kelly, A. E. (2000). Helping construct desirable identities: A self-presentational view of psychotherapy. *Psychological Bulletin, 126*, 475–494.

Kelly, A. E. (2002). *The psychology of secrets*. New York: Kluwer.

Kelly, A. E., & Achter, J. A. (1995). Self-concealment and attitudes toward counseling in university students. *Journal of Counseling Psychology, 42*, 40–46.

Kelly, A. E., & McKillop, K. J. (1996). Consequences of revealing personal secrets. *Psychological Bulletin, 120*, 651–665.

Kelly, A. E., & Yip, J. J. (2006). Is keeping a secret or being a secretive person linked to psychological symptoms? *Journal of Personality, 74*, 1349–1369.

Lane, J. D., & Wegner, D. M. (1995). The cognitive consequences of secrecy. *Journal of Personality and Social Psychology, 69*, 237–253.

Larson, D. G., & Chastain, R. L. (1990). Self-concealment: Conceptualization, measurement, and health implications. *Journal of Social and Clinical Psychology, 9*, 39–455.

Leary, M. R., & Kowalski, R. M. (1990). Impression management: A literature review and two-component model. *Psychological Bulletin, 107*, 34–47.

Maas, J., Wismeijer, A. A. J., Aquarius, A. E., & Van Assen, M. A. L. M. (2010). *The role of cognitive preoccupation in secrecy: Associations with physical and mental health.* Manuscript submitted for publication.

MacDonald, G., & Leary, M. R. (2005). Why does social exclusion hurt? The relationship between social and physical pain. *Psychological Bulletin, 131*, 202–223.

Margolis, G. J. (1974). Secrecy and identity. *International Journal of Psycho-Analysis, 47*, 517–522.

Nolen-Hoeksema, S. (2000). Further evidence for the role of psychosocial factors in depression chronicity. *Clinical Psychology: Science and Practice, 7*, 224–227.

Norton, R., Feldman, C., & Tafoya, D. (1974). Risk parameters across types of secrets. *Journal of Counseling Psychology, 21*, 450–454.

Olson, J. M., Barefoot, J. C., & Strickland, L. H. (1976). What the shadow knows: Person perception in a surveillance situation. *Journal of Personality and Social Psychology, 34*, 583–589.

Panksepp, J. (1998). *Affective neuroscience: The foundations of human and animal emotions.* London: Oxford University Press.

Pennebaker, J. W. (1989). Confession, inhibition, and disease. In L. Berkowitz (Ed.), *Advances in experimental social psychology* (pp. 211–244). New York: Academic.

Pennebaker, J. W., Colder, M., & Sharp, L. K. (1990). Accelerating the coping process. *Journal of Personality and Social Psychology, 58*, 528–537.

Petrie, K., Booth, R., & Pennebaker, J. (1995). Disclosure of trauma and immune response to a hepatitis B vaccination program. *Journal of Consulting and Clinical Psychology, 63*, 787–792.

Pennebaker, J. W., Hughes, C. F., & O´Heeron, R. C. (1987). The psychophysiology of confession: Linking inhibitory and psychosomatic processes. *Journal of Personality and Social Psychology, 52*, 781–793.

Ritz, T., & Dahme, B. (1996). Repression, self-concealment and rationality emotional defensiveness: The correspondence between three questionnaire measures of defensive coping. *Personality and Individual Differences, 20*, 95–102.

Roeling, M. P., Wismeijer, A. A. J., Waringa, R. A., & Van Assen, M. A. L. M. (2010). *Reasons for secrecy: exploring why people keep secrets.* Manuscript submitted for publication.

Schlenker, B. R., & Weigold, M. F. (1992). Interpersonal processes involving impression regulation and management. *Annual Review of Psychology, 43*, 133–168.

Smyth, J. M. (1998). Written emotional expression: Effect sizes, outcome types, and moderating variables. *Journal of Consulting and Clinical Psychology, 66*, 174–184.

Swinkels, A., & Giuliano, T. A. (1995). The measurement and conceptualization of Mood Awareness: Monitoring and labeling one's mood states. *Personality and Social Psychology Bulletin, 21*, 934–949.

Ullrich, P. M., Lutgendorf, S. K., Stapleton, J., & Horowitz, M. J. (2004). Self regard and concealment of homosexuality as predictors of CD4+ cell count over time among HIV seropositive gay men. *Psychology and Health, 19*, 183–196.

Vangelisti, A. L. (1994). Family secrets: Forms, functions, and correlates. *Journal of Social and Personal Relationships, 11*, 113–135.

Van Heck, G. L., & Vingerhoets, A. J. J. M. (2004). De helende kracht van de pen: soms voor sommigen of altijd voor iedereen? [The healing power of the pen: sometimes for some or always for everybody?] *Gedrag & Gezondheid, 32*, 108–114.

Van-Leeson, T., Totterdell, P., & Parkinson, B. (2006). Moderating effects of mood monitoring on premenstrual dysphoria. *Cognition and Emotion, 20*, 1236–1247.

Vittersø, J. (2001). Personality traits and subjective well-being: Emotional stability, not extraversion, is probably the most important predictor. *Personality and Individual Differences, 31*, 903–914.

Vrij, A., Nunkoosing, K., Paterson, B., Oosterwegel, A., & Soukara, S. (2002). Characteristics of secrets and the frequency, reasons, and effects of secrets keeping and disclosure. *Journal of Community and Applied Social Psychology, 12*, 56–70.

Wallace, B. C., & Constantine, M. G. (2005). Afrocentric cultural values, psychological help-seeking attitudes, and self-concealment in African American college students. *Journal of Black Psychology*, *31*, 369–385.

Warren, C., & Laslett, B. (1977). Privacy and secrecy: A conceptual comparison. *Journal of Social Issues*, *33*, 43–51.

Wegner, D. M. (1992). You can´t always think what you want: Problems in the suppression of unwanted thoughts. In M. P. Zanna (Ed.), *Advances in experimental social psychology* (pp. 193–225). New York: Academic.

Wegner, D. M. (1994). Ironic processes of mental control. *Psychological Review*, *101*, 34–52.

Wegner, D. M., & Gold, D. B. (1995). Fanning old flames: Emotional and cognitive effects of suppressing thoughts of a past relationship. *Journal of Personality and Social Psychology*, *68*, 782–792.

Wegner, D. M., & Lane, J. D. (1995). From secrecy to psychopathology. In J. W. Pennebaker (Ed.), *Emotion, disclosure, and health* (pp. 25–46). Washington: American Psychological Association.

Wegner, D. M., Lane, J. D., & Dimitri, S. (1994). The allure of secret relationships. *Journal of Personality and Social Psychology*, *66*, 287–300.

Wetzer, I. M. (2007). *Let's talk about it. Studies on the social sharing of emotions*. Unpublished doctoral dissertation, Tilburg: Tilburg University.

Wismeijer, A. A. J. (2008). *Self-concealment and secrecy: Assessment and associations with subjective well-being*. Unpublished doctoral dissertation. Tilburg: Tilburg University.

Wismeijer, A. A. J., Sijtsma, K., Van Assen, M. A. L. M., & Vingerhoets, A. J. J. M. (2008). A comparative study of the dimensionality of the Self-Concealment Scale using principal components analysis and Mokken scale analysis. *Journal of Personality Assessment*, *90*, 323–334.

Wismeijer, A. A. J., & Van Assen, M. A. L. M. (2008). Do neuroticism and extraversion explain the negative effect of self-concealment on subjective well-being? *Personality and Individual Differences*, *45*, 345–349.

Wismeijer, A. A. J., Van Assen, M. A. L. M., Sijtsma, K., & Vingerhoets, A. J. J. M. (2009). Is the negative association between self-concealment and subjective well-being mediated by mood awareness? *Journal of Clinical and Social Psychology*, *28*, 728–748.

Wismeijer, A. A. J., Van Assen, M. A. L. M., Sijtsma, K., & Vingerhoets, A. J. J. M. (2010a). *A 5-year longitudinal study of the relation between secrecy and subjective well-being: the differential roles of process and trait*. Manuscript submitted for publication.

Wismeijer, A. A. J., Van Assen, M. A. L. M., Sijtsma, K., & Vingerhoets, A. J. J. M. (2010b). *Development and testing of the Tilburg Secrecy Scale-25 (TSS25)*. Manuscript submitted for publication.

Wismeijer, A. A. J., & Vingerhoets, A. J. J. M. (2010). *Secrets uncovered. An overview of the multidisciplinary literature on secrecy*. Manuscript submitted for publication.

Yukawa, S., Tokuda, H., & Sato, J. (2007). Attachment style, self-concealment, and interpersonal distance among Japanese undergraduates. *Perceptual and Motor Skills*, *104*, 1255–1261.

Zech, E., Bradley, M. M., & Lang, P. J. (2002). Affective reactions when talking about emotional. events. *Psychophysiology*, *39*, S90.

**ERRATUM TO**

# From (Unconscious) Perception to Emotion: A Global-to-Specific Unfolding View of Emotional Responding

Kirsten I. Ruys, Diederik A. Stapel, and Henk Aarts

Utrecht University, Psychology Department, P.O. Box 80140,
3508 TC Utrecht, Netherlands
e-mail: k.i.ruys@uu.nl

Tilburg University, Tilburg, Netherlands

Utrecht University, Utrecht, Netherlands

I. Nyklíček et al. (eds.), *Emotion Regulation and Well-Being*,
DOI 10.1007/978-1-4419-6953-8_4, © Springer Science+Business Media, LLC 2011

**DOI 10.1007/978-1-4419-6953-8_20**

Reason:

This chapter has been retracted because the Editors were informed by the Levelt Committee that the chapter was based on falsified research and/or fabricated data.

The online version of the original Book can be found at
http://dx.doi.org/10.1007/978-1-4419-6953-8_4

# Index